The M____ _ealth Needs of Young Offenders

Forging _____ ___ ___ _ion and Rehabilitation

The majority of young people in the American juvenile justice system have diagnosable mental illnesses, including substance abuse, mental retardation, and learning disorders. However, these disorders often remain undetected and untreated. In this book, a team of experts examines the prevalence of mental disorders in this population and describes the means of screening for, diagnosing, and treating them effectively in a developmentally appropriate, culturally sensitive manner. They also examine psychopharmacologic and psychotherapeutic approaches; innovative community-based programs as an effective alternative to detention; the human and economic costs of detaining youth; the interrogation strategies that make young people particularly vulnerable to self-incrimination; and the alarming trend of disproportionate minority confinement. Their comprehensive coverage includes discussion of the ethical dilemmas that arise when mental health professionals practice in a forensic setting, and outlining the need for preventive strategies, and for integrated approaches involving judicial, law enforcement, educational, and mental health professionals. This book will be of interest to both mental health and juvenile justice professionals.

Carol L. Kessler is Assistant Clinical Professor in the Department of Psychiatry, Columbia University, New York.

Louis J. Kraus is the Womans Board Professor of Child and Adolescent Psychiatry and Chief, Department of Child and Adolescent Psychiatry, Rush University Medical Center, Chicago.

The Mental Health Needs of Young Offenders

Forging Paths toward Reintegration and Rehabilitation

Edited by

Carol L. Kessler, M.D., M.Div.
Louis J. Kraus, M.D.

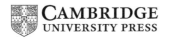

CAMBRIDGE
UNIVERSITY PRESS

CAMBRIDGE UNIVERSITY PRESS
Cambridge, New York, Melbourne, Madrid, Cape Town, Singapore, São Paulo

Cambridge University Press
The Edinburgh Building, Cambridge CB2 8RU, UK

Published in the United States of America by Cambridge University Press, New York

www.cambridge.org
Information on this title: www.cambridge.org/9780521612906

First published 2007

Printed in the United Kingdom at the University Press, Cambridge

A catalog record for this publication is available from the British Library

ISBN 978-0-521-61290-6 paperback

Cambridge University Press has no responsibility for the persistence or accuracy of URLs for external or
third-party internet websites referred to in this publication, and does not guarantee that any content on such
websites is, or will remain, accurate or appropriate.

Every effort has been made in preparing this publication to provide accurate and up-to-date information which
is in accord with accepted standards and practice at the time of publication. Although case histories are drawn
from actual cases, every effort has been made to disguise the identities of the individuals involved. Nevertheless,
the authors, editors, and publishers can make no warranties that the information contained herein is totally free
from error, not least because clinical standards are constantly changing through research and regulation. The
authors, editors, and publishers therefore disclaim all liability for direct or consequential damages resulting
from the use of material contained in this publication. Readers are strongly advised to pay careful attention to
information provided by the manufacturer of any drugs or equipment that they plan to use.

This work is dedicated to the memory of my mother, Rita Francesca Deppisch Kessler, who instilled in me respect for the potential of all human beings.

Contents

Contributors

Karen M. Abram, Ph.D.
Assistant Professor
Feinberg School of Medicine
Northwestern University
USA

William Arroyo, M.D.
LA County Department of Mental Health
Child, Youth and Family Administration
550 S. Vermont Avenue, Third Floor
Los Angeles, CA 90020
USA

Corinne Belsky, M.D.
98-A Cope Creek Rd.
Sylva, NC 28779
USA

Daniel Bober, D.O.
Forensic Psychiatry Fellowship
University of Massachusetts Medical School
55 Lake Avenue North, WSH 8B
Worcester, MA 01655
USA

Shiraz Butt, M.D.
Assistant Professor of Psychiatry
Rush University Medical Center
Marshall Field IV Building
1720 West Polk Street
Chicago, IL 60612
USA

David C. Clark, Ph.D.
Rush University Medical Center
Armour Academic Center
600 Paulina
Suite 529
Chicago, IL 60612
USA

Malika Closson, M.D.
University of Maryland
Department of Psychiatry
701 West Pratt Street
Baltimore, MD 21201
USA

Steven Drizin, J.D.
357 E. Chicago Avenue
Room 370 McCormick
Chicago, IL 60611
USA

Mina K. Dulcan, Ph.D.
Osterman Professor of Psychiatry,
Behavioral Sciences, and Pediatrics
Feinberg School of Medicine
Northwestern University
USA

David Fassler, M.D.
Otter Creek Associates
86 Lake Street
Burlington, VT 05401
USA

Peter Fink, M.D.
Assistant Professor of Psychiatry
Rush University Medical Center
Marshall Field IV Building
1720 West Polk Street
Chicago, IL 60612
USA

Thomas F. Geraghty, J.D.
Director of the Blum Legal Clinic
Northwestern University School of Law
357 E. Chicago Avenue
Chicago, IL 60611-8576
USA

Thomas Grisso, Ph.D.
Professor, Law and Psychiatry Program
Department of Psychiatry
University of Massachusetts
Medical School
55 Lake Avenue North, WSH 8B
Worcester, MA 01655
USA

Stephen K. Harper, J.D.
1320 N.W. 14th Street
Miami, FL 33125
USA

Niranjan S. Karnik, M.D., Ph.D.
Division of Child and Adolescent Psychiatry
Stanford University
401 Quarry Road
Stanford, CA 94305
USA

Carol L. Kessler, M.D., M.Div.
Assistant Clinical Professor in the
Department of Psychiatry
New York-Presbyterian
The University Hospital of Columbia
and Cornell
622 West 168 Street
Vanderbilt Clinic-Fourth Floor
New York, NY 10032
USA

Louis J. Kraus, M.D.
Womans Board Professor of Child and
Adolescent Psychiatry and Chief,
Department of Child and
Adolescent Psychiatry
Rush University Medical Center
Marshall Field IV Building
1720 West Polk Street
Chicago, IL 60612
USA

Ruth Kraus, Ph.D.
950 Skokie Boulevard
Suite 305
Northbrook, IL 60062
USA

Gary M. McClelland
Research Assistant Professor
Feinberg School of Medicine
Northwestern University
USA

Amy A. Mericle, Ph.D.
Postdoctoral Fellow
University of California, San Francisco
School of Medicine
Department of Psychiatry
USA

Robert E. Morris, M.D.
1192 Rancheros Place
Pasadena, CA 91103-2753
USA

Wade C. Myers, M.D.
Professor and Chief, Division of Child and
Adolescent Psychiatry
Director, Forensic Psychiatry Program
Department of Psychiatry, Silver CDC
University of South Florida
12901 Bruce B. Downs Blvd., MDC 102
Tampa, FL 33612
USA

Joseph V. Penn, M.D.
Director of Child and Adolescent Forensic
Psychiatry
Rhode Island Hospital
RI Training School Medical Clinic
300 New London Avenue
Cranston, RI 02920
USA

Kayla Pope, M.D., J.D.
University of Maryland/Sheppard Pratt
701 West Pratt Street,
Suite 476
Baltimore, MD 21201
USA

Allison D. Redlich, Ph.D.
Policy Research Association
345 Delaware Avenue
Delmar, NY 12054
USA

Kenneth M. Rogers, M.D.
University of Maryland
Department of Psychiatry
Section of Child and Adolescent Psychiatry
701 West Pratt Street
Baltimore, MD 21201
USA

Lilia Romero-Bosch, M.D.
Chief Resident
Hasbro and Rhode Island Hospitals
Providence, Rhode Island 02903
USA

Deborah R. Simkin, M.D.
4641 Gulfstarr Drive
Suite 106
Destin, FL 32541
USA

Amer Smajkic, M.D.
Rush University Medical Center
Marshall Field IV Building
1720 West Polk Street
Chicago, IL 60612
USA

Hollie Sobel, Ph.D.
Assistant Professor of Psychiatry and
Behavioral Sciences
Rush University Medical Center
Marshall Field IV Building
1720 West Polk Street
Chicago, IL 60612
USA

Marie V. Soller, M.D.
Resident in Psychiatry
San Mateo Medical Center
San Mateo, CA
USA

Hans Steiner, M.D.
Professor of Psychiatry and Behavioral
Sciences
Director of Education, Division of Child
and Adolescent Psychiatry
Co-Director, Center for Psychiatry
and the Law
Stanford University School of Medicine
401 Quarry Road
Stanford, CA 94305
USA

Linda A. Teplin, Ph.D.
Owen L. Coon Professor of Psychiatry
and Behavioral Sciences
Director, Psycho-Legal Studies Program
Feinberg School of Medicine
Northwestern University
710 N. Lake Shore Drive
Chicago, IL 60611
USA

Anna Terry, B.A.
Research Associate, Law & Psychiatry Program
Department of Psychiatry
University of Massachusetts Medical School
55 Lake Avenue North, WSH 8B
Worcester, MA 01655
USA

Christopher R. Thomas, M.D.
Professor of Psychiatry and Behavioral
Sciences
University of Texas
301 University Boulevard
Galveston, TX 77555
USA

Eric Trupin, Ph.D.
University of Washington
Public Behavioral Health
146 North Canal Street, Suite 100
Seattle, WA 98103
USA

Gina M. Vincent, Ph.D.
Department of Psychiatry
University of Massachusetts
Medical School
55 Lake Avenue North, WSH 8B
Worcester, MA 01655
USA

Jason J. Washburn
Research Assistant Professor
Feinberg School of Medicine
Northwestern University
USA

Julie Wolf, Ph.D.
Yale Child Study Center
230 South Frontage Road
New Haven, CT 06520
USA

Foreword

In 1995, as the Training Director of the Division of Child and Adolescent Psychiatry at Columbia University, I brought a group of psychiatric residents to a local juvenile detention center. What we found was a far cry from the mandate of the Juvenile Court, according to the Illinois Juvenile Court Act of 1899 that stated that the court was "to act as kind parents seeking to educate and rehabilitate rather than to punish." We found that the inmates were principally African-American or Hispanic inner city kids (white youngsters hired lawyers who kept them out of jail, at least until adjudication). These young people were either high school dropouts or far behind their expected level of academic achievement. Two thirds of the adolescents carried at least one psychiatric diagnosis. Rehabilitation and education was definitely not a part of the 1995 picture.

Four years later I was elected to the Presidency of the American Academy of Child and Adolescent Psychiatry. My first official act was to appoint a task force, headed by Dr. William Arroyo, to study the serious problems inherent in the juvenile justice system and to make recommendations for reform. The monograph resulting from the efforts of a group of dedicated members served as the model for this long-awaited book.

The mission of the committee that emerged from the task force states that the juvenile justice system "will become responsive to children and adolescents with mental disorders who are in the juvenile or adult justice system. It is imperative that a comprehensive continuum of mental health services are accessible to this population, that the system be strongly community-based, family centered, culturally competent, developmentally relevant, and well integrated with other child system components, including health education and child welfare" (Kraus & Arroyo, 2005).

This seminal work fulfills the mission of the committee. Their recommendations for mental health screening standards of care for juvenile detention facilities, and developmentally appropriate services are well defined and clearly stated.

I believe that everyone who reads this book will be convinced by the strong evidence presented for the need for a complete overhaul of the present system and that the time for change is now.

Clarice J. Kestenbaum, M.D.
Professor of Clinical Psychiatry
Columbia University College of
Physicians & Surgeons

Kraus, L. J. & Arroyo, W. (2005). *Recommendations for Juvenile Justice Reform, 2nd edn.* Washington, DC: American Academy of Child and Adolescent Psychiatry, Committee on Juvenile Justice Reform.

Acknowledgments

First and foremost I would like to acknowledge the young people and their families, with whom I have had the privilege to work as a child and adolescent psychiatrist. Their resilience in the face of innumerable psychosocial stressors is an inspiration to me. My hope is that communities will be motivated to provide supports, to prevent interventions that further their distress.

I would also like to thank the American Academy of Child and Adolescent Psychiatry, and more particularly, the leadership of Clarice Kestenbaum, M.D. during her tenure as president. She had the commitment to dedicate her term to the establishment of the Juvenile Justice Task Force that was instrumental in bringing together many of the authors in this book, in what has resulted in various creative ventures. Among those ventures was the publication of a monograph on Juvenile Justice Reform on the Academy's website. This monograph ultimately drew this publisher's attention to the urgency of mental health needs amongst justice-involved youth.

Cambridge University Press has had the vision to bring this work to press, and I particularly acknowledge the patience and encouragement of Pauline Graham, of Betty Fulford, and of Dawn Preston.

An overview of child and adolescent mental health needs in the juvenile justice system

Carol L. Kessler

Never doubt that a small group of thoughtful committed citizens can change the world; indeed it's the only thing that ever has.

Margaret Mead

The following pages reflect the dedication of a diverse group of professionals to the needs of an oft neglected population. Youth who become involved with the justice system, by committing delinquent acts and/or status offenses, present with a myriad of issues. It has become increasingly evident that their mental health, educational, and social needs have all too often been inadequately assessed or addressed. Punitive measures and detention create a population of repeat offenders and fail to respond to the root causes of antisocial behavior. With the realization that most justice-involved youth silently suffer from mental health problems, professionals have begun to seriously study both the prevalence of these disorders, and how they might effectively be treated.

We are fortunate to have the contributions of Teplin and colleagues (Chapter 2), who are leaders in an epidemiological approach to psychiatric diagnoses in the juvenile justice population. Their chapter reviews the existing literature, and presents the results of their Northwestern Juvenile Project, which they designed to address limitations of previous research. Prevalence rates of youth in Cook County detention are presented. They indicate high rates of mental illness and of co-morbidity, and point to the need to ensure that youth's right to care is met. They acknowledge the limitations of their method, which did not include those justice-involved youth who are not detained, and which measured symptomatology shortly after confinement, when distress may partly reflect adjustment reactions. They point to the need for further study of co-morbidity, of justice-involved young women, of the long-term outcome of detained youth, and of pathways from trauma-exposure to the development of posttraumatic stress disorder.

The disproportionate number of minority – African American, Asian American, Latino/Hispanic, Native American – youth confined to detention centers in the United States is the concern of Arroyo (Chapter 3). He reviews current research,

The Mental Health Needs of Young Offenders: Forging Paths toward Reintegration and Rehabilitation, eds. Carol L. Kessler and Louis J. Kraus. Published by Cambridge University Press. © Cambridge University Press 2007.

and points to the potential biases at various points along the path of juvenile justice processing. He also reports efforts by the Office of Juvenile Justice and Delinquency Prevention to address discriminatory practices through education, technical assistance, and research. Awareness of the problem of disproportionate minority confinement must be heightened so that its root causes can be further elucidated and addressed.

Redlich and Drizin (Chapter 4) define the interrogation room as a station along the path of juvenile justice processing where youth, especially with mental disorders, are vulnerable to false or coerced confessions and consequent wrongful detention and/or conviction. The specific techniques used by police officers in a global fashion, with young and old alike, are delineated. The authors present research that indicates how young people and those with mental disorders are liable to respond in a self-incriminating manner. They outline the advances that have been made in the handling of child witnesses and victims, and point out that these advances have not been translated to the interrogation process. Young people are at risk due to their concrete thinking and due to their limited knowledge and understanding of the legal system. They are unlikely to request an attorney. The authors point to the need to advocate for electronic recording of interrogations and for training of police in proper guidelines for the interrogation of youth.

Geraghty, Kraus, and Fink (Chapter 5) point to the role that attorneys and mental health professionals might play in advocating for those youth who inadvertently incriminate themselves during interrogation. Psychiatrists and/or psychologists may be enlisted as expert witnesses to determine whether an alleged offender was competent to waive his/her Miranda rights – the right to remain silent; the right to avoid self-incrimination; the right to legal counsel. Furthermore, mental health professionals may assist legal professionals in assessing whether a justice-involved youth is competent to stand trial. Such assessments are critical to ensure youth's right to a fair trial.

To examine the root causes of behaviors that lead to involvement of youth with the juvenile justice system, Pope and Thomas (Chapter 6) outline a comprehensive list of key factors that influence the development of antisocial acts. They mention genetics, prenatal toxin exposure, temperament, intelligence, and attachment. Later in childhood and adolescence, parenting style, academic achievement, peer relationships, media exposure, and the quality of the surrounding neighborhood become critical. Abuse and exposure to violence are further variables. The authors point to the need to understand how these factors interact with one another, and to determine their longitudinal impact.

Simkin (Chapter 7) focuses more specifically on those risk factors that lead youth toward substance use, an illegal behavior in and of itself. She introduces the notion that early identification of risk factors might lead to the development of strategies to transform risk into protective factors. Methods of assessing youth's stage of substance use and readiness for change are reviewed, as well as an overview of existing psychopharmacologic and therapeutic interventions. The need for early intervention and for coordination of services is emphasized.

Early intervention is a critical need to prevent the high rate of suicide amongst justice-involved youth. Studies are limited by their sole focus on detained youth. Smajkic and Clark (Chapter 8) point to the need for consistent suicide prevention policies to be developed and enforced in all detention centers. Early screening of youth, and training of staff could hopefully decrease significantly the loss of young lives, primarily to hanging.

A unique challenge is posed to the juvenile justice system by those youth who have been accused of sexual offenses. Belsky, Myers, and Bober (Chapter 9) present available demographic data regarding the scope of these offenses. They point to risk factors and theories as to how these factors evolve into sexual offending behavior. The particular challenges posed to the justice system by young sexual offenders are explored, as well as various legal strategies that are implemented. Tools to assess youth who sexually offend are presented, in the form of guided interviews, and categorization schemes. Treatment methods are surveyed, with the emphasis on management of a probable lifelong disorder that is frequently co-morbid with other mental illnesses.

The educational needs of justice-involved youth are explored by Closson and Rogers (Chapter 10). They point to deficiencies in the US educational system that lead to youth's disengagement from school, and consequent risk for involvement in delinquent behavior. Youth with learning disorders or intellectual challenges are at risk for school failure and dropout. Those with mental disorders are at risk of behavioral problems that tend to be reprimanded with suspension or expulsion – i.e., alienation from the school system. Youth who are detained tend not to receive appropriate educational services, and are liable to fall behind academically as a result of their interaction with the justice system. Standards of educational assessment and of individualized planning are presented to provide a map of adequate teaching for justice-involved youth.

Fassler and Harper (Chapter 11), psychiatrist and lawyer, point to the power of cross-discipline communication, as they highlight the contribution of medical, behavioral, and neurological sciences in abolishing the juvenile death penalty in the United States. The United States was one of the last countries to punish juveniles with death. To establish that young people are less culpable, and that a sentence of death would constitute cruel and unusual punishment, legislators relied not only on the emerging societal standard of decency, but more importantly, on the testimony of mental health professionals. These scientists presented evidence from imaging studies, that mature brain development, particularly in areas of impulse control and foresight, is not achieved until early adulthood. These insights informed groundbreaking legislation that saves children from the sentence of death.

Morris (Chapter 12) comprehensively delineates medical problems that may predispose to antisocial behavior, as well as illnesses that may result from participating in delinquent activity. Youth in contact with the justice system often have neglected their medical and dental health. Morris cites detention as a time when health needs can be assessed and addressed. He points to the need for health screening, physical examinations, treatment, as well as comprehensive planning for follow-up of chronic illnesses.

Means of screening for mental illness amongst justice-involved youth are reviewed by Vincent, Grisso, and Terry (Chapter 13). They emphasize the role of screening in identifying youth at risk of harming self or others, and youth in need of further mental health evaluation. Systematic screening also documents the level of need for mental health services within the juvenile justice system. The distinction between screening and assessment is delineated. Available screening tools are described that are intended for widespread implementation with minimal resources.

Ruth Kraus (Chapter 14) focuses on assessment tools utilized by psychologists to perform more thorough assessments of each youth's strengths and weaknesses that might inform an individualized treatment plan. She notes that there is a high incidence of neuropsychological deficits amongst juveniles in the juvenile justice system. Areas of executive functioning and verbal ability tend to be particularly compromised. These deficits likely contribute to poor academic functioning and consequent predisposition to delinquent behavior. Comprehensive assessment of cognitive functioning, intelligence, executive functioning, academic achievement, personality, language skills, and adaptive functioning would provide invaluable information that might tailor behavioral, educational, and psychiatric interventions to each youth's level of functioning.

Karnik, Soller, and Steiner (Chapter 15) provide an overview of psychopharmacologic treatment for youth offenders, and advocate for the use of medication only after a timely medical, psychiatric, and psychological assessment. Medication is seen as one tool that must be part of an integrated treatment plan. The chapter on psychopharmacology delineates acute or chronic aggression as a frequent target symptom; yet, medications aimed at a primary psychiatric disorder are the goal. It is recognized that it is often difficult to discern whether psychiatric problems have predisposed to delinquency, or have arisen as a result of detention. Risks and benefits must constantly be reassessed and weighed. Psychopharmacologic recommendations are based on clinical trials, and on practice guidelines, where they are available. However, the authors point to the need to establish evidence-based psychopharmacologic care for the disorders that are just recently being described amongst justice-involved youth.

Evidence-based psychotherapeutic care is the focus of Trupin (Chapter 16). They outline treatment strategies with documented efficacy that target risk factors as well as systemic and behavioral issues of youth and families. Both empirically supported and promising treatment programs are described at the level of prevention, community-based treatment, and transition from detention to aftercare. These programs are depicted via clinical vignettes; their strengths and weaknesses are identified. Treatment modalities include diversion programs, mentoring programs, multisystemic therapy, functional family therapy, and multidimensional therapeutic foster care. The authors point to key components of effective treatment programs, and they emphasize the need for legislative support and funding to translate evidence-based treatment interventions into a therapeutic reality for youth, their families, and their communities.

Thomas (Chapter 17) further emphasizes the promise of community alternatives to incarceration. He provides a historical context, and reviews existing meta-analyses of interventions with justice-involved youth. Evidence is provided that structured treatment modalities of sufficient duration can be effective in community-based work with youth who have committed serious, multiple offenses. Thomas also identifies popular programs that have been shown to have a negative impact, by increasing recidivism rates. He describes community-based multiagency programs, including his own Galveston Island Youth Program, whose outcome studies serve to justify the goal of community-based rehabilitation.

This writer – Kessler (Chapter 18) – describes creative means of transforming the adjudication process into a therapeutic experience. Court and mental health professionals leave their islands to develop a multidisciplinary team approach to justice-involved youth. The judge is at the center, and holds both youth and service providers accountable to the implementation of individualized treatment plans that strive to be developmentally appropriate, culturally sensitive, and gender specific. Plans emerge only after a comprehensive assessment that addresses both legal and clinical needs. Successful team functioning across disciplines depends on consistent cross-training. Implementation of plans depends on the existence of effective community-based systems of care. Alternatives to traditional adjudication – youth court; juvenile drug court; juvenile mental health court – aim to embody restorative, rather than punitive, justice. The goal is to restore right-relationship of youth with themselves, their families, and their communities.

Ethical principles of right-relationship that arise in the course of evaluation and treatment of justice-involved youth are the focus of Romero-Bosch and Penn (Chapter 19). They point to the need for clarity of role when a mental health professional enters into a relationship with a young offender. The need to distinguish between forensic evaluator and treating clinician is critical. The authors address youth's right to consent to or to refuse evaluation and/or treatment, and the issue of competency. The tension between a young person's right to confidentiality and a parent's right to know is explored. The notion of a young person's right to care for a mental illness in the least restrictive setting is introduced. The need for clear delineation of appropriate indications for seclusion and/or restraint is also emphasized.

Whereas Romero-Bosch and Penn (Chapter 19) highlight the boundaries of the relationship between forensic mental health evaluator and youth offender, Louis Kraus and Sobel (Chapter 20) outline the content of a post-adjudicatory evaluation. They point to the critical role mental health professionals have in educating the court regarding youth's mental health needs, and in providing recommendations for appropriate disposition. The post-adjudicatory evaluation ideally consists of interactions not only with the youth, but also teachers and family members. Relevant data concerning previous delinquent behavior, police reports, school records, educational and psychiatric evaluations, and clinic records need to be carefully reviewed. Referrals may need to be made for educational or psychological testing. The evaluator will be expected to provide both a sense of the youth's risk of harm to the community, as well as recommendations for appropriate means of addressing educational, vocational, and mental health needs. Kraus and Sobel (Chapter 20) point to community-based treatment as the most promising, though often unavailable due to inadequate funding.

This volume indicates the broad range of mental health needs present within those youth who present to the juvenile justice system. It points to strategies for screening and for assessing mental health issues, and it also indicates emerging evidence-based treatment interventions. The need for ongoing collaboration across disciplines – legal, correctional, educational, psychiatric – is evident. For paths toward rehabilitation and reintegration to be forged, and for knowledge to be translated into effective interventions, communities must commit resources to these at-risk youth.

2

Psychiatric disorders of youth in detention

Linda A. Teplin, Karen M. Abram, Gary M. McClelland, Amy A. Mericle, Mina K. Dulcan, Jason J. Washburn, and Shiraz Butt

The juvenile justice system faces a significant challenge in identifying and responding to the psychiatric disorders of detained youth. In 2003, over 96 000 juvenile offenders were in custody in juvenile residential placement facilities (Sickmund *et al.*, 2006). Despite the difficulty of handling such youth, providing them with psychiatric services may be critical to breaking the cycle of recidivism.

A comprehensive understanding of the prevalence of psychiatric disorders among juvenile detainees is an important step toward meeting their needs. Like adult prisoners, juvenile detainees with serious mental disorders have a constitutional right under the 8th and 14th Amendments to needed services (American Association of Correctional Psychology, 2000; The President's New Freedom Commission on Mental Health, 2005; Soler, 2002; Costello & Jameson, 1987). Without sound data on the prevalence of psychiatric disorders, however, defining the best means to use and enhance the juvenile justice system's scarce mental health resources is difficult.

Prior research

Although epidemiological data are key to understanding the psychiatric disorders of juvenile detainees, few empirical studies exist. Table 2.1 lists studies published in the United States since 1990 that examined the diagnostic characteristics of incarcerated and detained juveniles. These studies do not provide data that are comprehensive enough to guide juvenile justice policy. For example, although six studies present rates of multiple disorders, only four of those examine patterns of psychiatric comorbidity among juvenile detainees (Domalanta *et al.*, 2003; Duclos *et al.*, 1998; Pliszka *et al.*, 2000; Shelton, 2001). Furthermore, the results of the studies presented in Table 2.1 are inconsistent. For example, the prevalence of affective disorder in the studies varied from 5 percent (McCabe *et al.*, 2002) to 72 percent (Timmons-Mitchell *et al.*, 1997); substance use disorders from 20 percent (Atkins *et al.*, 1999)

The Mental Health Needs of Young Offenders: Forging Paths toward Reintegration and Rehabilitation, eds. Carol L. Kessler and Louis J. Kraus. Published by Cambridge University Press. © Cambridge University Press 2007.

Table 2.1. Published studies of psychiatric disorders in incarcerated, detained, and/or secured juvenile populations in the US, since 1990. [a]

Authors, year	Sample	Diagnostic measures	Major findings [b]
Davis et al., 1991	**Participants:** Youth in a state residential facility **N:** 173 **Age:** N/R **Sex:** N/R **Race/ethnicity:** " . . . fairly equally divided between white and non-white . . ." (p. 7).	Clinical interview (DSM-III-R criteria)	**Affective:** Dysthymia: 17%; MDD: 15% **SUD/AUD:** Alcohol Abuse Disorder: 34.1%; Alcohol Dependence Disorder: 12%; Drug Abuse Disorder: 45%; Drug Dependence Disorder: 19% **CD:** 81% **Other:** ADD: 19%; Adjustment Disorder: 18%; Any Developmental Disorder: 17%; Any PD: 17%; ODD: 5%
Forehand et al., 1991	**Participants:** Youth in a juvenile prison **N:** 52 **Age:** 16 years (mean) **Sex:** all males **Race/ethnicity:** African American: 63.4%; White: 36.5%	DISC-2	**Affective:** MDD: 33% **CD:** Group Delinquency: 58%; Solitary Aggression: 23% **Anxiety:** Overanxious: 40% **Other:** ADD: 27%
Eppright et al., 1993	**Participants:** Youth in a juvenile detention center **N:** 100 **Age:** 14.6 years (mean) **Sex:** 21 females; 79 males **Race/ethnicity:** African American: 32%; White: 68%	DICA-R; SCID-II	**CD:** 87% **Other:** Antisocial PD: 75%; Avoidant PD: 4%; Borderline PD: 27%; Dependent PD: 7%; Histrionic PD: 3%; Narcissistic PD: 8%; Obsessive-compulsive PD: 2%; Paranoid PD: 17%; Passive Aggressive PD: 14%; Schizoid PD: 1%; Schizotypal PD: 0%; Self-defeating PD: 2%

Study	Participants	Measure	Diagnosis	Lifetime	Current
Rohde et al., 1997	**Participants**: Youth in a secure detention facility **N**: 60 **Age**: 14.9 years (mean) **Sex**: 16 females; 44 males **Race/ethnicity**: African American: 1.7%; Asian/Pacific Islander: 1.7%; Hispanic: 6.8%; Native American: 5.1%; White: 83.1%; other: 1.7%	K-SADS-PL (additional items added for DSM-III-R criteria)	**Affective:**		
			Dysthymia:	8%	8%
			MDD:	40%	23%
			SUD/AUD:		
			Alcohol Abuse:	7%	2%
			Alcohol Dependence:	42%	18%
			Hard Drug Abuse:	7%	2%
			Hard Drug Dependence:	33%	17%
			Marijuana Abuse:	5%	3%
			Marijuana Dependence:	43%	23%
			CD:	73%	73%
			Anxiety:	18%	10%
			Other:		
			ADHD:	17%	13%
			ODD:	17%	2%
Steiner et al., 1997	**Participants**: Violent incarcerated youth **N**: 85 **Age**: 16.6 years (mean) **Sex**: all male **Race/ethnicity**: African American: 37.6%; Hispanic: 26.9%; White: 30.1%; other: 5.4%	Psychiatric Diagnostic Interview-Revised	**Anxiety**: 20% met "partial criteria" for PTSD; 31.7% met full criteria for PTSD.		

Table 2.1. (cont.)

Authors, year	Sample	Diagnostic measures	Major findings[b]	Males	Females

Timmons-Mitchell et al., 1997	**Participants:** Institutionalized delinquents
	N: 50
	Age: females: 15.7 years; males: 15.9 years (means)
	Sex: 25 females; 25 males
	Race/ethnicity: N/R
	Other: 50 subjects were administered the DISC out of the total sample of 173 subjects.
		DISC (modified)	**Psychosis:**
			Affective:
			SUD:
			CD:
			Anxiety:
			Other:
			  ADHD:
			  Eating Disorder:
			  Sleep Disorder:
				16%
				72%
				88%
				100%
				52%
				
				76%
				0%
				68%
					12%
					88%
					56%
					96%
					72%
					
					68%
					16%
					72%

Cauffman et al., 1998	**Participants:** Incarcerated wards **N:** 189 **Age:** females: 17.2 years; males: 16.6 years (mean) **Sex:** 96 females; 93 males **Race/ethnicity:** Males: 37.6% African American 26.9% Hispanic 30.1% White 5.4% Other Females: 21.1% African American 28.9% Hispanic 23.3% White 26.7% Other	Psychiatric Diagnostic Interview-Revised (PTSD module only)	**Anxiety:** PTSD:	Males 32%	Females 49%

Study	Details	Instrument		Males	Females	Total
Duclos et al., 1998	**Participants:** Youth in a detention facility **N:** 150 **Age:** 15 years (median) **Sex:** 65 females; 85 males **Race/ethnicity:** 100% Native American, specific group(s) N/R **Other:** 77% status offenders	DISC 2.3; CIDI	**Affective:** Dysthymia: MDD: **SUD/AUD:** **CD:** **Anxiety (any):** Generalized: Overanxious: PTSD: **Other:** ODD ADHD **Co-morbidity:** 21.4% had two or more disorders: Of those, 83% had SUD + DBD	0% 6% 37% 21% 2% 0% 0% 2% 1% 6% 17%	0% 16% 39% 11% 13% 8% 13% 0% 3% 11% 27%	0% 10% 38% 17% 7% 3% 5% 1% 2% 8% 21%
Atkins et al., 1999	**Participants:** Youth in a detention facility **N:** 75 **Age:** 15.5 years (mean) **Sex:** 4 females; 71 males **Race/ethnicity:** African American: 77.3%; Non-Hispanic White: 22.7%	DISC 2.3	**Psychosis:** 45% **Affective:** 24% **SUD:** 20% **CD:** 40% **Anxiety:** 33% **Other:** ODD: 15%; ADHD: 1% **Co-morbidity:** mean of 2.4 diagnoses per youth			
Erwin et al., 2000	**Participants:** Youth in a secure juvenile treatment facility **N:** 51 **Age:** 17.5 years (mean) **Sex:** all male **Race/ethnicity:** African American: 28%; Hispanic: 12%; White: 57%	Clinician Administered PTSD Scale for Children & Adolescents	**Anxiety:** lifetime PTSD: 45%; current PTSD: 18%			

Table 2.1. (cont.)

Authors, year	Sample	Diagnostic measures	Major findings [b]
Pliszka et al., 2000	**Participants:** Youth in a detention center N: 50 **Age:** 15.4 years (mean) **Sex:** 5 females; 45 males **Race/ethnicity:** N/R	DISC 2.3	**Affective (any):** 42%; MDD: 20%; Mania 20% **SUD:** Alcohol Dependence: 28%; Marijuana Dependence: 46%; other: 14% **CD:** 60% **Other:** ADHD: 18%; ODD: 24% **Co-morbidity:** Among those with Mania: 82% had CD; 36% had Alcohol Dependence; 64% had Marijuana Dependence; 45% had Other Substance Dependence. Among those with MDD: 80% had CD; 20% had Alcohol Dependence; 60% had Marijuana Dependence.

Aarons et al., 2001	**Participants:** Adjudicated youth
	N: 419
	Age: 16.9 years (mean)
	Sex: 66.3% male
	Race/ethnicity: African American: 20.7%; Asian/Pacific Islander: 9.4%; Hispanic: 28.8%; Non-Hispanic White: 34%; biracial: 4.2%; other: 3%
	Other: Participants from a subsample (N = 1036) of the larger study, "Patterns of Care;" Age & race based on the total subsample.
		CIDI (SUD module only)	**SUD/AUD (any):**
			
			                    Lifetime Past year
			AUD: 62% 37%
			Amphetamine: 49% 28%
			Cannabis: 23% 10%
			Cocaine: 46% 15%
			Hallucinogen: 2% 0.5%
			Opiate: 9% 3%
			                    0.5% 0%

Study	Instrument	Sample characteristics	Findings
Garland et al., 2001	Computer-assisted DISC-IV	**Participants:** Adjudicated youth N: 478 **Age:** 16.9 years (mean) **Sex:** 74 females; 404 males **Race/ethnicity:** African American: 21%; Asian/Pacific Islander: 6%; Hispanic: 26%; White: 39%; mixed: 5%; other: 3% **Other:** Participants from a subsample (N = 1,618) of the larger study, "Patterns of Care;" Age & race based on total subsample.	**Affective (any):** 7%; Dysthymia: 0%; Hypomania: 1%; MDD: 5%; Mania: 2% **CD:** 30% **Anxiety (any):** 9%; Generalized Anxiety: 1%; Obsessive-compulsive: 2%; Panic: 0%; PTSD: 3%; Separation Anxiety: 4%; Social Phobia: 2% **Other:** any DBD: 48%; ADHD: 13%; ODD: 15%
Shelton, 2001	DISC	**Participants:** Youth in commitment & detention facilities N: 312 **Age:** 12–20 years (mean or median N/R) **Sex:** 60 females; 252 males **Race/ethnicity:** African American: 57%; Hispanic & other: 17%; White: 26%	**Psychosis:** 32% **Affective:** 17% **SUD:** 37% **Anxiety:** 58% **Other:** any DBD: 40%; Misc. Disorders: 18% **Co-morbidity:** Anxiety + DBD: 27.5% Anxiety + Psychotic: 20.5% Anxiety + Affective: 13.8% Anxiety + SUD: 25.0% DBD + Psychotic: 14.1% DBD + Affective: 8.6% DBD + SUD: 18.6% Psychotic + Affective: 1.3% Psychotic + SUD: 14.7% Affective + SUD: 6.7%

Table 2.1. (cont.)

Authors, year	Sample	Diagnostic measures	Major findings[b]	Males	Females
McCabe et al., 2002	**Participants:** Adjudicated youth **N:** 625 **Age:** 16.2 years (mean) **Sex:** 112 females; 513 males **Race/ethnicity:** African American: 19.2%; Asian/Pacific Islander: 12.3%; Hispanic: 30.4%; White: 29%; biracial/other: 9.1% **Other:** Participants from the larger study, "Patterns of Care" (N = 1715).	Computer-assisted DISC-IV (selected modules); CIDI Substance Abuse Module	**Affective (any):**	5%	16%
			MDD	3%	14%
			Mania	1%	3%
			SUD:	37%	28%
			CD:	33%	38%
			Anxiety (any):	8%	15%
			PTSD	2%	7%
			Separation	4%	10%
			Other:		
			Any DBD	49%	64%
			ADHD:	15%	21%
			ODD:	30%	42%
			Co-morbidity (more than one disorder):	38%	28%
Wasserman et al., 2002	**Participants:** Youth in secure facilities **N:** 292 **Age:** 17 years (mean) **Sex:** male only **Race/ethnicity:** African American: 54%; Hispanic: 16%; White: 28%; other: 2%	Voice DISC-IV	**Affective (any):** 10%; Dysthymic: 1%; Hypomanic: 1%; MDD: 8%; Manic: 2% **SUD (any):** 50%; Alcohol Abuse: 17%; Alcohol Dependence: 13%; Marijuana Abuse: 15%; Marijuana Dependence: 26%; Other Substance Abuse: 4%; Other Substance Dependence: 13% **CD:** 32% **Anxiety (any):** 20%; Agoraphobia: 5%; Generalized Anxiety: 2%; Obsessive-compulsive: 5%; Panic: 5%; PTSD: 5%; Specific Phobia: 9%; Social Phobia: 2% **Other:** any DBD: 33%; ADHD: 2%		

			Males	Females
Domalanta et al., 2003	**Participants:** Youth in a detention center	Patient Health Questionnaire		
	N: 1024			
	Age: females: 14.9 years; males: 15.3 years (mean)			
	Sex: 274 females; 750 males			
	Race/ethnicity:			
	Males: 42.0% African American		**Affective (any):**	26%	31%
	35.3% Hispanic		MDD:	10%	10%
	18.5% White		Mood NOS:	12%	13%
	4.2% Other		Other Mood:	4%	8%
	Females: 32.8% African American		**Drug Abuse:**	43%	36%
	36.5%Hispanic		**Alcohol Abuse:**	27%	27%
	23.4% White		**Anxiety:**		
	7.3% Other		Other:	8%	12%
			Panic:	5%	8%
			Somatoform:	12%	22%

Co-morbidity (two or more disorders): 38%

Among those with MDD:

49% had Substance Abuse; 39% had Alcohol Abuse

Among those with Alcohol Abuse:

14.2 % had MDD; 83.3% had Substance Abuse

Among those with Substance Abuse:

11.7% had MDD; 54.5% had Alcohol Abuse

[a] Excludes treatment studies; only diagnoses reported by each study are displayed; percentages are rounded to the nearest whole number; arranged by year published and author; mean age is reported unless unavailable and otherwise indicated.

[b] ADD = Attention-Deficit Disorder; ADHD = Attention-Deficit/Hyperactivity Disorder; AUD = Alcohol Use Disorder; CD = Conduct Disorder; CIDI = Composite International Diagnostic Interview; DBD = Disruptive Behavior Disorders; DICA-R = Diagnostic Interview for Children and Adolescents-Revised; DISC = Diagnostic Interview Schedule for Children; DSM = Diagnostic and Statistical Manual of Mental Disorders; K-SADS-PL = Kiddie – Schedule for Affective Disorders, Present and Lifetime Version; MDD = Major Depressive Disorder; NOS = Not Otherwise Specified; N/R = Not Reported; ODD = Oppositional Defiant Disorder; PD = Personality Disorder; PTSD = Posttraumatic Stress Disorder; SCID = Structured Clinical Interview for DSM; SUD = Substance Use Disorder.

to 88 percent (Timmons-Mitchell *et al.*, 1997); and psychosis from 16 percent (Timmons-Mitchell *et al.*, 1997) to 45 percent (Atkins *et al.*, 1999). Differences in the methodology of these studies may account for the inconsistency in results.

- **Variations in sampling strategies**. Samples varied substantially among the studies presented in Table 2.1. Some studies used random samples. Others, however, relied on non-random samples, for example, consecutive admissions over a specified time period. Only a few studies examined racial/ethnic differences, and some studies did not report the racial or ethnic composition of the sample. Females were excluded entirely from some investigations.

- **Small samples**. Some severe disorders have low base rates in the general population, between one and four percent (Whitaker *et al.*, 1990). Low base rates require large sample sizes to generate reliable estimates (Cohen, 1998). Among the studies described in Table 2.1, sample sizes varied substantially, between 50 (Pliszka *et al.*, 2000; Timmons-Mitchell *et al.*, 1997) and 1024 subjects (Domalanta *et al.*, 2003). Many of the studies sampled too few subjects to generate reliable rates, even for the more common disorders. Most studies did not have enough participants in key demographic subgroups to compare rates by sex, race/ethnicity, or age.

- **Problems in measurement**. Some studies in Table 2.1 used non-standard or untested instruments, did not assess if the disorder impaired functioning, or reported data on only one category of diagnoses (e.g., substance use disorders, anxiety disorders, personality disorders).

The Northwestern Juvenile Project

The Northwestern Juvenile Project was designed to overcome these methodological limitations in two ways. First, it uses a random sample of juvenile detainees, 10–18 years old. Second, it uses a widely accepted and reliable diagnostic tool, the Diagnostic Interview Schedule for Children (DISC) to measure alcohol, drug, and psychiatric diagnoses (Shaffer *et al.*, 1996, 2003).

Methods

Subjects were a randomly selected sample of 1829 male and female youth who were arrested and subsequently detained at the Cook County Juvenile Temporary Detention Center (CCJTDC) between November 20, 1995, and June 14, 1998. The sample was stratified by sex, race/ethnicity (African American, non-Hispanic white, Hispanic), age (10–13 years old, or 14 and older), and legal status (processed as a juvenile or an adult). The final sample comprised 1172 males (64.1 percent) and 657 females (35.9 percent), 1005 African Americans (54.9 percent),

524 Hispanics (28.7 percent), 296 non-Hispanic whites (16.2 percent), and 4 from other racial/ethnic groups (0.2 percent). The mean age of participants was 14.9 years.

Like juvenile detainees nationwide (Sickmund *et al.*, 2006) approximately 90 percent of the detainees at CCJTDC are male and most are racial/ethnic minorities: African American (77.9 percent), non-Hispanic white (5.6 percent), Hispanic (16.0 percent), and other racial or ethnic groups (0.5 percent). The age and offense distributions of detainees at CCJTDC are also similar to detained juveniles nationwide (Sickmund *et al.*, 2006).

Although no single site can represent the entire country, Illinois' criteria for detaining juveniles are similar to other states (Grisso *et al.*, 1988; Illinois Criminal Justice Information Authority, 1997). Pretrial detention is allowed if a juvenile needs protection, is likely to flee, or is considered a danger to the community (Grisso *et al.*, 1988; Illinois Criminal Justice Information Authority, 1997).

Psychiatric diagnoses

The DISC Version 2.3 (Shaffer *et al.*, 1996; Bravo *et al.*, 1993) was used to assess affective disorders (major depression, dysthymia, mania, hypomania), anxiety disorders (panic, generalized anxiety, separation anxiety, obsessive-compulsive, and over-anxious disorder), behavioral disorders (conduct disorder, attention-deficit/hyperactivity disorder [ADHD], oppositional defiant disorder), psychosis, and substance use disorders (alcohol, marijuana, and drug use disorders other than marijuana) within the past six months.

Psychosis and ADHD required special management. The psychosis module of the DISC is a broad symptom screen and does not generate a specific diagnosis. Instead, this module flags subjects if they indicate any essential symptoms of psychosis or at least three associated symptoms. More than one-quarter of the subjects scored positive on the screen. To rule out false positive diagnoses, these subjects were counted as psychotic only if their symptoms persisted for at least one week; they had not used alcohol, drugs, or medication during this time; and the psychiatrist or clinical psychologist who reviewed the case judged that the symptoms were probably indicative of psychosis. Twelve subjects met these criteria. An additional eight subjects were counted as psychotic because, although they denied symptoms, they appeared to have auditory hallucinations, thought disorders, or delusions during their interviews.

ADHD among youth is difficult to assess via self-report (Schwab-Stone *et al.*, 1996) and is even more difficult to diagnose among delinquent youth (Thompson *et al.*, 1996). In addition, the DSM-III-R requires that ADHD symptoms be present before age seven. Most subjects who reported symptoms of ADHD could not remember when their symptoms began. To reduce the risk of underreporting

ADHD, rates were calculated by counting the disorder as present regardless of the reported age of onset, as long as the duration criterion was met.

Data on posttraumatic stress disorder (PTSD) were collected 13 months after the larger study began because PTSD was not included in the DISC 2.3. PTSD was measured with the DISC 4.0, which provided 12-month rates using DSM-IV criteria for PTSD. Data on PTSD diagnoses were examined using a sub-sample of 898 participants. The sub-sample comprised 532 males (59.2 percent) and 366 females (40.8 percent); 490 African Americans (54.6 percent), 154 non-Hispanic whites (17.1 percent), 252 Hispanic (28.1 percent), and 2 others (0.2 percent). Participants ranged in age from 10–18 years; the mean was 14.8 years; the median was 15 years. Data on PTSD are based on the youth's self-report because it was not feasible to interview caretakers. Like other measures of PTSD in children, there are still insufficient data on the DISC-IV's reliability and validity. Despite the lack of psychometric data on the PTSD module of the DISC-IV, we chose it for several reasons. The DISC is the most widely used diagnostic instrument for child and adolescent research. It is especially useful for large-scale epidemiologic studies because it is relatively brief; it can be administered by non-clinicians; it is designed to assess youth who have and have not been traumatized; and it generates DSM-IV disorders using computerized scoring.

Statistical analysis

Because the sample was stratified by sex, race/ethnicity, age, and legal status, prevalence estimates were weighted to reflect the detention center's population. Taylor series linearization was used to correct for sample design (Cochrane, 1977; Levy & Lemeshow, 1999).

Results

Table 2.2 shows that nearly two-thirds of males and nearly three-quarters of females met the diagnostic criteria for one or more of the disorders listed (Sickmund *et al.*, 2006). Overall rates excluding conduct disorder were also calculated because many of its symptoms are related to delinquent behaviors. Excluding conduct disorder, overall rates decreased only slightly. Rates of PTSD were omitted from the overall rates of disorder in Table 2.2 because PTSD was measured using DISC 4.0 with a subsample of youth.

Prevalence rates by sex

The most common disorders among males and females were substance use disorders and disruptive behavior disorders (oppositional-defiant disorder and

Table 2.2. Six-month prevalence and odds ratios of DSM III-R diagnoses by sex with and without diagnosis-specific impairment criteria[a]

DISORDER	MALE (%, 95% CI) (n = 1170)						FEMALE (%, 95% CI) (n = 656)						FEMALE TO MALE ODDS RATIOS (OR, 95% CI)					
	Diagnosis			Diagnosis with Impairment			Diagnosis			Diagnosis with Impairment			Diagnosis			Diagnosis with Impairment		
	%	LCI	UCI	%	LCI	UCI	%	LCI	UCI	%	LCI	UCI	OR	LCI	UCI	OR	LCI	UCI
ANY OF THE LISTED DISORDERS[b]	66.3	61.6	70.7	63.3	58.6	67.8	73.8	70.1	77.1	71.2	67.5	74.7	1.43	1.09	1.88	1.43	1.10	1.87
ANY EXCEPT CONDUCT DISORDER[b]	60.9	56.2	65.5	59.7	54.9	64.3	70.0	66.2	73.5	68.2	64.4	71.8	1.49	1.15	1.94	1.45	1.12	1.88
ANY AFFECTIVE DISORDER	18.7	15.2	22.8	16.1	12.8	20.0	27.6	23.6	32.0	22.9	19.0	27.2	1.66	1.20	2.29	1.55	1.09	2.20
Major depressive episode	13.0	10.0	16.6	11.0	8.3	14.5	21.6	17.8	25.9	18.9	15.2	23.2	1.85	1.27	2.70	1.88	1.25	2.82
Dysthymia	12.2	9.3	15.8	9.9	7.3	13.2	15.8	13.1	18.8	12.5	10.2	15.3	1.34	0.93	1.95	1.31	0.87	1.96
Manic episode	2.2	1.1	4.3	2.0	1.0	4.1	1.8	1.0	3.2	1.2	0.6	2.4	0.81	0.33	1.99	0.58	0.21	1.63
PSYCHOTIC DISORDERS	1.0	0.4	2.6	...			1.0	0.5	2.1	...			0.98	0.30	3.25	...		
ANY ANXIETY DISORDER	21.3	17.6	25.6	20.7	17.0	24.9	30.8	27.2	34.6	28.9	25.5	32.7	1.64	1.22	2.20	1.56	1.16	2.10
Panic disorder	0.3	0.1	0.6	0.1	0.0	0.4	1.5	0.8	2.7	1.0	0.5	2.0	5.65	2.04	15.65	8.13	2.01	32.85
Separation anxiety disorder	12.9	9.9	16.5	10.8	8.1	14.2	18.6	15.7	21.9	16.3	13.6	19.4	1.55	1.08	2.21	1.61	1.10	2.34
Overanxious disorder	6.7	4.6	9.7	5.9	4.0	8.7	12.3	9.9	15.1	11.5	9.2	14.2	1.95	1.23	3.10	2.06	1.27	3.35
Generalized anxiety disorder	7.1	4.9	10.2	6.4	4.3	9.4	7.3	5.6	9.6	6.8	5.1	9.0	1.03	0.63	1.69	1.07	0.64	1.79
Obsessive-compulsive disorder	8.3	6.1	11.3	...			10.6	8.4	13.2	...			1.31	0.86	2.00	...		

Table 2.2. (cont.)

DISORDER	MALE (%, 95% CI) (n = 1170)						FEMALE (%, 95% CI) (n = 656)						FEMALE TO MALE ODDS RATIOS (OR, 95% CI)					
	Diagnosis			Diagnosis with Impairment			Diagnosis			Diagnosis with Impairment			Diagnosis			Diagnosis with Impairment		
	%	LCI	UCI	%	LCI	UCI	%	LCI	UCI	%	LCI	UCI	OR	LCI	UCI	OR	LCI	UCI
ATTENTION-DEFICIT/ HYPERACTIVITY DISORDER^c	16.6	13.3	20.5	11.2	8.5	14.6	21.4	18.4	24.8	16.4	13.7	19.5	1.37	0.99	1.89	1.55	1.07	2.25
ANY DISRUPTIVE BEHAVIOR DISORDER	41.4	36.8	46.2	31.4	27.2	36.0	45.6	41.4	49.8	38.0	33.9	42.2	1.19	0.92	1.53	1.33	1.02	1.75
Oppositional-defiant disorder	14.5	11.4	18.2	12.6	9.8	16.2	17.5	14.7	20.6	15.1	12.5	18.1	1.25	0.89	1.76	1.23	0.86	1.76
Conduct disorder	37.8	33.3	42.6	24.3	20.5	28.5	40.6	36.5	44.8	28.5	24.6	32.8	1.12	0.86	1.46	1.24	0.92	1.67
ANY SUBSTANCE USE DISORDER	50.7	45.9	55.5	...			46.8	42.6	51.1	...			0.86	0.66	1.11	...		
Alcohol use disorder	25.9	21.9	30.4	...			26.5	22.6	30.9	...			1.03	0.76	1.40	...		
Marijuana use disorder	44.8	40.1	49.6	...			40.5	36.8	44.4	...			0.84	0.65	1.08	...		
Other substance use disorder	2.4	1.7	3.4	...			6.9	4.1	11.4	...			3.00	1.57	5.74	...		
Both alcohol and other drug use disorders	20.7	17.0	24.9	...			20.9	18.0	24.2	...			1.01	0.75	1.38	...		

[a] CI indicates confidence interval. Ellipses indicate that diagnosis and diagnosis with impairment are identical because the diagnostic criteria for psychotic disorders, obsessive-compulsive disorder, and substance use disorders include impairment.

[b] Rates of PTSD are presented in the text and were omitted from analyses of overall rates of disorder.

[c] Attention-deficit/hyperactivity disorder is reported without the criterion of onset before age seven years because caretaker information is not available and self-report of symptoms before age seven years is unreliable.

Although not included in Table 2.2, combined prevalence rates of major depressive episode and dysthymia were 17 percent for males and 24 percent for females.

conduct disorder). One-half of males and almost one-half of females met criteria for a substance use disorder; more than 40 percent of males and females met the criteria for disruptive behavior disorders. More than one-fourth of females and almost one-fifth of males met criteria for one or more affective disorders.

Table 2.2 also reports the female-to-male odds ratios. The odds ratios show the relative likelihood of having a disorder for one group compared to another group. For the female-to-male odds ratios, odds ratios greater than 1.0 indicate that females had higher odds of having a specific disorder than males; ratios less than 1.0 show that females had lower odds of having the disorder. Females had significantly higher odds than males of having any disorder, any disorder except conduct disorder, any affective disorder, a major depressive episode, any anxiety disorder, panic disorder, separation anxiety disorder, overanxious disorder, and substance use disorder other than alcohol or marijuana.

Significantly more females (56.5 percent) than males (45.9 percent) met criteria for two or more of the following disorders: major depressive, dysthymic, manic, psychotic, panic, separation anxiety, overanxious, generalized anxiety, obsessive-compulsive, ADHD, conduct, oppositional-defiant, alcohol, marijuana, and other substance. Approximately one-fifth (17.3 percent) of females and males (20.4 percent) had only one disorder.

Figures 2.1 and 2.2 show substantial comorbidity for females and males. Psychosis was omitted from analyses of co-morbidity because there were so few cases; PTSD was omitted from the analyses of co-morbidity because it was assessed using the DISC 4.0 with a subsample of youth. Patterns of overlap differ somewhat by sex. Nearly one-third of females (29.5 percent) and males (30.8 percent) had both substance use disorders and ADHD or behavioral disorders; approximately half of these also had anxiety disorders, affective disorders, or both. Significantly more females (47.8 percent) than males (41.6 percent) had two or more of the following types of disorders: affective, anxiety, substance use, and ADHD or behavioral. Significantly more females (22.5 percent) than males (17.2 percent) had three or more types of disorders. Further information is available in Abram, Teplin, McClelland and Dulcan (2003).

Prevalence rates by race/ethnicity

Tables 2.3 and 2.4 show the prevalence rates of disorders for males and females by race/ethnicity. Table 2.3 indicates that among males, non-Hispanic whites had the highest rates for many disorders and African Americans had the lowest. Compared with African Americans, non-Hispanic whites had significantly higher rates of any disorder, any disorder except conduct disorder, any disruptive behavior disorder,

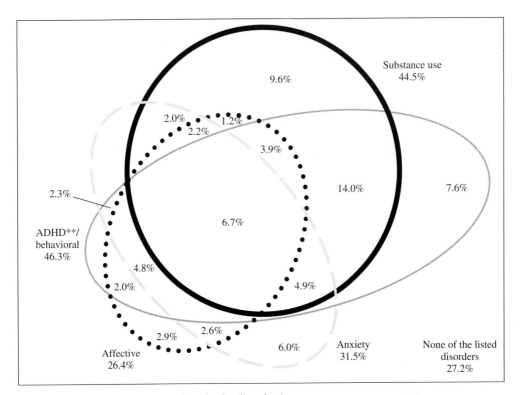

Figure 2.1   Co-morbidity among females by disorder.*
  * Percents may not sum to 100% due to rounding error.
  ** ADHD indicates attention-deficit/hyperactivity disorder.

conduct disorder, any substance use disorder, and substance use disorder other than alcohol or marijuana. The only disorder for which African Americans had significantly higher rates than non-Hispanic whites was separation anxiety disorder. Hispanics had significantly higher rates than non-Hispanic whites of any anxiety disorder and separation anxiety disorder. Compared with African Americans, Hispanics had higher rates of panic disorder, obsessive-compulsive disorder, and substance use disorder other than alcohol or marijuana. Non-Hispanic whites had higher rates than Hispanics of any disorder, any disruptive behavior disorder, conduct disorder, and substance use disorder other than alcohol or marijuana.

Table 2.4 compares rates by race/ethnicity for females. Compared with African American females, non-Hispanic white females had significantly higher rates of any disorder, any disorder except conduct disorder, any disruptive behavior disorder, conduct disorder, and all substance use disorders. Compared with Hispanic females, non-Hispanic white females had higher rates of any disorder except conduct disorder. Hispanic females had higher rates of generalized anxiety disorder than either African American or non-Hispanic white females. Compared

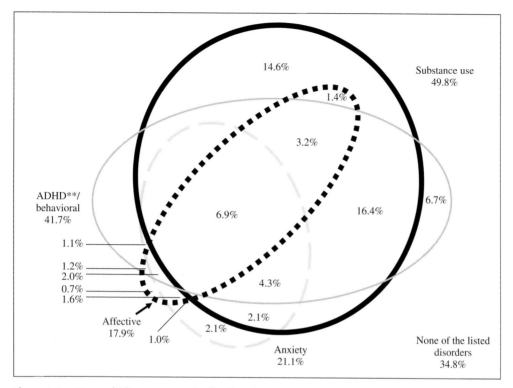

Figure 2.2.   Co-morbidity among males by disorder.*
          * Percents may not sum to 100% due to rounding error.
          ** ADHD indicates attention-deficit/hyperactivity disorder.

with African American females, Hispanic females had higher rates of all disruptive behavior disorders, alcohol use disorder, substance use disorder other than alcohol or marijuana, and alcohol and drug use disorders.

  Among females, significantly more non-Hispanic whites (63.1 percent) had two or more types of disorders than African Americans (42.6 percent). (Detailed statistical findings are presented in Abram *et al.*, 2003.) Among males, significantly more non-Hispanic whites (53.1 percent) had two or more types of disorders than African Americans (40.7 percent). The odds of having co-morbid disorders are higher than expected by chance for most racial/ethnic subgroups, except when base rates of disorders were already high or when cell sizes were small.

Prevalence rates by age

Tables 2.5 and 2.6 indicate the prevalence of disorders for males and females by age. Table 2.5 indicates that among males, the youngest age group had the lowest rates of many disorders. This group had significantly lower rates than both older

Table 2.3. Six-month prevalence of DSM III-R diagnoses for males by race/ethnicity[a]

	African-American (n = 574)			Non-Hispanic White (n = 207)			Hispanic (n = 386)			Overall significance	Protected Tests[b]
	%	LCI	UCI	%	LCI	UCI	%	LCI	UCI		
ANY OF THE LISTED DISORDERS[c]	64.6	58.8	69.9	82.0	76.2	86.7	70.4	63.3	76.7	<.001	White > African American; White > Hispanic
ANY EXCEPT CONDUCT DISORDER[c]	59.4	53.5	65.0	72.9	66.5	78.6	65.3	58.1	71.9	0.009	White > African American
ANY AFFECTIVE DISORDER	18.6	14.4	23.6	13.8	9.6	19.5	21.5	15.3	29.3	0.19	
Major depressive episode	12.5	9.1	17.0	9.5	6.0	14.6	16.6	10.8	24.7	0.20	
Dysthymia	12.2	8.8	16.7	9.5	6.1	14.5	13.3	8.4	20.6	0.53	
Manic episode	2.5	1.2	5.2	0.5	0.1	3.7	1.4	0.6	3.2	0.27	
PSYCHOTIC DISORDERS	1.0	0.3	3.2	2.6	1.1	6.2	0.7	0.2	2.6	0.19	
ANY ANXIETY DISORDER	20.9	16.5	26.1	14.4	10.1	20.2	25.5	18.7	33.7	0.046	Hispanic > White
Panic disorder	0.1	0.0	0.4	0.5	0.1	3.7	1.0	0.3	3.1	0.04	Hispanic > African American
Separation anxiety disorder	12.7	9.3	17.2	5.9	3.3	10.3	15.5	9.8	23.6	0.02	African American > White; Hispanic > White
Overanxious disorder	6.9	4.4	10.7	2.9	1.3	6.6	7.0	3.6	13.0	0.16	
Generalized anxiety disorder	7.5	4.8	11.4	2.5	1.0	5.9	7.2	3.7	13.3	0.08	

Obsessive-compulsive disorder	6.5	4.2	10.0	9.3	5.8	14.4	17.0	10.7	25.9	0.01	Hispanic > African American
ATTENTION-DEFICIT/ HYPERACTIVITY DISORDER[d]	17.0	13.0	21.9	20.9	15.8	27.3	13.7	9.4	19.5	0.18	
ANY DISRUPTIVE BEHAVIOR DISORDER	39.8	34.2	45.7	60.3	53.3	66.9	43.3	36.1	50.8	<.001	White > African American; White > Hispanic
Oppositional-defiant disorder	14.4	10.7	19.1	19.4	14.4	25.6	13.6	9.3	19.5	0.23	
Conduct disorder	35.6	30.1	41.5	59.9	53.0	66.5	41.7	34.5	49.2	<.001	White > African American; White > Hispanic
ANY SUBSTANCE USE DISORDER	49.1	43.2	55.0	62.6	55.7	69.0	55.4	47.8	62.7	0.01	White > African American
Alcohol use disorder	24.6	19.8	30.2	30.1	24.0	36.9	30.8	24.1	38.5	0.28	
Marijuana use disorder	44.4	38.6	50.4	53.8	46.8	60.6	45.4	38.0	52.9	0.11	
Other substance use disorder	0.5	0.1	2.8	21.1	15.9	27.4	6.0	3.9	9.1	<.001	White > African American; White > Hispanic; Hispanic > African American
Both alcohol and other drug use disorders	20.4	16.0	25.7	24.0	18.5	30.6	21.7	16.5	28.0	0.65	

[a] CI indicates confidence interval. Two cases of "other" Race/ethnicity are excluded from this table.

[b] Protected tests are performed only if the alpha for the overall test is less than .05.

[c] Rates of PTSD are presented in the text and were omitted from analyses of overall rates of disorder.

[d] Attention-deficit/hyperactivity disorder is reported without the criterion of onset before the age of seven years because caretaker information is not available and self-report of symptoms before the age of seven years is unreliable.

Table 2.4. Six-month prevalence DSM III-R diagnoses for females by Race/ethnicity[a]

	African American (n = 430)			Non-Hispanic White (n = 89)			Hispanic (n = 136)			Overall significance	Protected Tests[b]
	%	LCI	UCI	%	LCI	UCI	%	LCI	UCI		
ANY OF THE LISTED DISORDERS[c]	70.9	66.4	75.0	86.1	77.1	92.0	75.9	67.9	82.5	0.01	White > African American
ANY EXCEPT CONDUCT DISORDER[c]	67.4	62.8	71.6	83.9	74.6	90.3	69.5	61.2	76.7	0.01	White > African American; White > Hispanic
ANY AFFECTIVE DISORDER	26.2	22.2	30.5	23.4	15.8	33.4	28.7	21.8	36.9	0.68	
Major depressive episode	19.7	16.2	23.7	19.0	12.1	28.5	22.8	16.5	30.5	0.70	
Dysthymia	15.5	12.4	19.2	17.9	11.2	27.3	17.2	11.8	24.5	0.80	
Manic episode	1.9	0.9	3.7	1.1	0.2	7.5	2.1	0.7	6.4	0.85	
PSYCHOTIC DISORDERS	0.9	0.4	2.5	0.0			2.1	0.7	6.3	.29[d]	
ANY ANXIETY DISORDER	31.2	27.0	35.8	30.0	21.4	40.3	32.6	25.2	40.9	0.92	
Panic disorder	0.9	0.4	2.5	3.4	1.1	10.0	2.8	1.0	7.1	0.17	
Separation anxiety disorder	18.9	15.5	22.9	14.5	8.6	23.4	21.7	15.5	29.4	0.41	
Overanxious disorder	12.5	9.7	16.0	11.1	6.1	19.5	13.2	8.4	20.1	0.90	
Generalized anxiety disorder	6.6	4.6	9.4	4.4	1.7	11.3	13.1	8.4	19.9	0.03	Hispanic > African American; Hispanic > White
Obsessive-compulsive disorder	10.3	7.8	13.6	12.4	7.0	21.1	10.6	6.5	16.9	0.84	
ATTENTION-DEFICIT/HYPERACTIVITY DISORDER[e]	20.0	16.5	24.1	22.2	14.7	32.0	29.3	22.2	37.5	0.08	

ANY DISRUPTIVE BEHAVIOR DISORDER	39.4	34.9	44.1	61.6	51.0	71.1	56.5	47.9	64.6	<.001	White > African American; Hispanic > African American
Oppositional-defiant disorder	15.8	12.7	19.6	17.8	11.1	27.1	26.2	19.5	34.3	0.03	Hispanic > African American
Conduct disorder	34.3	29.9	38.9	58.9	48.3	68.7	50.2	41.8	58.6	<.001	White > African American; Hispanic > African American
ANY SUBSTANCE USE DISORDER	42.3	37.6	47.1	61.9	51.2	71.6	51.7	43.1	60.1	0.002	White > African American
Alcohol use disorder	21.2	17.5	25.3	39.2	29.5	49.9	34.0	26.4	42.5	<.001	White > African American; Hispanic > African American
Marijuana use disorder	37.8	33.3	42.5	53.4	42.9	63.6	44.7	36.3	53.3	0.02	White > African American
Other substance use disorder	0.9	0.4	2.5	20.0	12.9	29.6	14.7	9.7	21.5	<.001	White > African American
Both alcohol and other drug use disorders	17.2	13.9	21.1	35.1	25.7	45.8	28.3	21.2	36.7	<.001	White > African American; Hispanic > African American

[a] CI indicates confidence interval. Two cases of "other" Race/ethnicity are excluded from this table.

[b] Protected tests are performed only if the alpha for the overall test is less than 0.05.

[c] Rates of PTSD are presented in the text and were omitted from analyses of overall rates of disorder.

[d] Test computed with 1 df because of empty cells.

[e] Attention-deficit/hyperactivity disorder is reported without the criterion of onset before the age of seven years because caretaker information is not available and self-report of symptoms before the age of seven years is unreliable.

Table 2.5. Six-month prevalence of DSM III-R diagnosis for males by age[a]

	Age $<=$ 13 Years (n = 315)			Age 14 and 15 Years (n = 361)			Age $>=$ 16 Years (n = 494)			Overall	Protected Tests[b]
	%	LCI	UCI	%	LCI	UCI	%	LCI	UCI	Significance	
ANY OF THE LISTED DISORDERS[c]	52.7	46.5	58.8	68.0	60.3	74.8	67.3	60.3	73.7	0.001	14 and 15 years > 13 years and younger; 16 years and older > 13 years and younger
ANY EXCEPT CONDUCT DISORDER[c]	44.9	38.9	51.0	63.4	55.6	70.6	61.8	54.7	68.5	<.001	14 and 15 years > 13 years and younger; 16 years and older > 13 years and younger
ANY AFFECTIVE DISORDER	13.0	9.4	17.6	21.2	15.4	28.4	17.7	12.9	23.7	0.09	
Major depressive episode	7.5	4.9	11.4	14.8	10.0	21.5	12.4	8.5	17.8	0.06	
Dysthymia	7.3	4.7	11.3	14.5	9.7	21.1	11.2	7.4	16.4	0.08	
Manic episode	1.6	0.7	4.0	2.6	0.9	7.2	2.0	0.7	5.1	0.80	
PSYCHOTIC DISORDERS	0.0			2.1	0.7	6.0	0.3	0.2	0.8	0.01[d]	14 and 15 years > 16 years and older
ANY ANXIETY DISORDER	17.7	13.6	22.9	23.0	16.9	30.4	20.6	15.5	26.7	0.42	
Panic disorder	0.8	0.2	3.3	0.1	0.0	0.9	0.3	0.1	0.9	0.25	
Separation anxiety disorder	10.0	6.9	14.3	14.5	9.7	21.1	12.0	8.1	17.5	0.40	
Overanxious disorder	4.8	2.8	8.0	5.1	2.6	9.9	8.4	5.1	13.5	0.25	

Disorder										p	Age differences
Generalized anxiety disorder	1.3	0.5	3.4	5.9	3.1	11.0	9.2	5.8	14.4	0.001	14 and 15 years > 13 years and younger; 16 years and older > 13 years and younger
Obsessive-compulsive disorder	6.0	3.7	9.7	9.4	5.7	15.0	7.8	4.9	12.2	0.43	
ATTENTION-DEFICIT/ HYPERACTIVITY DISORDER[e]	12.5	9.1	16.9	20.9	15.1	28.0	13.8	9.7	19.2	0.06	
ANY DISRUPTIVE BEHAVIOR DISORDER	32.9	27.5	38.8	43.5	35.9	51.3	41.2	34.5	48.2	0.06	
Oppositional-defiant disorder	10.7	7.5	14.9	18.2	12.8	25.1	12.1	8.3	17.3	0.08	
Conduct disorder	30.8	25.6	36.6	41.1	33.6	49.1	36.4	30.0	43.3	0.10	
ANY SUBSTANCE USE DISORDER	28.3	23.1	34.0	51.3	43.5	59.1	54.4	47.3	61.3	<.001	14 and 15 years > 13 years and younger; 16 years and older > 13 years and younger
Alcohol use disorder	12.9	9.5	17.4	25.6	19.3	33.0	28.7	22.8	35.4	<.001	14 and 15 years > 13 years and younger; 16 years and older > 13 years and younger
Marijuana use disorder	25.1	20.3	30.5	46.9	39.1	54.8	46.8	39.8	53.9	<.001	14 and 15 years > 13 years and younger; 16 years and older > 13 years and younger
Other substance use disorder	0.8	0.4	1.7	2.5	1.2	5.0	2.6	1.9	3.6	0.01	14 and 15 years > 13 years and younger; 16 years and older > 13 years and younger

Table 2.5. (cont.)

	Age <= 13 Years (n = 315)			Age 14 and 15 Years (n = 361)			Age >= 16 Years (n = 494)			Overall	
	%	LCI	UCI	%	LCI	UCI	%	LCI	UCI	Significance	Protected Tests[b]
Both alcohol and other drug use disorders	10.2	7.2	14.3	21.5	15.7	28.7	22.0	16.7	28.3	<.001	14 and 15 years > 13 years and younger; 16 years and older > 13 years and younger

[a] CI indicates confidence interval.

[b] Protected tests are performed only if the alpha for the overall test is less than 0.05.

[c] Rates of PTSD are presented in the text and were omitted from analyses of overall rates of disorder.

[d] Test computed with 1 *df* because of empty cells.

[e] Attention-deficit/hyperactivity disorder is reported without the criterion of onset before the age of seven years because caretaker information is not available and self-report of symptoms before the age of seven years is unreliable.

Table 2.6. Six-month prevalence of DSM III-R diagnosis for females by age[a]

	Age <= 13 Years (n = 56)			Age 14 and 15 Years (n = 353)			Age >= 16 Years (n = 247)			Overall	
	%	LCI	UCI	%	LCI	UCI	%	LCI	UCI	Significance	Protected Tests[b]
ANY OF THE LISTED DISORDERS[c]	66.7	53.2	77.9	72.2	67.2	76.7	77.6	71.6	82.7	0.18	
ANY EXCEPT CONDUCT DISORDER[c]	64.7	51.2	76.2	67.4	62.2	72.1	74.8	68.6	80.2	0.13	
ANY AFFECTIVE DISORDER	20.7	12.0	33.3	27.9	23.5	32.9	28.8	21.2	37.8	0.50	
Major depressive disorder	13.0	6.5	24.2	21.6	17.6	26.3	23.4	16.0	32.9	0.27	
Dysthymia	10.4	4.7	21.4	15.6	12.2	19.8	17.2	12.8	22.6	0.46	
Manic episode	3.9	1.0	14.4	1.4	0.6	3.3	1.9	0.8	4.7	0.45	
PSYCHOTIC DISORDERS	0.0			0.6	0.2	2.5	1.8	0.7	4.3	0.21[d]	
ANY ANXIETY DISORDER	26.6	16.7	39.7	32.6	27.8	37.7	29.2	23.4	35.7	0.55	
Panic disorder	1.9	0.3	12.4	1.7	0.8	3.6	1.0	0.3	3.2	0.75	
Separation anxiety disorder	18.1	10.0	30.6	19.7	15.8	24.2	17.2	12.9	22.7	0.77	
Overanxious disorder	7.1	2.7	17.7	13.8	10.5	17.8	11.4	7.9	16.1	0.34	
Generalized anxiety disorder	3.8	1.0	14.1	7.1	4.9	10.3	8.4	5.5	12.7	0.51	
Obsessive-compulsive disorder	10.4	4.7	21.5	11.8	8.8	15.7	8.8	5.8	13.1	0.51	

Table 2.6. (cont.)

	Age <= 13 Years (n = 56)			Age 14 and 15 Years (n = 353)			Age >= 16 Years (n = 247)			Overall Significance	Protected Tests[b]
	%	LCI	UCI	%	LCI	UCI	%	LCI	UCI		
ATTENTION-DEFICIT/ HYPERACTIVITY DISORDER[e]	26.6	16.6	39.7	22.7	18.6	27.4	18.5	14.0	24.0	0.30	
ANY DISRUPTIVE BEHAVIOR DISORDER	44.7	32.2	57.9	50.0	44.8	55.2	39.6	32.0	47.8	0.11	
Oppositional-defiant disorder	30.5	19.9	43.6	20.2	16.4	24.7	10.7	7.3	15.2	<.001	13 years and younger > 16 years and older; 14 and 15 years > 16 years and older
Conduct disorder	33.0	22.0	46.3	45.3	40.2	50.5	35.7	28.1	44.2	0.06	
ANY SUBSTANCE USE DISORDER	30.5	19.9	43.7	45.8	40.6	51.2	52.0	44.5	59.4	0.02	14 and 15 years > 13 years and younger; 16 years and older > 13 years and younger
Alcohol use disorder	16.7	9.1	28.6	25.4	21.1	30.3	30.3	22.7	39.2	0.16	
Marijuana use disorder	24.8	15.3	37.5	41.3	36.2	46.6	43.3	37.1	49.7	0.04	14 and 15 years > 13 years and younger; 16 years and older > 13 years and younger

Other substance use disorder	5.9	2.2	14.9	5.3	3.5	7.8	9.5	3.7	22.2	0.52
Both alcohol and other drug use disorders	11.5	5.5	22.5	21.8	17.7	26.4	22.0	17.2	27.6	0.20

[a] CI indicates confidence interval.

[b] Protected tests are performed only if the alpha for the overall test is less than 0.05.

[c] Rates of PTSD are presented in the text and were omitted from analyses of overall rates of disorder.

[d] Test computed with 1 df because of empty cells.

[e] Attention-deficit/hyperactivity disorder is reported without the criterion of onset before the age of seven years because caretaker information is not available and self-report of symptoms before the age of seven years is unreliable.

age groups of any disorder, any disorder except conduct disorder, generalized anxiety disorder, and all the substance use disorders. The 14–15 age group had higher rates of psychotic disorders than the 16-and-older age group. Significantly more males aged 16 years and older (41.2 percent) had two or more types of disorders than males aged 13 years and younger (27.0 percent). Similarly, significantly more males aged 14 and 15 years (45.3 percent) had two or more types of disorders than males aged 13 years and younger.

Table 2.6 indicates somewhat different patterns of disorders for females. The oldest age group had significantly lower rates of oppositional-defiant disorder than the younger age groups. Compared with the older age groups, the youngest age group had significantly lower rates of any substance use disorder and marijuana use disorder. Among females, there were no significant age differences in the overall prevalence of co-morbid types of disorder.

Prevalence rates of trauma and PTSD

Most participants experienced at least one trauma (92.5 percent). Significantly more males (93.2 percent) than females (84.0 percent) reported a traumatic experience. There were no significant differences in overall prevalence of trauma across race/ethnicity for males and females. More than one-tenth (11.2 percent) of participants had PTSD in the past year; 10.9 percent of males and 14.7 percent of females had PTSD. There were no significant differences in PTSD diagnosis by sex or across race/ethnicity for males and females (Abram *et al.*, 2004).

Co-morbidity of substance use disorders and major mental disorders

More than one tenth of males (10.8 percent) and 13.7 percent of females had both a major mental disorder (psychosis, manic episode, or major depressive episode) and a substance use disorder. We examined these disorders in depth because detention centers are mandated to treat major mental disorders and because co-morbidity complicates treatment.

Rates of substance use disorders among youth with major mental disorders

Compared with participants with no major mental disorder, both females and males with any major mental disorder had significantly greater odds of having substance use disorders. We also examined two subcategories of major mental disorder: psychosis or manic episode (combined because there were too few cases to analyze separately and because these disorders present similarly) and major depressive episode. Most odds ratios for these subcategories were statistically significant, except when cell sizes were small.

Sex differences

Among youth with major mental disorders (n = 305), more than half of females and nearly three-quarters of males had any substance use disorder. Differences between females and males (and the corresponding odds ratios) were not statistically significant. This analysis is available from the authors.

Racial/ethnic differences

Among females with major mental disorders, significantly more non-Hispanic whites and Hispanics had both drug and alcohol use disorders than did African Americans (50.0 percent and 43.4 percent, respectively vs. 21.3 percent); significantly more Hispanic females had alcohol use disorders than did African Americans (52.5 percent vs. 26.6 percent). Among males with major mental disorders, there were no significant differences by race/ethnicity. These analyses are available from the authors.

Age differences

Among females with major mental disorders, there were no significant differences by age. Among males, nearly 90 percent aged 16 years and older who had a major mental disorder also had a substance use disorder, significantly more than males 10–13 years and 14–15 years of age (55.2 percent and 60.6 percent, respectively). These analyses are available from the authors.

Rates of major mental disorder among youth with substance use disorders

Nearly 30 percent of females and more than 20 percent of males with any substance use disorder also had a major mental disorder. Among youth with both drug and alcohol use disorders, more than one-third of females and more than one-quarter of males had a major mental disorder. There were no significant differences by sex, race/ethnicity, or age (analyses are available from the authors).

Compared with participants with no substance use disorder (the residual category), both females and males with any substance use disorder had significantly greater odds of having any major mental disorder, and its subcategory, major depressive episode. Among males, odds ratios for psychosis or a manic episode were significant for some subcategories of substance use disorders.

Relative onset of major mental disorders and substance use disorders

One-quarter of both females (27.2 percent) and males (25.0 percent) reported that their major mental disorder preceded their substance use disorder by more than one year. One-tenth of females (9.8 percent) and 20.7 percent of males reported that their substance use disorder preceded their major mental disorder by more than one year. Nearly two-thirds of females (63.0 percent) and 54.3 percent of males developed their disorders within the same year. Findings were similar for subcategories of disorders. (Analyses are available from the authors.)

Discussion

This study indicates that youth with psychiatric disorders pose a challenge for the juvenile justice system. Even when conduct disorder was excluded, nearly 60 percent of male and 70 percent of female juvenile detainees met diagnostic criteria and had diagnosis-specific impairment for one or more psychiatric disorders. Co-morbidity was common. To the extent that Cook County is typical, our findings suggest that on an average day, there may be as many as 72 000 detained youth with at least one psychiatric disorder; 47 000 detained youth who have two or more types of psychiatric disorder; and more than 12 000 detained youth who have both a major mental disorder and a substance use disorder.

These findings may underestimate the prevalence among youth entering the juvenile justice system for two reasons. First, the sample included only detainees; it excluded youth who were not detained because their charges were less serious, because they were immediately released, or because they were referred directly to the mental health system. Second, underreporting of symptoms and impairments by youth is common, especially for disruptive behavior disorders (Schwab-Stone *et al.*, 1996).

Comparing these findings with studies of youth in the general population is difficult because published estimates for the latter vary widely depending on the sample, the method, the source of data (subject or collaterals), and whether functional impairment was required for diagnosis (Roberts *et al.*, 1998). Despite these differences, the overall rates presented here are substantially higher than the median rate (15 percent) reported by Roberts, Attkisson, and Rosenblatt (1998) and the rates of other recent investigations, including the Great Smoky Mountains Study (20 percent) (Costello *et al.*, 1996), the Virginia Twin Study of Adolescent Behavioral Development (142 cases per 1000 persons) (Simonoff *et al.*, 1997), the Methods for the Epidemiology of Child and Adolescent Mental Disorders (6 percent) (Shaffer *et al.*, 1996), and the Miami-Dade County Public School Study (38 percent) (Turner & Gil, 2002). Our rates of co-morbidity are also substantially higher than those reported in community samples (Costello *et al.*, 1996; Angold *et al.*, 1999; Costello *et al.*, 1999; Kessler & Walters, 1998; Lewinsohn *et al.*, 1995). Moreover, the 12-month prevalence of PTSD among detained youth exceeds *lifetime* estimates of PTSD reported in community samples of youth and young adults (3.5–9.2 percent) (Breslau *et al.*, 1991; 1998; Kessler *et al.*, 1995; Giaconia *et al.*, 1995).

Of particular concern are the high rates of depression and dysthymia among detained youth (The President's New Freedom Commission on Mental Health, 2005), which are also higher than rates in the general population (Costello *et al.*, 1996; Simonoff *et al.*, 1997; Turner & Gil, 2002; Costello *et al.*, 1999; Kessler & Walters, 1998; Garrison *et al.*, 1997; McGee *et al.*, 1992). Depressive disorders, which are a risk factor for suicide and attempted suicide, are difficult to detect and treat in the corrections milieu. Overall, the prevalence rates presented here are comparable to rates in other high-risk populations, such as maltreated or runaway youth (Famularo *et al.*, 1992; Feitel *et al.*, 1992).

The co-morbidity of substance use disorders is also of particular concern. Among the disorders assessed, detainees are more likely to have substance use plus ADHD or behavioral disorders than any other combination. Half of these detainees also have an affective or anxiety disorder. Among adolescent substance users, these internalizing disorders are associated with more severe substance use (Riggs *et al.*, 1999; Whitmore *et al.*, 1997) but better treatment outcomes (Randall *et al.*, 1999).

The data highlight an important paradox regarding race and ethnicity. More than one-half of the youth in the juvenile justice system are African American or Hispanic. Therefore, most delinquent youth with psychiatric disorders are minorities. The prevalence of many single and co-morbid disorders, however, is highest among non-Hispanic whites. Thus, white youth in the juvenile justice system may, on average, be more dysfunctional (have greater psychiatric morbidity) than minorities.

Females had higher rates than males of many single and co-morbid psychiatric disorders, including major depressive episodes, some anxiety disorders, and substance use disorders other than alcohol and marijuana (e.g., cocaine and hallucinogens). These findings confirm those of prior studies of adult female detainees and conduct-disordered females that find females have higher rates of psychiatric disorders than males (Lewis *et al.*, 1991; Teplin *et al.*, 1996; Wasserman *et al.*, 2005). The youngest age group (13 and younger) had the lowest prevalence rates of most disorders, consistent with studies of youth in the general population (Simonoff *et al.*, 1997; Cohen *et al.*, 1993; Kandel *et al.*, 1997; Newman *et al.*, 1996). Many youth in the juvenile justice system may develop new or additional disorders as they grow older. Although co-morbidity of major mental and substance use disorders is more prevalent among older detainees, we found no dominant sequence of onset. This suggests that there are multiple pathways to disorders.

Limitations

This study provides a snapshot of the subjects' psychopathology immediately after arrest and detention. It cannot show whether mental disorder causes delinquency, increases the likelihood of arrest and detention, or is merely a frequent trait among delinquent youth. Some symptoms may be a reaction to detention. Moreover, the rates might differ somewhat using DSM-IV rather than DSM-III-R criteria. The findings are drawn from one site only and may pertain only to youth in urban detention centers with a similar demographic composition. Finally, because interviewing caretakers was not feasible, the data are subject to the limitations of self-reporting. Despite these constraints, the study has implications for research on delinquent youth and for the juvenile justice system as a whole.

Future research

Four directions for future research are recommended:

1. **Pathways to co-morbidity.** We need to determine the most common pathways to co-morbidity, critical periods of vulnerability, and how these differ by sex, race/ethnicity, and age. Longitudinal studies that identify the most common developmental sequences will demonstrate when primary and secondary preventive interventions may be most beneficial (Nottlemann & Jensen, 1995).

2. **Studies of females in the juvenile justice system.** Females are increasingly arrested for violent crimes, and they make up an increasing proportion of delinquent youth (Snyder, 2005). Earlier studies of conduct-disordered youth (many of whom will become delinquent) suggest that females have a greater persistence of emotional disorder and worse outcomes than males (Loeber & Stouthamer-Loeber, 1998; Zoccolillo, 1992). Moreover, female problem behaviors often persist beyond adolescence. As they grow older, females may become suicidal, addicted to alcohol or drugs, enmeshed in violent relationships, and unable to care for their children (Lewis *et al.*, 1991; Zoccolillo, 1992). Delinquent females also engage in sexual activity at an earlier age than non-offenders, placing them at greater risk for unwanted pregnancy and the human immunodeficiency virus (Gender-Specific Programming for Girls Advisory Committee, 1998). Understanding psychiatric morbidity and associated risk factors among delinquent females could help improve treatment and reduce the cycle of disorder and dysfunction.

3. **Longitudinal studies.** Many youth in the juvenile justice population will develop new disorders as they grow older. Risk factors for the development of disorders are common among delinquent youth (Werner, 1989). These factors include physical and sexual abuse, a troubled family environment, parental substance abuse, poverty, poor education, neighborhood disintegration, and neglect (Buckner & Bassuk, 1997; Dembo *et al.*, 1993; Leventhal & Brooks-Gunn, 2000; Lewis *et al.*, 1994; National Research Council, 1993). Delinquent youth have few protective factors to offset these risks (Cocozza, 1992). Thus, most youth in the juvenile justice system are at great risk for psychopathology,

problem behaviors, and even early death (Teplin *et al.*, 2005; Lattimore *et al.*, 1997; Loeber *et al.*, 1999). Longitudinal studies are needed to examine why some delinquent youth develop new psychopathology and others do not, to investigate protective factors, and to determine how vulnerability and risk differ by key variables such as sex and race/ethnicity.

4. **Studies of vulnerability to PTSD in high-risk youth.** Although more than 90 percent of our sample were exposed to one or more traumas, only 11.2 percent of the sample met criteria for PTSD in the past year. We need to determine the relative risk of PTSD for types of trauma (e.g., witnessing murder, being shot, witnessing ongoing domestic violence, sudden loss of a loved one) among youth who are frequently exposed to trauma and violence, such as our participants. Such studies could document factors that increase resilience to PTSD among high-risk youth and guide prevention strategies (Miller *et al.*, 1999; Kliewer *et al.*, 1998).

Implications for juvenile justice

Research findings indicate that a substantial number of youth in detention need mental health services. As previously mentioned, youth with serious mental disorders have a constitutional right to receive needed treatment while detained. Providing mental health services to youth in detention and redirecting them to the mental health system after release may help prevent their returning to the correctional system (Dembo *et al.*, 1997; National Research Council and Institute of Medicine, 2001). However, providing services within the juvenile justice system poses a number of challenges:

1. **Screening for mental health needs.** Identifying youth who need mental health services is an important first step. Experts recommend that youth be screened for psychiatric problems within 24 hours of admission to a juvenile facility (Wasserman *et al.*, 2003). At a minimum, screening should address acute mental health problems, including psychosis, risk for suicide or harm to self, psychiatric medications, substance abuse, and risk for assaultive behavior (Wasserman *et al.*, 2003). Youth who disclose such information should have appropriate legal protections (Wasserman *et al.*, 2003). Many detention centers do not routinely screen for psychiatric problems (Goldstrom *et al.*, 2001). Only recently have specialized screening tools been developed to assess the needs of youth entering the juvenile justice system (Dembo *et al.*, 1996; Grisso *et al.*, 2001); these instruments need further testing and evaluation.

2. **Providing services.** Youth in need of mental health services require access to them while in detention (Costello & Jameson, 1987; Wasserman *et al.*, 2003). Detention centers should train personnel to detect mental disorders that are

overlooked at intake or that arise during incarceration (Dembo *et al.*, 1997; Hayes, 2000; Ulzen & Hamilton, 1998).

Although fewer in number, females in detention have even greater service needs than males. Earlier studies indicate that females with problem behaviors may have worse outcomes than males (Lewis *et al.*, 1991; Loeber & Stouthamer-Loeber, 1998; Zoccolillo, 1992). Services should be developed to address the unique needs of this growing population.

3. **Community linkages**. Most detainees return to their communities within two weeks (Snyder & Sickmund, 1999). Ideally, those with mental disorders should be linked to community mental health services prior to their release (Cocozza, 1992; Faenza *et al.*, 2000). However, youth in the juvenile justice system are disproportionately minority, impoverished, and poorly educated, and many lack social networks, characteristics known to limit the type and scope of mental health services provided to youth (Kataota *et al.*, 2002; McKay *et al.*, 1996). Juvenile justice administrators need to form collaborative relationships with education, child welfare, mental health, and substance abuse service systems to ensure that youth have adequate access to care after their release.

4. **Avoid retraumatizing youth**. The conditions of confinement often exacerbate symptoms of mental disorder, including PTSD (Coalition for Juvenile Justice, 2000). Juvenile justice providers must also reduce the likelihood that youth will be retraumatized during routine processing. Symptoms of PTSD may be exacerbated by such common practices as handcuffs and searches (Prescott, 1998; Veysey, 1998). In detention centers, psychiatric crises are often handled by isolating and restraining symptomatic detainees. These practices can trigger or escalate symptoms of PTSD (e.g., severe anxiety, aggression, and numbing of emotions) (Prescott, 1998; Veysey, 1998). Psychiatrists can help to develop strategies to manage emergencies more humanely – and, ultimately, more cost-effectively.

Many youth in detention suffer from psychiatric disorders and pose a challenge to the juvenile justice system. Research is needed to better understand the comorbidity of psychiatric disorders, psychiatric disorders among females involved in the juvenile justice system, and the long-term outcomes of detained youth with mental disorders. These youth will continue to overburden the juvenile justice system and eventually the adult system until it is better able to detect them and offer an integrated system of appropriate services during detention and after their release.

Acknowledgments

Linda A. Teplin, Ph.D., is the Owen L. Coon Professor of Psychiatry and Behavioral Sciences and Director, Psycho-Legal Studies Program, Feinberg

School of Medicine, Northwestern University. Karen M. Abram, Ph.D., is Assistant Professor, Feinberg School of Medicine, Northwestern University. Gary M. McClelland is Research Assistant Professor, Feinberg School of Medicine, Northwestern University. Amy A. Mericle, Ph.D., is Postdoctoral Fellow, University of California, San Francisco, School of Medicine, Department of Psychiatry. Mina K. Dulcan, Ph.D., is the Osterman Professor of Psychiatry and Behavioral Sciences and Pediatrics, Feinberg School of Medicine, Northwestern University, and Head of Child and Adolescent Psychiatry, Children's Memorial Hospital. Jason J. Washburn is Research Assistant Professor, Feinberg School of Medicine, Northwestern University. Shiraz Butte, M. D., is Assistant Professor of Psychiatry, Rush University Medical Center and Director, Mental Health Division, Cook County Juvenile Detention Center.

References

Aarons, G. A., Brown, S. A., Hough, R. L., Garland, A. F. & Wood, P. A. (2001). Prevalence of adolescent substance use disorders across five sectors of care. *Journal of the American Academy of Child and Adolescent Psychiatry*, **40**, 419–426.

Abram, K. A., Teplin, L. A., McClelland, G. M. & Dulcan, M. K. (2003). Comorbid psychiatric disorders in youth in juvenile detention. *Archives of General Psychiatry*, **60**, 1097–1108.

Abram, K. M., Teplin, L. A., Charles, D. R., Longworth, S. L., McClelland, G. M. & Dulcan, M. K. (2004). Posttraumatic stress disorder and trauma in youth in juvenile detention. *Archives of General Psychiatry*, **661**, 403–410.

American Association of Correctional Psychology. (2000). Standards for psychology services in jails, prisons, correctional facilities, and agencies. *Criminal Justice and Behavior*, **27**, 433–494.

Angold, A., Costello, E. & Erkanli, A. (1999). Comorbidity. *Journal of Child Psychology and Psychiatry*, **40**, 57–87.

Atkins, D. L., Pumariega, A. J., Rogers, K. *et al.* (1999). Mental health and incarcerated youth. I: Prevalence and nature of psychopathology. *Journal of Child and Family Studies*, **8**, 193–204.

Bravo, M., Woodbury-Farina, M., Canino, G. J. & Rubio-Stipec, M. (1993). The Spanish translation and cultural adaptation of the Diagnostic Interview Schedule for Children (DISC) in Puerto Rico. *Culture Medicine and Psychiatry*, **17**, 329–344.

Breslau, N., Davis, G. C., Andreski, P. & Peterson, E. (1991). Traumatic events and posttraumatic stress disorder in an urban population of young adults. *Archives of General Psychiatry*, **48**, 216–222.

Breslau, N., Kessler, R. C., Chilcoat, H. D. *et al.* (1998). Trauma and posttraumatic stress disorder in the community: The 1996 Detroit area survey of trauma. *Archives of General Psychiatry*, **55**, 626–632.

Buckner, J. C. & Bassuk, E. L. (1997). Mental disorders and service utilization among youths from homeless and low-income housed families. *Journal of the American Academy of Child and Adolescent Psychiatry*, **36**, 890–900.

Cauffman, E., Feldman, S., Waterman, J. & Steiner, H. (1998). Posttraumatic stress disorder among female juvenile offenders. *Journal of the American Academy of Child and Adolescent Psychiatry*, **37**, 1209–1216.

Coalition for Juvenile Justice. (2000). *Handle with Care: Serving the Mental Health Needs of Young Offenders*. Washington, DC.

Cochran, W. G. (1977). *Sampling Techniques*, 3rd edn. New York: John Wiley & Sons.

Cocozza, J. J. (1992). *Responding to the Mental Health Needs of Youth in the Juvenile Justice System*. Seattle, WA: National Coalition for the Mentally Ill in the Criminal Justice System.

Cohen, J. (1998). *Statistical Power Analysis for the Behavioral Sciences*, 2nd edn. Hillsdale, NJ: Lawrence Earlbaum Associates.

Cohen, P., Cohen, J. & Brook, J. (1993). An epidemiological study of disorders in late childhood and adolescence – II. Persistence of disorders. *Journal of Child Psychology and Psychiatry*, **34**, 869–877.

Costello, J. C. & Jameson, E. J. (1987). Legal and ethical duties of health care professionals to incarcerated children. *Journal of Legal Medicine*, **8**, 191–263.

Costello, E., Angold, A., Burns, B. J. *et al.* (1996). The Great Smoky Mountains Study of youth: goals, design, methods, and the prevalence of DSM-III-R disorders. *Archives of General Psychiatry*, **53**, 1129–1136.

Costello, E., Erkanli, A., Federman, E. & Angold, A. (1999). Development of psychiatric comorbidity with substance abuse in adolescents: effects of timing and sex. *Journal of Clinical Child Psychology*, **28**, 298–311.

Davis, D. L., Bean, G. J., Schumacher, J. E. & Stringer, T. L. (1991). Prevalence of emotional disorders in a juvenile justice institutional population. *American Journal of Forensic Psychology*, **9**, 5–17.

Dembo, R., Williams, L. & Schmeidler, J. (1993). Gender differences in mental health service needs among youths entering a juvenile detention center. *Journal of Prison and Jail Health*. **12**, 73–101.

Dembo, R., Schmeidler, J., Borden, P. *et al.* (1996). Examination of the reliability of the Problem Oriented Screening Instrument for Teenagers (POSIT) among arrested youths entering a juvenile assessment center. *Substance Use and Misuse*, **31**, 785–824.

Dembo, R., Schmeidler, J., Pacheco, K., Cooper, S. & Williams, L. W. (1997). The relationships between youth's identified substance use, mental health or other problems at a juvenile assessment center and their referrals to needed services. *Journal of Child and Adolescent Substance Abuse*, **6**, 23–54.

Domalanta, D. D., Risser, W. L., Roberts, R. E. & Risser, W. L. (2003). Prevalence of depression and other psychiatric disorders among incarcerated youths. *Journal of the American Academy of Child and Adolescent Psychiatry*, **42**, 477–484.

Duclos, C. W., Beals, J., Novins, D. K. *et al.* (1998). Prevalence of common psychiatric disorders among American Indian adolescent detainees. *Journal of the American Academy of Child and Adolescent Psychiatry*, **37**, 866–873.

Eppright, T. D., Kashani, J. H., Robison, B. D. & Reid, J. C. (1993). Comorbidity of conduct disorder and personality disorders in an incarcerated juvenile population. *American Journal of Psychiatry*, **150**, 1233–1236.

Erwin, B. A., Newman, E., McMackin, R. A., Morrissey, C. & Kaloupek, D. G. (2000). PTSD, malevolent environment, and criminality among criminally involved male adolescents. *Criminal Justice and Behavior*, **27**, 196–215.

Faenza, M., Siegfried, C. & Wood, J. (2000). *Community Perspectives on the Mental Health and Substance Abuse Treatment Needs of Youth Involved in the Juvenile Justice System*. Alexandria, VA: National Mental Health Association and the Office of Juvenile Justice and Delinquency Prevention.

Famularo, R., Fenton, T., Kinscherff, R. *et al.* (1992). Differences in neuropsychological and academic achievement between adolescent delinquents and status offenders. *American Journal of Psychiatry*, **149**, 1252–1257.

Feitel, B., Margetson, N., Chamas, J. & Lipman, C. (1992). Psychosocial background and behavioral and emotional disorders of homeless and runaway youth. *Hospital and Community Psychiatry*, **43**, 155–159.

Forehand, R., Frame, C. L., Wierson, M., Armistead, L. & Kempton, T. (1991). Assessment of incarcerated juvenile delinquents: agreement across raters and approaches to psychopathology. *Journal of Psychopathology and Behavioral Assessment*, **13**(1), 17–25.

Garland, A. F., Hough, R. L., McCabe, K. M. *et al.* (2001). Prevalence of psychiatric disorders in youths across five sectors of care. *Journal of the American Academy of Child and Adolescent Psychiatry*, **40**, 409–418.

Garrison, C. Z., Waller, J. L., Cuffe, S. P. *et al.* (1997). Incidence of major depressive disorder and dysthymia in young adolescents. *Journal of the American Academy of Child and Adolesent Psychiatry*, **36**, 458–465.

Gender-Specific Programming for Girls Advisory Committee. (1998). *Guiding Principles for Promising Female Programming*. Washington, DC: Office of Juvenile Justice and Delinquency Prevention.

Giaconia, R. M., Reinherz, H. Z., Silverman, A. B. *et al.* (1995). Traumas and posttraumatic stress disorder in a community population of older adolescents. *Journal of the American Academy of Child and Adolesent Psychiatry*, **34**, 1369–1380.

Goldstrom, I., Jaiquan, F., Henderson, M., Male, A. & Manderscheid, R. W. (2001). The availability of mental health services to young people in juvenile justice facilities: a national study. In R. W. Manderscheid and M. J. Henderson, eds., *Mental Health, United States, 2000*. Rockville: USDHHS, Center for Mental Health Services; pp. 248–268.

Grisso, T., Tomkins, A. & Casey, P. (1988). Psychosocial concepts in juvenile law. *Law and Human Behavior*, **12**, 403–437.

Grisso, T., Barnum, R., Fletcher, K. E., Cauffman, E. & Peuschold, D. (2001). Massachusetts Youth Screening Instrument for mental health needs of juvenile justice youths. *Journal of the American Academy of Child and Adolescent Psychiatry*, **40**, 541–548.

Hayes, L. M. (2000). Suicide prevention in juvenile facilities. *Juvenile Justice*, **7**, 24–32.

Illinois Criminal Justice Information Authority. (1997). *Trends and Issues 1997*. Chicago, IL: Illinois Criminal Justice Information Authority.

Kandel, D. B., Johnson, J. G., Bird, H. R. *et al.* (1997). Psychiatric disorders associated with substance use among children and adolescents: findings from the Methods for the Epidemiology of Child and Adolescent Mental Disorders (MECA) Study. *Journal of Abnormal Child Psychology*, **25**, 121–132.

Kataoka, S. H., Zhang, L. & Wells, K. B. (2002). Unmet need for mental health care among U.S. children: variation by ethnicity and insurance status. *American Journal of Psychiatry*, **159**, 1548–1555.

Kessler, R. C. & Walters, E. E. (1998). Epidemiology of DSM-III-R major depression and minor depression among adolescents and young adults in the National Comorbidity Survey. *Depression and Anxiety*, **7**, 3–14.

Kessler, R. C., Sonnega, A., Bromet, J., Hughes, M. & Nelson, C. B. (1995). Posttraumatic stress disorder in the National Comorbidity Survey. *Archives of General Psychiatry*, **52**, 1048–1060.

Kliewer, W., Lepore, S. J., Oskin D. & Johnson, P. D. (1998). The role of social and cognitive processes in children's adjustment to community violence. *Journal of Consulting and Clinical Psychology*, **66**, 199–209.

Lattimore, P. K., Linster, R. L. & MacDonald, J. M. (1997). Risk of death among serious young offenders. *Journal of Research in Crime and Delinquency*, **34**, 187–209.

Leventhal, T. & Brooks-Gunn, J. (2000). The neighborhoods they live in: the effects of neighborhood residence on child and adolescent outcomes. *Psychological Bulletin*, **126**, 309–337.

Levy, P. S. & Lemeshow, S. (1999). *Sampling of Populations: Methods and Applications*, 3rd edn. New York: John Wiley and Sons.

Lewinsohn, P. M., Gotlib, I. H. & Seeley, J. R. (1995). Adolescent psychopathology: IV. Specificity of psychosocial risk factors for depression and substance abuse in older adolescents. *Journal of the American Academy of Child and Adolescent Psychiatry*, **34**, 1221–1229.

Lewis, D. O., Yeager, C. A., Cobham-Portorreal, C. S. *et al.* (1991). A follow-up of female delinquents: maternal contributions to the perpetuation of deviance. *Journal of the American Academy of Child and Adolescent Psychiatry*, **30**, 197–201.

Lewis, D. O., Yeager, C. A., Lovely, R., Stein, A. & Cobham-Portorreal, C. S. (1994). A clinical follow-up of delinquent males: ignored vulnerabilities, unmet needs, and the perpetuation of violence. *Journal of the American Academy of Child and Adolescent Psychiatry*, **33**, 518–528.

Loeber, R. & Stouthamer-Loeber, M. (1998). Development of juvenile aggression and violence. *The American Psychologist*, **53**, 242–259.

Loeber, R., DeLamatre, M., Tita, G. *et al.* (1999). Gun injury and mortality: the delinquent backgrounds of juvenile victims. *Violence and Victims*, **14**, 339–352.

McCabe, K. M., Lansing, A. E., Garland, A. & Hough, R. (2002). Gender differences in psychopathology, functional impairment, and familial risk factors among adjudicated delinquents. *Journal of the American Academy of Child and Adolescent Psychiatry*, **41**, 860–867.

McGee, R., Feehan, M., Williams, S. & Anderson, J. (1992). DSM-III disorders from age 11 to age 15 years. *Journal of the American Academy of Child and Adolescent Psychiatry*, **31**, 50–59.

McKay, M. M., McCadam, K. & Gonzales, J. (1996). Addressing the barriers to mental health services for inner city children and their caretakers. *Community Mental Health Journal*, **32**, 353–361.

Miller, L. S., Wasserman, G. A., Neugebauer, R., Gorman-Smith, D. & Kamboukos, D. (1999). Witnessed community violence and antisocial behavior in high-risk, urban boys. *Journal of Clinical Child Psychology*, **28**, 2–11.

National Research Council (1993). *Losing Generations: Adolescents in High-Risk Settings*. Washington, DC: National Academy Press.

National Research Council and Institute of Medicine. (2001). *Juvenile Crime Juvenile Justice.* Washington, DC: National Academy Press.

Newman, D. L., Moffitt, T. E., Caspi, A. *et al.* (1996). Psychiatric disorder in a birth cohort of young adults: prevalence, comorbidity, clinical significance, and new case incidence from ages 11 to 21. *Journal of Consulting and Clinical Psychology*, **64**, 552–562.

Nottlemann, E. D. & Jensen, P. S. (1995). Comorbidity of disorders in children and adolescents. *Advances in Clinical Child Psychology*, **17**, 109–155.

Pliszka, S. R., Sherman, J. O., Barrow, M. V. & Irick, S. (2000). Affective disorder in juvenile offenders: a preliminary study. *American Journal of Psychiatry*, **157**, 130–132.

Prescott, L. (1998). *Improving Policy and Practice for Adolescent Girls with Co-Occurring Disorders in the Juvenile Justice System.* Delmar, NY: The GAINS Center.

Randall, J., Henggeler, S. W., Pickrel, S. G. & Brondino, M. J. (1999). Psychiatric comorbidity and the 16-month trajectory of substance-abusing and substance-dependent juvenile offenders. *Journal of the American Academy of Child and Adolescent Psychiatry*, **38**, 1118–1124.

Riggs, P. D., Mikulich, S. K., Whitmore, E. A. & Crowley, T. J. (1999). Relationship of ADHD, depression, and non-tobacco substance use disorders to nicotine dependence in substance-dependent delinquents. *Drug and Alcohol Dependence*, **54**, 195–205.

Roberts, R. E., Attkisson, C. & Rosenblatt, A. (1998). Prevalence of psychopathology among children and adolescents. *American Journal of Psychiatry*, **155**, 715–725.

Rohde, P., Mace, D. E. & Seeley, J. R. (1997). The association of psychiatric disorders with suicide attempts in a juvenile delinquent sample. *Criminal Behavior and Mental Health*, **7**, 187–200.

Schwab-Stone, M. E., Shaffer, D., Dulcan, M. K. *et al.* (1996). Criterion validity of the NIMH Diagnostic Interview Schedule for Children Version 2.3 (DISC-2.3). *Journal of the American Academy of Child and Adolescent Psychiatry*, **35**, 878–888.

Shaffer, D., Fisher, P., Dulcan, M. K. & Davies, M. (1996). The NIMH Diagnostic Interview Schedule for Children Version 2.3 (DISC-2.3): description, acceptability, prevalence rates, and performance in the MECA study. *Journal of the American Academy of Child and Adolescent Psychiatry*, **35**, 865–877.

Shaffer, D., Fisher, P. & Lucas, C. (2003). The Diagnostic Interview Schedule for Children (DISC). In M. J. Hilsenroth and D. L. Segal, eds., *Comprehensive Handbook of Psychological Assessment* (Vol. 2). Hoboken, NJ: John Wiley & Sons, 256–270.

Shelton, D. (2001). Emotional disorders in young offenders. *Image Journal of Nursing Scholarship*, **33**, 259–263.

Sickmund, M., Sladky, T. J. & Kang, W. (2006). Census of Juveniles in Residential Placement Databook. http://www.ojjdp.ncjrs.org/ojstatbb/cjrp/. Accessed January 9, 2006.

Simonoff, E., Pickles, A., Meyer, J. M. *et al.* (1997). The Virginia Twin Study of Adolescent Behavioral Development: Influences of age, sex, and impairment on rates of disorder. *Archives of General Psychiatry*, **54**, 801–808.

Snyder, H. N. (2005). *Juvenile Arrests 2003.* Washington, DC: Office of Juvenile Justice and Delinquency Prevention. NCJ209735.

Snyder, H. N. & Sickmund, M. (1999). *Juvenile Offenders and Victims: 1999 National Report.* Washington, DC: Office of Juvenile Justice and Delinquency Prevention.

Soler, M. (2002). Health issues for adolescents in the justice system. *Journal of Adolescent Health,* **31**, 321–333.

Steiner, H., Garcia, I. G. & Mathews, Z. (1997). Posttraumatic stress disorder in incarcerated juvenile delinquents. *Journal of the American Academy of Child and Adolescent Psychiatry,* **36**(3), 357–365.

Teplin, L. A., Abram, K. M. & McClelland, G. M. (1996). Prevalence of psychiatric disorders among incarcerated women: I. Pretrial jail detainees. *Archives of General Psychiatry,* **53**, 505–512.

Teplin, L. A., McClelland, G. M., Abram, K. M. & Mileusnic, D. (2005). Early violent death among delinquent youth: a prospective longitudinal study. *Pediatrics,* **115**, 1586–1593.

The President's New Freedom Commission on Mental Health. (2005). Subcommittee on Criminal Justice: Background Paper. http://www.mentalhealthcommission.gov/reports/FinalReport/downloads/FinalReport.pdf. Accessed January 9, 2005.

Thompson, L. L., Riggs, P. D., Mikulich, S. K. & Crowley, T. J. (1996). Contribution of ADHD symptoms to substance problems and delinquency in conduct-disordered adolescents. *Journal of Abnormal Child Psychology,* **24**, 325–347.

Timmons-Mitchell, J., Brown, C., Schulz, S. C. *et al.* (1997). Comparing the mental health needs of female and male incarcerated juvenile delinquents. *Behavioral Sciences and the Law,* **15**, 195–202.

Turner, R. J. & Gil, A. G. (2002). Psychiatric and substance use disorders in South Florida: Racial/ethnic and gender contrasts in a young adult cohort. *Archives of General Psychiatry,* **59**, 43–50.

Ulzen, T. P. M. & Hamilton, H. (1998). The nature and characteristics of psychiatric comorbidity in incarcerated adolescents. *Canadian Journal of Psychiatry,* **43**, 57–63.

Veysey, B. M. (1998). Specific needs of women diagnosed with mental illnesses in U.S. jails. In B. L. Levin, A. K. Blanch and A. Jennings, eds., *Women's Mental Health Services: A public health perspective.* Thousand Oaks, CA: Sage, pp. 368–389.

Wasserman, G. A., McReynolds, L. S., Lucas, C. P., Fisher, P. & Santos, L. (2002). The voice DISC-IV with incarcerated male youths: prevalence of disorder. *Journal of the American Academy of Child and Adolescent Psychiatry,* **41**(3), 314–321.

Wasserman, G. A., Jensen, P., Ko, S. J. *et al.* (2003). Mental health assessments in juvenile justice: report on the Consensus Conference. *Journal of the American Academy of Child and Adolescent Psychiatry,* **42**, 751–761.

Wasserman, G. A., McReynolds, L. S., Ko, S. J., Katz, L. M. & Carpenter, J. R. (2005). Gender differences in psychiatric disorders at juvenile probation intake. *American Journal of Public Health,* **95**, 131–137.

Werner, E. E. (1989). High-risk children in young adulthood: a longitudinal study from birth to 32 years. *American Journal of Orthopsychiatry,* **59**, 72–81.

Whitaker, A., Johnson, J., Shaffer, D. *et al.* (1990). Uncommon troubles in young people: prevalence estimates of selected psychiatric disorders in a nonreferred adolescent population. *Archives of General Psychiatry,* **47**, 487–496.

Whitmore, E. A., Mikulich, S. K., Thompson, L. L. *et al.* (1997). Influences on adolescent substance dependence: conduct disorder, depression, attention deficit hyperactivity disorder and gender. *Drug and Alcohol Dependence*, **47**, 87–97.

Zoccolillo, M. (1992). Co-occurrence of conduct disorder and its adult outcomes with depressive and anxiety disorders: a review. *Journal of the American Academy of Child and Adolescent Psychiatry*, **31**, 547–556.

3

Disproportionate minority confinement

William Arroyo

Disproportionate minority confinement generally refers to the disproportionate percentage of minority youth or one group of youth confined in juvenile detention facilities relative to the percentage of youth found in the local or surrounding jurisdiction. The term, disproportionate minority confinement (DMC), has been the preferred term in the juvenile justice system since the late 1980s. When the reauthorization of the Juvenile Justice Delinquency and Prevention (JJDP) Act (2002) was passed, the Act mandated states to address: "juvenile delinquency prevention efforts and system improvement efforts designed to reduce, without establishing or requiring numerical standards or quotas, the disproportionate number of juvenile members of minority groups who come into *contact* with the juvenile justice system." This is different from the previous act in that the requirement is broadened from "confinement" to "contact" by requiring states to examine possible disproportionate representation of minority youth at all decision points along the juvenile justice system continuum.

Other terms used to refer to this pattern of practice include "overrepresentation," "disparity," and "discrimination." Overrepresentation exists when, at various stages of the juvenile justice system, the proportion of a certain population exceeds its proportion in the general population. Disparity refers to a situation in which different groups have different probabilities that certain outcomes will occur. Disparity may in turn lead to overrepresentation. Discrimination refers to differential decision-making among juvenile justice professionals affecting different groups of juveniles based on their gender, racial, and/or ethnic identity.

The JJDP Act, also, requires multipronged strategies of interventions that not only include juvenile delinquency prevention efforts but, also, system improvement efforts to assure equal treatment of all youth. This Act was linked to the Title I Formula B Grants Program; those states that were out of compliance with any of the four core requirements of the Act including DMC were at risk of losing 25 percent of this funding.

The Mental Health Needs of Young Offenders: Forging Paths toward Reintegration and Rehabilitation, eds. Carol L. Kessler and Louis J. Kraus. Published by Cambridge University Press. © Cambridge University Press 2007.

The groups of minority youth to which DMC pertains are those identified by the federal government, namely, African American youth, Latino or Hispanic youth, Asian American youth, and American Indian youth.

Literature review

The research in this field has varied extensively in regard to sampling, jurisdictions, hypotheses, data collection, and other aspects of methodology. Two reviews of this body of literature (Pope, Lovell & Hsia, 2002; Pope & Feyerherm, 1990) examine 80 publications. Although virtually all of these publications pre-date the broadening of DMC in the 2002 reauthorization Act, many address various decision-making points within the juvenile justice system. However, one of the major problems with the body of literature is the fact that the studies focus on different decision-making points in many instances.

In the earlier research analysis of 46 published studies (Pope & Feyerherm, 1990), the authors demonstrated that there were indeed substantial differences in the various juvenile justice systems insofar as the juvenile processing was concerned. It was clear that there were factors other than legal characteristics to which the differences could be attributed. The youth's racial status was the factor in approximately two-thirds of the reviewed research that made a difference at various decision-making points along the continuum. Differential outcomes were found at various stages of juvenile processing. In some instances, differential outcomes were cumulative, that is, for example, racial differences became more pronounced the further the youth penetrated the system.

In the more recent analysis (Pope, Lovell & Hsia, 2002) of 34 studies, the minority group that garnered the most discussion was that of African American youth in 27 studies, Hispanic or Latino in 11 studies, American Indian in 4 studies, and Asian American in 2 studies. The majority of studies focused on more than one minority group of youth. A handful of studies aggregated data in an "other" category to refer to minority youth, while another small group of studies referred to a more general category of "non-white" youth in their analysis. Disposition, in 20 studies, and petition, in 13 studies, proved to be the most frequent decision-making points that were studied. A multivariate analytic method was used in more than 80 percent of the studies. The more salient findings of this analysis of research studies were that the majority of the studies, 25 of 34, concluded that race affects the processing of youth. It should be noted, however, that in some of the studies race effects were apparent for certain types of offenders or certain offenses and, in other instances, race was important at some decision points but not at others. The conclusions of this analysis is similar to the analysis of a prior period of research; however, in the latter analysis, there appears to be a broader range of decision-making points where race is a factor in addition to the factor of type of offense.

These research findings strongly support the claim of disparities and potential biases in juvenile justice processing. The causes and mechanisms of these disparities and biases are very complex. Some of the more important contributing factors appear to be an "inherent system bias, effects of local policies and practices, and social conditions (such as inequality, family situation, or underemployment) that may place youth at risk. Further overrepresentation may result from the interaction of factors. Also, the most significant factors may vary by jurisdiction" (Pope, Lovell & Hsia, 2002, p. 5). Some of the research gaps include police decision-making, attitudes of youth and their relationship of those attitudes to the decisions of officials, studies on decision-making points and varying practices within the same jurisdiction (such as urban vs. suburban), and limited number of studies on Asian American youth and Native American youth.

Current state of DMC

Residential placement

The latest national data regarding youth in residential placement are drawn from the Census of Juveniles in Residential Placement (CJRP), which is administered by the U.S. Bureau of the Census for the Office of Juvenile Justice and Delinquency Prevention program (OJJDP) (Sickmund, 2004). These data reflect a one-day count in October, 1999; such data is collected biennially. All data reflect the population in residential placement who are younger than 21, are charged with an offense or court adjudicated for an offense, and are in residential placement because of the offense. These data do not capture data reflecting youth held in adult prisons or jails, nor data relevant to youth placed by criminal courts in juvenile facilities.

These data strongly support the practice of disproportionate placement of minority youth in residential settings. Although minority youth accounted for only 34 percent of the US juvenile population in 1999, 62 percent of youth in custody were of a minority group (Table 3.1). In addition, minority youth were more frequently placed in public rather than private facilities despite being a majority in both categories.

Minorities accounted for more than 70 percent of the total population of juvenile offenders in nine states and the District of Columbia (Table 3.2).

Custody rates for African American youth are highest among all four minority groups of youth (Table 3.3). Nationally, for every 100 000 non-Hispanic African American juveniles living in the U.S., 1004 were in a residential placement facility. The rate was 485 for Hispanics and 212 for non-Hispanic whites.

Table 3.1. Racial profile of juvenile offenders in residential placement, 1999

Race/ethnicity	Facility operation		
	Total	Public	Private
Total	100%	100%	100%
White	38	35	45
Minority	62	65	55
Black	39	40	38
Hispanic	18	21	12
American Indian	2	2	2
Asian	2	2	2

Source: Office of Juvenile Justice and Delinquency Prevention (1998, 2001)

Table 3.2. State racial profile of juvenile offenders in residential placement, 1999

State of offense	Juvenile population	Total CJRP
US total	34%	62%
California	59	79
Connecticut	25	77
District of Columbia	86	97
Hawaii	75	91
Louisiana	44	78
Maryland	40	70
Mississippi	47	73
New Jersey	37	84
New Mexico	62	78
Texas	52	74

Source: Office of Juvenile Justice and Delinquency Prevention (1999, 2001)

Other decision-making points in the juvenile justice continuum

Although reliable national data for various decision-making points relevant to all four minority groups do not exist, there are some national data relevant to African American youth (Snyder & Sickmund, 2000) (Table 3.4) that illustrate some of the challenges for jurisdictions. The racial composition of the national juvenile population in 2001 was 78 percent white, 17 percent black, 4 percent Asian/Pacific Islander, and 1 percent American Indian. Latino youth were generally included

Table 3.3. Partial list of states' racial profile of juvenile offenders in residential placement, 1999

State of offense	Custody Rate (per 100 000)				
	White	Black	Hispanic	American Indian	Asian
US total	212	1004	485	632	182
Alabama	208	588	249	314	93
California	269	1666	623	612	238
Delaware	203	1143	304	0	0
District of Columbia	173	855	369	0	0
Georgia	273	878	163	861	72
Illinois	152	1005	271	590	37
Maryland	136	575	131	0	12
Michigan	243	1058	1112	428	215
Oklahoma	194	821	297	343	56
Oregon	353	1689	478	1074	270

Source: Office of Juvenile Justice and Delinquency Prevention (1999, 2001)

Table 3.4. Black juveniles are overrepresented at all stages of the juvenile justice system compared with their proportion in the population

Year of data sets	1990–1	1998–9
US population ages 10–17	15%	16%
Violent juvenile offenders reported by victims	34	28
All juvenile arrests	26	25
Juvenile arrests for Violent Crime Index offenses	49	41
Delinquency cases in juvenile court	31	29
Delinquency cases involving detention	40	35
Petitioned delinquency cases	37	33
Adjudicated delinquency cases	36	35

Source: Sickmund, 2004

with whites in this data set. In contrast to their representation in the population, black youth were overrepresented in juvenile arrests for violent crimes, and, to a lesser extent, property crimes. In regard to arrests for violent crimes, 55 percent involved white youth, 43 percent involved black youth, 1 percent involved Asian youth, and 1 percent involved American Indian youth. The proportions for property crime arrests were 68 percent white youth, 28 percent black youth, 2 percent Asian youth, and 1 percent American Indian youth.

The Violent Crime Index arrest rate (i.e., arrests/100 000 juveniles in the racial group) in 2001 for black juveniles was more than three times the rate for American Indian juveniles and white juveniles; and nearly seven times the rate for Asian juveniles (Snyder, 2003). For Property Crime Index arrests, the rate for black juveniles was 40 percent greater than the rate for American Indian juveniles, about double the rate for white juveniles, and more than three times the rate for Asian juveniles. Over the period from 1980–2001, the black-to-white disparity in juvenile arrest rates for violent crimes declined. In 1980, the black juvenile Violent Crime Index arrest rate was 6.3 times the white rate; in 2001, the rate disparity had declined to 3.6. This reduction in arrest rate disparities between 1980–2001 was primarily the result of the decline in black-to-white arrest disparities for robbery (from 11.5 in 1980 to 6.8 in 2001), which was greater than the decline for aggravated assault (3.2 to 2.8).

Recent detention data also suggest racial disparities. In 1996, secure detention was twice as likely for black youth as compared to white youth even after controlling for offense (Snyder & Sickmund, 2000; Poe-Yamagata & Jones, 2000). Detention was least likely for cases involving whites that dealt with property crimes. Detention was more likely for black youth when an offense involved drugs compared to white youth (Snyder & Sickmund, 2000; Poe-Yamagata & Jones, 2000). Black youth were also disproportionately represented in the delinquency caseload (30 percent) and general detention caseload (45 percent).

In regard to waivers, there was a disparity among white and black youth especially in regard to person and drug offenses (Poe-Yamagata & Jones, 2000). For offenses against persons, white youth were petitioned 57 percent of the time and waived to adult court 45 percent of the time; black youth, however, were petitioned 40 percent of the time while waived 50 percent of the time. For drug offenses rate of petitioning and waived for whites was 59 percent and 35 percent respectively, while for black youth the rates were 39 percent and 63 percent.

An analysis of transfers of youth to the criminal justice system in California using 1996–9 data also strongly suggests racial disparities (Males & Macallair, 2000). This study is the first analysis of racial and ethnic disparity in the transfer of youths to adult court and sentencing to California Youth Authority (CYA) facilities in California. (California has both a county-based system of detention facilities and a state-based system, which is generally used for youth who commit more serious violent offenses.) Minority youths are 8.3 times more likely than white youths to be sentenced by an adult court to imprisonment in a California Youth Authority facility. Two factors appear to contribute in roughly equal measure to this discrepancy. First, minority youths are 2.7 times more likely than white youths to be arrested for a violent felony (the crimes most likely to result in transfer to adult court). Second, once in the system, minority juvenile violent crime arrestees are 3.1 times more likely than white juvenile violent crime arrestees to be transferred to adult court and sentenced to confinement in a CYA prison. While it is debatable whether the disproportionate minority youth arrests are a reflection of race-based violent crime differentials or racially biased policing and charging policies, the discriminatory treatment of minority youth arrestees accumulates within the justice system and accelerates measurably if the youth is transferred to adult court. The limited analysis of Los Angeles County data reveals that the major factor in the large racial disparities in sentencing lies in the much more frequent transfer of minority juveniles to adult court where harsher sentences of minority offenses is common. The reasons for these disparities remain unclear. Minority offenders remain 1.4 times more likely to be sentenced to CYA confinement by adult courts than are similarly offending white youth, even when each group's respective contribution to the homicide volume in California is factored.

Data regarding admissions to state prisons also suggest racial disparities. More than three-quarters of youth newly admitted to state prisons were minority youth in 1996 (Snyder & Sickmund, 2000). Minorities accounted for a greater proportion of new court commitments to prisons involving youth under age 18 than older age groups. The minority proportions varied by offense, with drug offenses accounting for the greater proportions of minority admissions in both youth groups, under 18 and over 18.

An analysis of the FBI's National Incident-Based Reporting System (NIBRS) data did not find any evidence of racial bias in the overall likelihood of arrest of white juveniles vs. non-white juveniles for violent crimes. (Both groups included Latino youth while the non-white group also included black, American Indian, Asian, and Pacific Islander) (Pope & Snyder, 2002).

Recent analysis of National Crime Victimization Survey data for 1980–1998 compared the rates of offending for black and white youth as reported by victims (Lynch, 2002). This data indicates that the offending rate for black youth was, on average, 4.1 times the offending rate for white youth. However, the black-to-white ratio of arrest rates for these same offenses shows that, during this same period, the arrest rate was 5.7 times higher for black youth than white youth. These findings cannot be generalized to non-violent or less serious offenses.

Latino youth are now the largest segment of youth in the US. Despite the fact that Latino youth are one of the four minority groups identified by the federal government to which reduction of DMC is applicable, there is limited data collected by federal, state, and local governments. It's impossible to develop strategies to reduce DMC if data is limited or non-existent. "The failure to collect separate data on Latino youth also inflates the incarceration rate of non-Hispanic whites further masking disparities" (Villaruel & Walker, 2002). Cultural and linguistic differences between the youth and the juvenile justice system further compounds the challenges for both youth and jurisdictions. Any coordination of efforts or direct reporting of information to the Immigration and Naturalization Service expands the mound of challenges for some of these youth and their families.

National strategies to address and resolve DMC

The Coalition for Juvenile Justice first brought the issue of DMC to national attention in 1988 when it submitted its annual report to Congress entitled, *A Delicate Balance*. Congress amended the Juvenile Justice and Delinquency Prevention (JJDP) Act of 1974, which mandates states to address their efforts to reduce the proportions of youth of minority background that were detained or placed in secure detention facilities, secure correctional facilities, jails, and lockups if this proportion exceeded the proportion of each of the groups relative to the general population.

The federal government through the Office of Juvenile Justice and Delinquency Prevention program began to launch a series of technical assistance efforts designed to help states with DMC and to sponsor specialized training (national and regional) in relevant areas. These efforts included the convening of advisory groups to develop technical assistance in 1989, publication of a *DMC Technical Assistance Manual* in 1990 (Community Research Associates, 1990) and 2000 (OJJDP, 2000), and contracting with various organizations to expand technical assistance to states.

In 1991, five states (Arizona, Florida, Iowa, North Carolina, and Oregon) were competitively selected to be part of a DMC initiative for a three-year period in which these states would test approaches to assessing and reducing DMC. In 1992, Congress amended the JJDP Act to establish DMC as a core requirement with future funding eligibility (Formula Grants allocations) contingent on state compliance with this additional core requirement. The Office of Juvenile Justice and Delinquency Prevention was to review states' three-year comprehensive JJDP plans, and plan updates to determine whether or not states were complying with this DMC core requirement. Monitoring has been better some years than others depending on OJJDP resources, among other factors.

In 1995–6, OJJDP issued 11 discretionary grants to states to refine previous assessment findings and improve their data systems, develop new innovations to reduce DMC, develop model DMC programs, and encourage multidisciplinary collaborations at the community level to reduce DMC.

The Office of Juvenile Justice and Delinquency Prevention has contracted with technical assistance centers to assist states in reducing DMC. In 1997, OJJDP entered into a cooperative agreement with Research and Evaluation Associates (REA) (www.reducingdmc.com/index.html) to develop further training, provide technical assistance, and to disseminate information to states around DMC. Research and Evaluation Associates established listservs to facilitate the exchange of information, conducted DMC training of trainers, reviewed data collection instruments, and compiled state-by-state status reports. In 1999 REA began its DMC Intensive Technical Assistance Project with five states (Delaware, Kentucky, Massachusetts, New Mexico, and South Carolina) and later expanded to include three others (California, Arkansas, and Tennessee) in 2001. The Juvenile Justice Evaluation Center (JJEC) (http://www.jrsainfo.org/jjec/about/index.html) is also providing technical assistance to states around DMC especially in the areas of evaluation capacity. It is also helping states and local agencies to form partnerships to assess their state's initiatives to reduce DMC. The Juvenile Justice Evaluation Center has also published a guide, *Seven Steps to Evaluate Strategies to Reduce Disproportionate Minority Confinement* (Nellis, 2005) (http://www.jrsainfo.org/jjec/about/dmc_guidebook.html) to assist states and local jurisdictions. Another technical assistance center that is helping states reduce DMC is the Development Services Group (www.dsgonline.com).

The Office of Juvenile Justice and Delinquency Prevention joined forces with various foundations, including Annie E. Casey, MacArthur, Rockefeller, and Ford Foundations in 1998 among other organizations, to launch the Building Blocks for Youth Initiative which was led by the Youth Law Center. Its goals were to protect minority youth in the juvenile justice system and to promote rational policies relevant to juvenile justice. A five-pronged approach was established consisting of conducting new research, analyzing decision-making in the juvenile justice system, directing advocacy for minority youth, building a constituency for change at the local, state, and national levels, and developing communications, media, and other public education strategies.

The Office of Juvenile Justice and Delinquency Prevention established a catalog of state DMC reports (www.ojjdp.ncjrs.org/dmc/tools/index.html) and a DMC website (www.ojjdp.ncjrs.org/dmc/index.html) in 2000.

The Office of Juvenile Justice and Delinquency Prevention convened a group of research consultants in large part to establish a DMC research agenda in 2002. In 2003, OJJDP convened research consultants to review the methodology for calculating DMC. Since 1988 the Disproportionate Representation Index (DRI) was being used to calculate disproportionate representation and had increasingly become problematic. Thus the adoption of a new method, DMC Relative Rate Index (RRI), took place.

The Youth Law Center was given a two-year award to develop new and accurate data collection methods relevant to Latino youth at two sites, and to implement activities to reduce DMC at critical points at these two sites.

The Office of Juvenile Justice and Delinquency Prevention has sponsored several seminal publications relevant to DMC during the past decade. These include DMC research summaries in 1993 (Pope & Feyerherm, 1990) and 2002 (Pope, Lovell & Hsia, 2002); DMC Updates in 1997 (Hsia & Hamparian, 1998), and in 2002 (Hsia, Bridges & McHale, 2004); DMC Technical Assistance Manuals (Community Research Associates, 1990; OJJDP, 2000).

State strategies to reduce DMC

In addition to OJJDP, and to the technical assistance provided by Service Group Associates, REA, and JJEC, some states have received assistance from various foundations and other organizations such as the Haywood Burns Institute (www.burnsinstitute.com) in their efforts to assess and reduce DMC.

The degree of success among states has been variable due to a myriad of factors. A survey of states in 2000 identified factors contributing to DMC (Hsia, Bridges & McCale, 2004). The most frequently cited areas in which factors were identified were in: the juvenile justice system, the educational system, the socioeconomic conditions, and the family. Within the *juvenile justice system*, contributing were: (1) racial stereotyping and cultural sensitivity on the part of police and other decision makers, (2) demeanor and attitude of minority youth, which often contributed to negative treatment and a more severe disposition; (3) lack of alternative to detention and incarceration especially in urban areas where detention centers simply become "convenient" placements; (4) misuse of discretionary authority in implementing laws and policies by police, probation officers, and even school system personnel; and (5) lack of culturally and linguistically appropriate services. Factors within the *educational system* that contributed to DMC were the failure of schools to engage students/families, ineffective school dropout prevention strategies, and failure of students/families to participate in the educational system. The *socioeconomic* factors included poverty, substance abuse, poor job market, local high crime rates, targeting of high crime areas by law enforcement, limited good role models for youth, more serious crime committed by minority youth, and very limited community resources to support normal youth development. *Family* factors included disproportionate number of minority youth from single parent households in which the parent had unsteady and low paying employment, family disintegration, diminished traditional family values, parental substance abuse, insufficient family/adult supervision, and noncompliance by minority youth with diversion requirements.

States have resorted to several actions to address DMC as a result of technical assistance among other reasons. The most frequently adopted strategies have been community-based prevention, intervention, and diversion programs, and cultural sensitivity training. Examples of community-based prevention and intervention efforts in minority communities include establishing a minority family advocate, probation advocate, parenting projects for Spanish speaking parents, Latino case managers in elementary schools to improve school attendance, an Elder-Mentor program for American Indian families, and many after-school and evening programs. Alternatives to incarceration include home detention, intensive supervision, electronic monitoring, emergency shelters, and transition and aftercare programming. In attempts to address cultural competency, states have instituted cultural sensitivity training for personnel of all relevant agencies, recruitment of minority staff and promotional efforts relevant to minority staff, establishing minority internship programs, publication of relevant materials in other languages, recruitment of minority representatives to community accountability boards, reduction of barriers to advocacy, adding juvenile court probation staff in tribal juvenile courts, and annual state conferences on DMC. Community empowerment efforts include supporting better relationships between the juvenile justice system and minority communities; and engagement of minority communities in planning services. In order to combat racial bias, some states have adopted standardized screening instruments to achieve more objective decision-making; they have also adopted standardized risk and needs assessment classification systems, model intake screenings, mandated prosecutorial standards, and standardized diagnostic tools. Some states have strengthened state leadership by establishing DMC subcommittees at high state levels, strategies to prioritize funding to reduce DMC, and established state DMC coordinator positions. Some states are systematically collecting and monitoring DMC data. Two states, Oregon and Washington, have institutionalized efforts through legislation. Oregon passed a law requiring cultural competency of all state agencies. Washington state has adopted prosecutorial standards, developed experimental programs implementing prosecutorial guidelines to reduce racial inequality in the prosecution of youth, established a requirement for state agencies monitoring youth to report annually on minority representation, and has established local juvenile justice advisory committees to monitor and report annually on proportionality and to review/report on citizen complaints regarding bias or disparity within juvenile justice. Research on the effectiveness of most of these methods has yet to be launched.

Challenges for states remain. These include: some states not having identified factors contributing to DMC, inadequate data systems, ongoing state monitoring of DMC efforts and trends, limited systems change in order to reduce DMC, and limited institutionalization of mechanisms to ensure reduction of DMC.

Summary

Adequate resolution of the problem of DMC is a core requirement of the reauthor-ization of the Juvenile Justice Prevention and Delinquency Act. The pattern of DMC is evident in research and practice. There are multiple points in juvenile justice processing where DMC can occur. DMC does not occur in all decision-making points in all jurisdictions. Some states have made adequate assessments of their systems and others have developed strategies to address the problem. More strategic efforts must be developed and adopted nationally and adapted on a state-by-state basis. The failure to resolve this challenge, not only has adverse implications in minority communities, but, also, in the future of our society in general.

References

Community Research Associates (1990). *Disproportionate Minority Confinement, Technical Assistance Manual*. Washington, DC: US Department of Justice, Office of Justice Programs, Office of Juvenile Justice and Delinquency Prevention.

Hsia, H. M. & Hamparian, D. (1998). *Disproportionate Minority Confinement, 1997*. Washington, DC: US Department of Justice, Office of Justice Programs, Office of Juvenile Justice and Delinquency Prevention.

Hsia, H. M., Bridges, G. S. & McHale, R. (2004). *Disproportionate Minority Confinement, Update 2002*. Washington, DC: US Department of Justice, Office of Justice Programs, Office of Juvenile Justice and Delinquency Prevention.

Juvenile Justice Delinquency Prevention (JJDP) Act of 1974 (1992, 2002) (P.L. 93-415, 42 USC 5601 *et seq.*) as amended.

Lynch, J. (2002). *Trends in Juvenile Violent Offending: An Analysis of Victim Survey Data*. Bulletin. Washington, DC: US Department of Justice, Office of Justice Programs, Office of Juvenile Justice and Delinquency Prevention.

Office of Juvenile Justice and Delinquency Prevention (1998, 2001). *Census of Juveniles in Residential Placement 1997 and 1999*. Washington, DC: US Bureau of the Census.

Office of Juvenile Justice and Delinquency Prevention (2000). *Disproportionate Minority Confinement Technical Assistance Manual*, 2nd edn. Washington, DC: US Department of Justice, Office of Justice Programs, Office of Juvenile Justice and Delinquency Prevention.

Males, M. & Macallair, D. (2000). *The Color of Justice: An Analysis of Juvenile Adult Court Transfers in California*. Washington, DC: Building Blocks for Youth.

Nellis, A. M. (2005). *Seven Steps to Develop and Evaluate Strategies to Reduce Disproportionate Minority Confinement*. Washington, DC: Justice Research and Statistics Association, Juvenile Justice Evaluation Center.

Poe-Yamagata, E. & Jones, M. (2000) *And Justice for Some: Differential Treatment of Minority Youth in the Justice System*. Washington, DC: Youth Law Center.

Pope, C. E. & Feyerherm, W. (1990) Minority status and juvenile justice processing. *Criminal Justice Abstracts*, **22**(2), 327–336 (part I); **22**(3), 527–542 (part II).

Pope, C. E. & Snyder, H. (2002). *Race As a Factor in Juvenile Arrests*. Bulletin. Washington, DC: US Department of Justice, Office of Justice Programs, Office of Juvenile Justice and Delinquency Prevention.

Pope, C. E., Lovell, R. & Hsia, H. M. (2002) *Disproportionate Minority Confinement: A Review of the Research Literature From 1989 Through 2001*. Bulletin. Washington, DC: US Department of Justice, Office of Justice Programs, Office of Juvenile Justice and Delinquency Prevention.

Sickmund, M. (2004). *Juveniles in Corrections*. Bulletin. Washington, DC: US Department of Justice, Office of Justice Programs, Office of Juvenile Justice and Delinquency Prevention.

Snyder, H. N. (2003). *Juvenile Arrests 2001*. Bulletin. Washington, DC: US Department of Justice, Office of Justice Programs, Office of Juvenile Justice and Delinquency Prevention.

Snyder, H. N. & Sickmund, M. (2000). *Minorities in the Juvenile Justice System, 1999*. Washington, DC: US Department of Justice, Office of Justice Programs, Office of Juvenile Justice and Delinquency Prevention.

Villaruel F. A. & Walker, N. E. (2002). *Donde Esta la Justicia? A Call to Action on Behalf of Latino and Latina Youth in the U.S. Justice System*. Washington, DC: Building Blocks for Youth.

4

Police interrogation of youth

Allison D. Redlich and Steven Drizin

In legal parlance, "double jeopardy" refers to being held responsible twice for substantially the same crime. The Fifth Amendment of the US Constitution disallows this, essentially holding that the state only gets one bite at the apple. The term "double jeopardy" has also been used to describe several situations in which two characteristics or two circumstances place people at risk in the legal system, perhaps because of the double entendre. For example, Professor Thomas Grisso (2004) recently published a book, entitled *Double Jeopardy: Adolescent Offenders with Mental Illness*, citing that the combination of young age and the presence of mental health problems among justice-involved youth pose special problems for treatment in custodial settings, due process, and public safety. Similarly, a recent report to Congress was entitled *Double Jeopardy: Persons with Mental Illness in the Criminal Justice System* (CMHS, 1995), examining the double-sided problem of the reactions of people with mental illness to the criminal justice system and the reactions of the system to this population.

In the present chapter, our focus is on two vulnerability characteristics – young age and mental health – that can place people in jeopardy in the interrogation room. The jeopardy that exists, and for which there are not suitable safeguards, is the risk of police eliciting false and coerced confessions. Moreover, once confessions or other guilty-knowledge statements are made, the risk of further miscarriages of justice, such as wrongful incarcerations and wrongful convictions, increases substantially.

To understand why youthfulness and mental disorder can place people at risk in the interrogation room, we first describe current police interrogation methods, which rely heavily on psychological manipulation. Next, we examine the unique characteristics of youth and mental illness in the context of current interrogation techniques, and indicate how the potential for miscarriages of justice are intensified. And we then conclude with recommendations and ideas for future research.

Before describing current police interrogation techniques, there are several points that should be explicitly stated and that serve as a basis underlying this

The Mental Health Needs of Young Offenders: Forging Paths toward Reintegration and Rehabilitation, eds. Carol L. Kessler and Louis J. Kraus. Published by Cambridge University Press. © Cambridge University Press 2007.

chapter. First, the number of juveniles (in most states, people aged 17 years or younger) who interact with the police formally and informally is quite impressive. In 2002, 2.3 million juveniles were formally arrested, accounting for 17 percent of all arrests (Snyder, 2004). A countless number of other juveniles interacted with and were questioned by the police on a less formal basis. Indeed, in a study of police–juvenile suspect interactions, Myers (2002) reported the police made the decision to arrest in only 13 percent of the encounters.

Second, there is a wealth of recent research, including chapters in the present book, indicating that justice-involved youth are more likely to have mental health and substance use problems in comparison to non-justice-involved youth (e.g., Teplin *et al.*, Chapter 2). According to the National Center for Mental Health and Juvenile Justice (2005), between 65 and 100 percent of these youth have a diagnosable mental disorder, and 20 percent have a serious mental disorder (see also Cocozza & Skowyra, 2000). Related is the prevailing fact that many justice-involved youth have cognitive and language deficits, educational difficulties, and learning disabilities (Heide, 1997).

Third, the treatment of juvenile offenders in the United States became increasingly harsh beginning in the 1990s (Grisso, 1996; Grisso & Schwartz, 2000, Tanenhaus & Drizin, 2003). A shift in focus from rehabilitation to punishment for the juvenile justice system could be seen, as reflected in the increased number of juveniles tried as adults (and the concomitant facilitation of prosecutorial waivers), the lax in confidentiality requirements, and the use of blended and mandatory sentences. In large part, these reforms were due to a short-lived increase in violent juvenile crime. Although violent juvenile crime has steadily decreased since 1994, the newer controversial reforms remain today. Of relevance here, and of particular irony, is that one of the major cases that led to the notion of juvenile "super-predators" and subsequently to these controversial reforms was the 1989 Central Park Jogger case (Hancock, 2003). Today, the Central Park Jogger case is recognized as a well-known case of false confessions; the five juvenile defendants falsely confessed to their involvement in the brutal rape and attack of a young woman and were convicted and imprisoned on the basis of these false confessions (Kassin, 2002). Instead of the case highlighting the violent and antisocial nature of some juveniles (i.e., "super-predators"), it now highlights juveniles' vulnerability to false confessions.

Contemporary police interrogations

In the United States, interrogation methods rely on psychological methods to elicit confessions and other statements against one's interest (Davis & O'Donohue, 2003; Gudjonsson, 2003; Inbau *et al.*, 2001; Kassin & Gudjonsson, 2004; Leo, 2004).

Of importance, all of the available evidence indicates that the police use the same interrogation tactics with juvenile and adult suspects, and with people with and without mental deficiencies (Inbau *et al.*, 2001; Meyer, 2005; Redlich *et al.*, 2004). Unlike other areas of forensic investigation and legal proceedings that discriminate by age and degree of mental competence, interrogators are trained to interrogate suspects of all ages and all mental abilities in the same manner.

Police interrogations are a multistage process in which these methods of "getting inside the suspect's head" are apparent at every stage. The stages include (1) the pre-interrogation interview, (2) the obtaining of Miranda waivers, and (3) the formal interrogation itself. The foremost police interrogation technique is referred to as the "Reid technique" and its manual by Inbau and colleagues (2001) is in its fourth edition. To date, more than 300 000 law enforcement and security personnel have been trained on the Reid technique (www.reid.com).

Pre-interrogation interview

Before the police formally *interrogate* a suspect, they first conduct an interview, during which they decide whether the suspect is guilty or innocent. If the police perceive the suspect to be deceptive (or in other words, guilty) during this pre-interrogation interview, the police will go forward with the formal interrogation. Because this interview is technically non-custodial, non-accusatory, and non-coercive, the police need not inform persons of their Constitutional Miranda rights at this point. Indeed, a distinguishing feature between the pre-interrogation interview and the formal interrogation is the reading of the Miranda warning. Table 4.1, which is derived directly from Inbau *et al.* (2001), delineates the distinctions between the police interview and the police interrogation.

To some, the difference between the pre-interrogation *interview* and the *interrogation* is a matter of semantics. During the interview, the police establish rapport with suspects (e.g., citing commonalities between the police officer and suspect), may claim the person is not a suspect but merely a witness, and may even take the stance that the police need this person's help in solving the crime. In this manner, the police are able to gather more information about the suspect's knowledge and involvement in the crime in a seemingly innocuous situation.

In addition to relying on oral information to make determinations of deceptiveness, the police will also rely on non-verbal, behavioral cues. Inbau *et al.* (2001, p. 6) state, "During an interview the investigator should closely evaluate the suspect's behavioral responses to interview questions. The suspect's posture, eye contact, facial expression, and word choice, as well as response delivery may reveal signs of truthfulness or deception. Ultimately, the investigator must make an assessment of the suspect's credibility when responding to investigative questions." However, these signs are also indicators of stress (Zimbardo & Leippe,

Table 4.1. Interview versus interrogation

	Interview	Interrogation
Accusatory style	Non-accusatory	Accusatory
Purpose	To gather information	To learn the truth
When	May be conducted early during an investigation	Only conducted when the investigator is reasonably certain of the suspect's guilt
Where	May be conducted in a variety of environments	Controlled environment
Structure	Free flowing and relatively unstructured	Active persuasion
Note-taking	Investigator should take written notes	Investigator should not take any notes until after the suspect has told the truth and is fully committed to that position

Source: Adapted from Inbau *et al.* (2001), pp. 5–9

1991) and are likely to appear more frequently with juveniles and persons with mental illness because of their young age (e.g., general teen angst), or because of their illness or the medications they are taking. This analysis, called the "Behavior Symptoms Analysis" (Inbau *et al.*, 2001) is quite controversial as the social science evidence indicates that people, even trained and experienced police officers, are poor at deception detection (Ekman & O'Sullivan, 1991; Kassin, 2005). In a meta-analysis, Meissner and Kassin (2002) found that police did not fare better than chance or naïve controls. Rather, number of years of experience and training were negatively related to accuracy, such that police officers who had been on the job longer were more likely to judge people deceptive but not do so accurately.

Thus, during this interview phase, the police determine whether to proceed with the formal interrogation, and this determination is based on what the suspect says and what the suspect does (behaviorally). As shown in Table 4.1, whereas the tone of the interview is non-accusatory, when the interrogation begins, the interrogator switches to an accusatory tone and uses "active persuasion" to obtain self-incriminating statements. However, it is important to emphasize that the friendly rapport established between police officer and suspect during the interview is carried over to the interrogation. In other words, although the two phases are distinct, they cannot be considered separate and apart as one is heavily contingent upon the other.

In addition to switching the tone and purpose of questioning, another way to distinguish between the interview and interrogation phase is the issuance of the Miranda warning. In the landmark 1966 decision (*Miranda v. Arizona*), the US

Supreme Court, recognizing the "inherent coercion" in interrogations, made it mandatory for the police to inform suspects of their rights to silence and to counsel before being questioned. Today, some have argued that the Miranda warning offers little protection, in part due to the manner in which they are presented (see Leo, 1996a; White, 2003).

Issuance of Miranda warning

There is a strong motivation for the police to obtain waivers of Miranda rights: if suspects invoke their rights to silence and/or counsel, the police cannot proceed with the interrogation at all, or at least not in the manner they would with an attorney present. Thus, over the 40 years Miranda has been in place, the police have developed methods to obtain these waivers. Leo (1996a) likens the process to a confidence game. Based on extensive research, Leo noted that some interrogators will (1) precede the Miranda warning with a discussion of the importance of truth telling, (2) read the warning while nodding (thereby cueing the suspect to nod along as well indicating agreement), (3) pass the warning off as a mere formality, and/or (4) inform the suspect that this is his one and only chance to tell his side of the story. Using methods such as these, the police are quite successful in obtaining waivers: approximately 75 percent of US suspects will give up their rights and talk to the police (Leo, 1996a).

For Miranda waivers to be valid, they must be made knowingly, intelligently, and voluntarily. Much of the research that has been done on Miranda has focused on the understanding and appreciation of these rights; that is, the knowing and intelligent portions. Beginning with Grisso's seminal research (1981) on juvenile's comprehension of Miranda, studies examining this topic have revealed a consistent picture: juveniles younger than age 15 have significantly less understanding and appreciation than older teens and adults (see also Redlich, Silverman & Steiner, 2003). Younger teens often don't appreciate the adversarial nature of interrogations and have difficulties understanding abstract concepts, such as "rights." Further, not surprisingly, persons with mental disabilities also have been found to have significant deficits in comprehension (Everington & Fulero, 1999; Viljoen, Roesch & Zapf, 2002).

Less attention has been paid to the voluntary portion of the Miranda waiver. Recent research by Kassin and Norwick (2004) demonstrated that when placed in a mock criminal situation, innocent people (81 percent) are much more likely to waive their rights than guilty people (36 percent). When questioned why they gave up their rights, the innocents often offered explanations indicating that they had nothing to hide, and that by invoking their rights police suspicion would increase. Although the Kassin and Norwick study involved young adults, it is likely that minors and persons with mental impairments would be even more likely to (incorrectly) believe that innocent people have no use for their constitutionally afforded rights. This is likely due to deficits in abstract thinking, inabilities to think long term (Steinberg & Cauffman, 2001), and defining traits of mental disorders, such as disorganization of thought and deficits in executive functioning.

The interrogation

After the police interrogator (1) determines that the person is guilty, and (2) has obtained a waiver of rights, the formal interrogation can proceed. By all accounts, contemporary police interrogation tactics rely on psychological (as opposed to physical) manipulation (Davis & O'Donohue, 2003; Leo, 1996b; 2004).

In the Inbau *et al.* (2001) police interrogation training manual, nine steps are delineated, culminating in a written confession. These nine steps are: (1) direct positive confrontation; (2) theme development; (3) handling denials; (4) overcoming objections; (5) keeping the suspect's attention; (6) handling the suspect's passive mood; (7) presenting the alternative question; (8) bringing the suspect into the conversation; and (9) the written confession. In order to appreciate the stressful, adversarial nature of interrogations, these steps must be understood (see Davis & O'Donohue, 2003 for a more detailed review of these steps).

The formal interrogation begins with the direct positive confrontation, i.e., the "I know you did it" statement. As such, interrogations are necessarily guilt-presumptive. The interrogation then proceeds from "I know you did it, but now let's discuss how (or why) you did it." This is where step 2, theme development, begins. The importance of these themes cannot be underestimated. These themes take the form of moral "outs" for the crime, whereby blame is placed elsewhere (e.g., the victim, co-suspect, society, alcohol) providing an outlet for the suspect to admit to the crime in a non-judgmental atmosphere. Referred to as "minimization" tactics (Kassin, 1997), Russano and her colleagues (Russano *et al.*, 2005) tested the influence of these tactics in a mock crime. When this tactic was used alone, the false confession rate was 18 percent; when the minimization technique was combined with an offer of leniency, the false confession rate increased to 43 percent. In many false confession cases, it is apparent that after many intense hours of interrogation, the beleaguered suspect gave in and accepted the themed scenario created by the police (Kassin & Gudjonsson, 2004).

Steps 3–6 are about not allowing the suspect to deny what the police officer already knows to be "true," but at the same time keeping the suspect focused on the ultimate goal, confession. These steps are accomplished by the interrogator speaking in lengthy monologues, and interrupting and disallowing protestations from the suspect, all of which serves to heighten the frustration, anxiety, and feelings of hopelessness of the suspect. Another technique embedded in these steps is lying to, or otherwise deceiving suspects, by telling them evidence exists against them when in fact there is no such evidence. For example, police interrogators may tell suspects that an eyewitness saw them near the victim's house or that their finger-prints are on the weapon. This technique is commonly used and is considered legal (*Frazier v. Cupp*, 1969). In addition, this technique of lying contributes to feelings of hopelessness and despair and has been noted as a major contributor to false confessions in certain cases.

Step 7 concerns the "alternate question," which is a question whose possible answers only point to guilt. An example question is, "Was this the first time, or has it happened many times before?" (Inbau *et al.*, 2001, p. 214). This question is only posed when the interrogator feels the suspect is ready to answer it, i.e., confess guilt, which are steps 8 and 9.

Overall, the contemporary interrogation process is a well-established art that has been in practice for more than 50 years (see Leo, 2004). Some interrogators receive training and this process should not be confused with some haphazard everyone-does-it-differently process. Indeed, in a situation where it is against all suspects' best interest to confess, an estimated two-thirds of suspects partially or fully admit guilt (Leo, 1996b). Confession rates among juveniles are higher with one study reporting an 84 percent confession rate (Ruback & Vardman, 1997). Confession rates among persons with mental illness have yet to be empirically examined, but it is expected that, like juveniles, their rates of confession would be higher than individuals with-out mental illness (Redlich, 2004).

Police interrogation of youths and persons with mental illness

The characteristics and defining traits of juveniles and persons with mental illness place them at risk of coerced and false confessions in the interrogation room. The current tactics, described above, have been found to produce false confessions from adults without mental impairments (Drizin & Leo, 2004). When incomplete cognitive, social, emotional, and moral development, and impairments in mental functioning are considered in the context of high-pressure interrogation tactics, the risks of false admissions of guilt become even greater. In the following, we describe research surrounding the police interrogation of youths and persons with mental impairments. The majority of the research highlights the deficiencies of these two populations, deficiencies that contribute to their increased susceptibility to false confession.

Youthfulness

The latest generation of studies on children involved in the legal system has been ongoing for more than two decades (Goodman, 1984). As such, the literature database of empirical research is extensive, but the majority of the research has focused on the capabilities and perceptions of young children as victims of and witnesses to crime. This extensive database on child victims/witnesses has consistently shown that younger children have less legal knowledge and understanding (Carter, Bottoms & Levine, 1996; Saywitz, Jaenicke & Camparo, 1990), and are more suggestible than older children and adults (Bruck & Melnyk, 2004; Ceci & Bruck, 1993; Quas *et al.*, 2000). Further, these limitations have significant legal implications, such as not understanding the oath to tell the truth in the courtroom, and providing false allegations to the police.

More recent research has focused on the abilities of children involved in the legal system as offenders, and one particular area of concentration has been the interrogation of youth. As mentioned above, police interrogators are trained to treat youths and adults the same – this fact cannot be overemphasized because it stands in the face of 100 years of developmental theory and knowledge, and in the face of the 20 or so years of child victim/witness research, which has determined the ways children should and should not be interviewed. More specifically, in the context of forensic interviewing of alleged child victims/witnesses, it has been established that age-appropriate questions *should be* used (see Poole & Lamb, 1998), and that assumptions, single hypothesis-testing, reinforcements, and co-witness ploys (see Garven, Wood & Malpass, 2000; Garven *et al.*, 1998) *should not be* used. That is, the very techniques that operationally define police interrogations – presumption of guilt, blaming co-suspects, lying – are the techniques specifically proscribed against when interviewing same-aged children alleged to be victims or witnesses. The extant research on youth's abilities in the interrogation room is beginning to bear this out: the techniques found to be dangerous with child victims/witnesses (in terms of generating false reports) can also be dangerous with child suspects (e.g. Billings *et al.*, 2007).

Because the ages of child victims/witnesses and child suspects often overlap, the two groups can theoretically share the same developmental limitations. Indeed, research has shown that like younger victims/witnesses, younger offenders have less legal knowledge, understanding, and appreciation than older offenders, particularly those younger than 15 years (Grisso, 1981; Grisso *et al.*, 2003; Redlich *et al.*, 2003). There have been three study methodologies examining juveniles' abilities in the interrogation room and potential for false confession. The first type has examined juveniles' responses to hypothetical scenarios. For example, Grisso *et al.* (2003) examined minor and young adults' responses to a hypothetical mock-interrogation situation, specifically, whether they would confess to the police, remain silent, or deny the offense. Compared to individuals aged 16 and older, those between the ages of 11–15 years were more likely to report that they would confess to the police. Similarly, Goldstein *et al.* (2003) investigated male juvenile offenders' self-reported likelihood of providing false confessions across multiple hypothetical interrogation scenarios. Their findings revealed that younger age significantly predicted likelihood of false confession. Moreover, 25 percent reported they would definitely falsely confess to at least one of the hypotheticals.

The second type of study methodology is similar to asking for self-reported behavior in hypothetical situations, but instead examines what juveniles and young adults would do in response to a mock crime/interrogation situation involving slight deception. Using the Kassin and Kiechel (1996) design of crashing the computer and determining if people are willing to sign a statement falsely taking responsibility for this, Redlich and Goodman (2003) found that in comparison to young adults, 12- to 16-year-olds were more likely to falsely confess, particularly when the ploy of presenting false evidence (i.e., lying to suspects) was used. Redlich and Goodman also found that youths were less likely to question the authority of the researcher/interrogator, with 50 percent not uttering a word before signing the false confession. As noted above, interrogators actively attempt to disallow denials, because denials disrupt the flow of the interrogation. When suspects do not deny guilt, assert their innocence, or otherwise "speak up," the interrogator is able to wield more control and more authority.

The third type of study methodology is asking juvenile suspects to describe their encounters with the police. Unlike the first and second methodologies, this method assesses what juveniles say they have done in response to actual situations. Viljoen and colleagues' research (2005) involving detained pre-trial juveniles aged 11–17 years, found that 73 percent of the defendants who confessed were aged 15 years or younger. Age was also a factor in requests for attorneys. Among Viljoen et al.'s entire sample of juveniles questioned by the police, only 10 percent had asked for a lawyer (all of whom were aged 15 or older), and only one then had an attorney present. Viljoen et al. also reported that about one in five juveniles questioned by police were high or intoxicated during the interrogation, which is another known risk factor for false confession (see also Redlich et al., 2004).

Finally, Viljoen et al. (2005) asked the youths if they had ever falsely confessed to the police – 6 percent said they had. Research on the prevalence of self-reported false confessions has ranged from 1 to 4 percent among young adults (Gudjonsson et al., 2004a; Gudjonsson, Sigurdsson & Einarsson, 2004b) to 12 percent among adult Icelandic prisoners (Sigurdsson & Gudjonsson, 1996a).

In summary, across the three study methodologies, findings indicate that younger juveniles are at higher risk for providing both true and false confessions than older juveniles and young adults (see also Drizin & Colgan, 2004; Redlich et al., 2004). Indeed, Drizin and Leo (2004) reported that 33 percent of their proven false confessor sample was juveniles. In contrast, juveniles make up 17 percent of those arrested (Snyder, 2004). Overall, both the empirical and case evidence has shown that youths are at risk in the interrogation room. Because an estimated two-thirds of these youths have a diagnosable mental disorder

(NCMHJJ, 2005), we now turn to the research on mental illness, police interrogations, and false confessions.

Mental illness

When compared to prevalence rates in the general population, both youths and adults with mental illness are overrepresented in the criminal justice system (Lamb & Weinberger, 1998; Teplin *et al.*, 2002). More than 800 000 adult offenders with serious mental illness are booked into jails annually (National GAINS Center, 2001). And, although persons with mental illness (PMI) are commonly cited for misdemeanors (Teplin, 1990), there is a subgroup who commit serious and violent crimes (Monahan & Steadman, 1994). For example, of the persons incarcerated for violent crimes in prison, approximately 10–17 percent are mentally ill (Lamb & Weinberger, 1998). In addition, in comparison to persons without mental illness, PMI are (1) more likely to get arrested, (2) once arrested, more likely to be detained in jail (as opposed to released on own recognizance or have the case dismissed), and (3) once jailed, stay incarcerated 2½ to 8 times longer. Thus, the number of minors and adults with mental illness who get arrested and are subject to police interrogation and detention is quite significant.

Certainly, persons with mental illness are a heterogeneous group. Serious mental illness usually refers to three diagnoses: (1) schizo-spectrum diagnoses, such as schizophrenia; (2) bipolar disorder; and (3) major depression. Persons with these disorders may experience delusions, hallucinations, disorganized speech, and feelings of grandiosity, mania, and intense depression. There are also "negative symptoms," such as flat affect associated with these disorders that can be less apparent to the untrained eye. Recent studies estimate 20 percent of justice-involved youth have a serious mental illness (NCMHJJ, 2005). However, all mental disorders, not only the ones categorized as "serious," can certainly cause impairments in social and other important areas of functioning, as well as in the interrogation context. In an extensive review of the interrogation process, Davis and O'Donohue (2003) list 15 mental disorders (e.g., communication disorders, separation anxiety disorder, personality disorders) and describe how each disorder could contribute to the production of a false confession.

Generally, the police have not had adequate training in determining who is and is not mentally unstable. The symptoms and classic characteristics of mental illness are not always easily recognized by non-trained professionals. Lamb, Weinberger and DeCuir (2002, p. 1267) state "A person who seems to be mentally ill to a mental health professional may not seem so to police officers – who despite their practical experience have not had sufficient training in dealing with this population." Similarly, Wellborn (1999, p. 6) states, "Police officers receive training in law enforcement, not necessarily in interacting with individuals with mental illness." Unlike age, which is usually a simple determination, determining whether someone has a mental disorder is more difficult. In addition, juveniles who have mental disorders may be even harder to recognize given that symptoms may be mistaken for "normal" teenage behavior.

If mental problems are suspected, the police should call trained professionals for advice on how to proceed. For example, Crisis Intervention Teams (CIT), which are increasing in number around the nation, are based on the notion that the police are not adequately trained to handle mental health crises by themselves. Rather, the police and trained mental health professionals work in concert (see Cochran, Deane & Borum, 2000). In regard to interrogation, however, the police interrogators seemingly get little training surrounding mental illness and how to question this population. In the Inbau *et al.* (2001) training manual, they recommend proceeding cautiously and offer the advice below:

A suspect with legitimate mental disabilities generally lacks assertiveness and experiences diminished self-confidence. In many cases he will have a heightened respect for authority and experience inappropriate self-doubt. Each of these traits, *if actually present*, may make the suspect more susceptible to offering a false admission when exposed to active persuasion. On the other hand, such suspects are not skilled or confident liars and will often reveal the truth through the interviewing process. (Inbau *et al.*, 2001, pp. 431–432)

In other words, Inbau *et al.* contend that a false confession from a PMI will be readily apparent as such. However, there are proven false confession cases that contradict this. In a recent study of 340 exonerations of defendants from 1989–2003, Gross *et al.* found at least ten exonerees with mental illness, seven of whom falsely confessed (Gross *et al.*, 2005). One such case involved Eddie Joe Lloyd, a man who was interrogated in a mental hospital and who spent 17 years wrongfully imprisoned (Wilgoren, 2002). Moreover, if the police cannot recognize mental illness, this advice offered by Inbau *et al.* is ineffectual. Because the police are not trained to recognize mental illness, safeguards and alterations in current police interrogation practices should be imposed. For example, controversial techniques such as lying to suspects should be disallowed.

To date, the empirical database concerning confessions and mental impairment is lacking. However, it stands to reason that individuals with fragile mental states will be more vulnerable to the psychologically oriented interrogation techniques described above. Like juveniles, there is a wealth of data indicating that PMI have less legal comprehension, including less understanding and appreciation of their Miranda rights (Everington & Fulero, 1999; Poythress *et al.*, 1994; Viljoen, Roesch & Zapf, 2002). Pearse *et al.* (1998) examined whether "vulnerable" suspects were more likely to (truly) confess than "non-vulnerable" suspects. They did not find a significant difference between the two groups, but there are several reasons to view this finding as preliminary and non-conclusive. First, the method of separating the vulnerable from the non-vulnerable suspects was made on the basis of a "brief clinical interview" during which participants were asked about mental state in the last seven days and investigators observed functioning during the interview. Of the eight mental states (e.g., crying, sleeping badly) and one observed functioning (agitation) assessed, the vulnerable and non-vulnerable groups only differed significantly on two. Second, the authors describe the types of crime as "run of the mill" (over 60 percent arrested for property crimes) and themselves state the need to retest their hypothesis with a sample of serious cases. Third, the sample size in Pearse *et al.* may not have been sufficient to detect significant differences. The vulnerable sample comprised 28 subjects.

Of relevance to the present chapter, Viljoen *et al.* (2005) examined whether three forms of psychopathology impacted juvenile interrogation decision-making. The three forms were depression-anxiety, psychomotor excitation, and behavior problems. Although none influenced decisions to confess, deny, or remain silent, psychomotor excitation did influence requests for counsel. Specifically, juveniles who scored higher in terms of excitation were less likely to request an attorney.

In regard to false confessions, Sigurdsson and Gudjonsson (1996a; 1996b) found that alleged false confessors had higher rates of personality disorders, were more compliant and more emotionally labile, and were more likely to be serious drug users than those who never claimed to have falsely confessed. As noted, persons with mental limitations are overrepresented among proven false confessors. The promoters of the most well-known Innocence (DNA exoneration) Project note that "truly startling is the number of false confession cases involving the mentally impaired and the mentally ill" and "Police interrogation in the[se] cases reveals a lack of training and a disregard for mental disabilities." In Drizin and Leo's (2004) research, of a combined total of 125 proven false confession cases, 30 percent of the false confessors had been described as mentally impaired in some way (this is likely to be an underestimate as this trait was not systematically studied or reported in the authors' resources).

To summarize, evidence is amassing indicating that persons with mental disorders are at increased risk for false confession. Like youths, the limitations and traits that define mental disorders must be examined in the context of contemporary police interrogation techniques that are designed to "trick" the guilty into admitting guilt. Regardless of whether it is fair to "trick" minors and persons with mental illness who are guilty, minors and persons with mental illness who are innocent are not suitably protected.

Conclusions and recommendations

The police have developed arguably successful methods to (1) determine a person's guilt, (2) get the person to waive their Constitutional rights, and (3) procure confessions. However, the problem with these methods is the potential for false confession. With the advent of DNA testing and other technological advances, the number of identified false confessions is increasingly growing (e.g., Drizin & Leo, 2004). A number of factors – both internal to the suspect and external – have been identified that are commonly present in these types of false confession cases, though certainly no one factor has been identified as sufficient to produce a false confession (see Kassin & Gudjonsson, 2004). The present chapter focused on the factors of youthfulness and mental impairment.

Although the research bases on these two factors as separate vulnerability characteristics continues to grow, more research is needed on whether and how the two combined *exponentially* increase the risk of false confession and wrongful conviction and imprisonment. There are several known specifics that lead to the conclusion that the two factors place people in double jeopardy in the inter-rogation room. First, on a yearly basis, millions of youths and persons with mental illness are subject to police questioning. Second, justice-involved youths have significantly higher rates of mental disorders, have multiple diagnoses (Steiner & Redlich, 2002; Teplin et al., 2002), and intellectual disabilities. Third, common police interrogation techniques, such as lying to suspects and minimizing the seriousness of the crime, are controversial even when juveniles and persons with mental illness are not involved. And, finally, the protection of Miranda does not protect all juveniles and all PMI, and thus should be considered as wholly unreliable.

Although some states require the presence of an attorney at juvenile interro-gations, most do not (Huang, 2001; Kaban & Tobey, 1999). However, this per se requirement, while perhaps making juvenile interrogation more difficult logisti-cally, can only serve to protect the rights of youths accused of crimes. Another advocated method of protecting suspects during the interrogation process is mandating that the entire process is electronically recorded (Drizin & Reich, 2004). A recent Wisconsin Supreme Court decision (*In re Jerrell, C. J.* 2005) mandated that all juvenile interrogations be electronically recorded. To date, six states and the District of Columbia now mandate the electronic recording of interrogations in their entirety, including Illinois, Maine, and New Mexico, by legislation, and Minnesota, Alaska, and New Jersey, by state Supreme Court decisions or rules. Because the detection of mental illness is more difficult than age recognition, requiring that all interrogations be taped is a viable solution to enhancing protection.

The research findings in regard to child victims/witnesses have been translated into policy changes, including the use of standardized forensic interviews (e.g., Poole & Lamb, 1998), and special courtroom accommodations (Goodman et al., 1999). Findings in regard to youthful offenders stand in stark contrast to the policies concerning treatment of juveniles accused of crimes, such as zero-tolerance attitudes and waivers to adult criminal court (see Fagan & Zimring, 2000). Currently, the US has no standardized guidelines on the interrogation of persons at risk. In contrast, Great Britain enacted the Police and Criminal Evidence Act (PACE), which mandates that psychologically vulnerable suspects (which includes juveniles and mentally disordered/handicapped persons), may only be interviewed by the police within the presence of an "appropriate adult" (Home Office, 1995). The reasoning behind the PACE mandate is that persons at risk "may without knowing or wishing to do so, be particularly prone in certain circumstances to provide information which is unreliable, misleading, or self-incriminating" (Home Office, 1995).

Clearly, more research is needed on how the combination of mental illness and youthful status contribute to coerced and false confessions. But, because each characteristic on its own is an identified risk factor for miscarriages of justice, changes need to occur in regard to the interrogation of these two overlapping populations. Two worthy and relatively easy-to-implement changes are increases in police training and electronic recording. As it currently stands, youths with mental illness are in double jeopardy in the interrogation room without adequate protection.

References

Billings, F. J. *et al.* (2007). Can reinforcement induce children to falsely incriminate themselves? *Law and Human Behavior*, **31**, 125–139.

Bruck, M. & Melnyk, L. (2004). Individual differences in children's suggestibility: a review and synthesis. *Applied Cognitive Psychology*, **18**, 947–996.

Carter, C. A., Bottoms, B. L. & Levine, M. (1996). Linguistic and socioemotional influences on accuracy of children's reports. *Law and Human Behavior*, **20**, 335–358.

Ceci, S. J. & Bruck, M. (1993). Suggestibility of the child witness: a historical review and synthesis. *Psychological Bulletin*, **113**, 403–439.

CMHS (1995). Double jeopardy: persons with mental illnesses in the criminal justice system. A report to Congress. Rockville, MD: U.S. Department of Health and Human Services, Substance Abuse and Mental Health Services Administration, Center for Mental Health Services.

Cochran, S., Deane, M. W. & Borum, R. (2000). Improving police response to mentally ill people. *Psychiatric Services*, **51**, 1315–1316.

Cocozza, J. J. & Skowyra, K. R. (2000). Youth with mental health disorders: issues and emerging responses. *Juvenile Justice*, **7**, 3–13. Washington, DC: Office of Juvenile Justice and Delinquency Prevention.

Davis, D. & O'Donohue, W. (2003). The road to perdition: "Extreme influence" tactics in the interrogation room. In W. O'Donohue, P. Laws and C. Hollin, eds., *Handbook of Forensic Psychology*. New York: Basic Books, pp. 897–996.

Drizin, S. & Colgan, B. (2004). Tales from the juvenile confession front: a guide to how standard police interrogation tactics can produce coerced and false confessions from juvenile suspects. In G. D. Lassiter, ed., *Interrogations, Confessions, and Entrapment.* New York: Kluwer Academic/Plenum Publishers, pp. 127–162.

Drizin, S. A. & Leo, R. A. (2004). The problem of false confessions in the post-DNA world. *North Carolina Law Review,* **82,** 891–1008.

Drizin, S. A. & Reich, M. J. (2004). Heeding the lessons of history: the need for mandatory recording of police interrogations to accurately assess the reliability and voluntariness of confessions. *Drake Law Review,* **52,** 619–646.

Ekman, P. & O'Sullivan, M. (1991). Who can catch a liar? *American Psychologist,* **46,** 913–920.

Everington, C. & Fulero, S. M. (1999). Measuring understanding and suggestibility of defendants with mental retardation. *Mental Retardation,* **37,** 212–220.

Fagan, J. & Zimring, F. E. (2000). *The Changing Borders of Juvenile Justice: Transfer of Adolescents to the Criminal Court.* Chicago, IL: University of Chicago Press.

Frazier v. Cupp, 394 U.S. 731 (1969).

Garven, S., Wood, J. M., Malpass, R. S. & Shaw, J. S. (1998). More than suggestion: the effect of interviewing techniques from the McMartin preschool case. *Journal of Applied Psychology,* **83,** 347–359.

Garven, S., Wood, J. M. & Malpass, R. S. (2000). Allegations of wrongdoing: the effects of reinforcement on children's mundane and fantastic claims. *Journal of Applied Psychology,* **85,** 38–49.

Goldstein, N., Condie, L., Kalbeitzer, R., Osman, D. & Geier, J. (2003). Juvenile offenders' Miranda rights comprehension and self-reported likelihood of offering false confessions. *Assessment,* **10,** 359–369.

Goodman, G. S. (1984). The child witness (special issue). *Journal of Social Issues,* **40,** 1–176.

Goodman, G. S., Quas, J. A., Bulkley, J. & Shapiro, C. (1999). Innovations for child witnesses: A national survey. *Psychology, Public Policy, and the Law,* **5,** 255–281.

Grisso, T. (1981). *Juvenile's Waiver of Rights: Legal and Psychological Competence.* New York: Plenum.

Grisso, T. (1996). Society's retributive response to juvenile violence: a developmental perspective. *Law and Human Behavior,* **20,** 229–247.

Grisso, T. (2004). *Double Jeopardy: Adolescent Offenders with Mental Illness.* Chicago, IL: University of Chicago Press.

Grisso, T. & Schwartz, R. (2000). *Youth on Trial: A Developmental Perspective on Juvenile Justice.* Chicago, IL: University of Chicago Press.

Grisso, T., Steinberg, L., Woolard, J. *et al.* (2003). Juveniles' competence to stand trial: a comparison of adolescents' and adults' capacities as trial defendants. *Law and Human Behavior,* **27,** 333–363.

Gross, S., Jacoby, K., Matheson, D., Montgomery, N. & Patil, S. (2005). Exonerations in the United States, 1989 through 2003. *Journal of Criminal Law and Criminology,* **95,** 523–556.

Gudjonsson, G. H. (2003). *The Psychology of Interrogations and Confessions.* Chichester: Wiley.

Gudjonsson, G. H., Sigurdsson, J. F., Bragason, O. O., Einarsson, E. & Valdimarsdottir, E. B. (2004a). Confessions and denials and the relationship with personality. *Legal and Criminological Psychology,* **9,** 121–133.

Gudjonsson, G. H., Sigurdsson, J. F. & Einarsson, E. (2004b). The role of personality in relation to confessions and denials. *Psychology, Crime, and Law*, **10**, 125–135.

Hancock, L. (2003). Wolf pack: the press and the Central Park jogger. *Columbia Journalism Review*, January/February, 1–11.

Heide, K. M. (1997). Juvenile homicide in America: how can we stop the killing? *Behavioral Sciences and the Law*, **15**, 203–220.

Home Office (1995). *The Police and Criminal Evidence Act 1984 (s. 66), Codes of Practice* (revised edn.), London: HMSO.

Huang, D. T. (2001). "Less unequal footing": state courts' per se rules for juvenile waivers during interrogations and the case for their implementation. *Cornell Law Review*, **86**, 437–477.

In re Jerrell, C. J., 699 N.W.2d 110 (Wis. 2005).

Inbau, F. E., Reid, J. E., Buckley, J. P. & Jayne, B. C. (2001). *Criminal Interrogation and Confessions*, 4th edn. Gaithersburg, MD: Aspen Publishers, Inc.

Kaban, B. & Tobey, A. E. (1999). When police question children: are protections adequate? *Journal of the Center for Children and the Courts*, **1**, 151–160.

Kassin, S. M. (1997). The psychology of confession evidence. *American Psychologist*, **52**, 221–233.

Kassin, S. M. (2002). False confessions and the jogger case. (Opinion Editorial) *New York Times*, November 2002.

Kassin, S. M. (2005). On the psychology of confessions: does innocence put innocents at risk? *American Psychologist*, **60**, 215–228.

Kassin, S. M. & Gudjonsson, G. H. (2004). The psychology of confessions: a review of the literature and issues. *Psychological Science in the Public Interest*, **5**, 33–67.

Kassin, S. M. & Kiechel, K. L. (1996). The social psychology of false confessions: compliance, internalization, and confabulation. *Psychological Science*, **7**, 125–128.

Kassin, S. M. & Norwick, R. J. (2004). Why people waive their Miranda rights: the power of innocence. *Law and Human Behavior*, **28**, 211–221.

Lamb, H. R. & Weinberger, L. E. (1998). Persons with severe mental illness in jails and prisons: a review. *Psychiatric Services*, **49**, 483–492.

Lamb, H. R., Weinberger, L. E. & DeCuir, W. J. (2002). The police and mental health. *Psychiatric Services*, **53**, 1266–1271.

Leo, R. A. (1996a). Miranda's revenge: police interrogation as a confidence game. *Law and Society Review*, **30**, 259–288.

Leo, R. A. (1996b). Inside the interrogation room. *Journal of Criminal Law and Criminology*, **86**, 266–303.

Leo, R. A. (2004). The third degree and the origins of psychological interrogation in the United States. In G. D. Lassiter, ed., *Interrogations, Confessions, and Entrapment*. New York: Kluwer Academic/Plenum Publishers, pp. 37–84.

Meissner, C. A. & Kassin, S. M. (2002). He's guilty!: Investigator bias in judgements of truth and deception. *Law and Human Behavior*, **26**, 469–480.

Meissner, C. A. & Kassin, S. M. (2004). "You're guilty, so just confess!" Cognitive and behavioral confirmation biases in the interrogation room. In G. D. Lassiter, ed., *Interrogations, Confessions, and Entrapment*. New York: Kluwer Academic/Plenum Publishers, pp. 85–106.

Meyer, J. (2005). The effect of coercive and deceptive interrogation techniques on the reliability of young suspects' reports. Paper presented in N. D. Reppucci (chair), *Testimony and Interrogation of Minors: Assumptions about Maturity and Morality*. La Jolla, CA: American Psychology-Law Society.

Miranda v. Arizona, 384 U.S. 436 (1966).

Monahan, J. & Steadman, H. J. (1994). *Violence and Mental Disorder: Developments in Risk Assessment*. Chicago: University of Chicago Press.

Myers, S. M. (2002). Police encounters with juvenile suspects: Explaining the use of authority and provision of support. Final report to the National Institute of Justice, Project # 2000-IJ-CX-0039. Washington, DC: U.S. Department of Justice.

National Center for Mental Health and Juvenile Justice. (2005). http://www.ncmhjj.com/about/default.asp. Retrieved October 17, 2005.

National GAINS Center for People with Co-Occurring Disorders in the Justice System (2001). The prevalence of co-occurring mental illness and substance use disorders in jails. Fact sheet series. Delmar, NY: The National GAINS Center.

Pearse, J., Gudjonsson, G. H., Clare, I. C. H. & Rutter, S. (1998). Police interviewing and psychological vulnerabilities: predicting the likelihood of a confession. *Journal of Community and Applied Social Psychology*, **8**, 1–21.

Poole, D. A. & Lamb, M. E. (1998). *Investigative Interviews of Children: A Guide for Helping Professionals*. Washington, DC: American Psychological Association.

Poythress, N. G., Bonnie, R. J., Hoge, S. K., Monahan, J. & Oberlander, L. B. (1994). Client abilities to assist counsel and make decisions in criminal cases: findings from three studies. *Law and Human Behavior*, **18**, 437–452.

Quas, J. A., Goodman, G. S., Ghetti, S. & Redlich, A. D. (2000). Questioning the child witness: what can we conclude from the research thus far? *Trauma, Abuse, and Violence*, **1**, 223–249.

Redlich, A. D. (2004). Mental illness, police interrogations, and the potential for false confession. *Psychiatric Services*, **55**, 19–21.

Redlich, A. D. & Goodman, G. S. (2003). Taking responsibility for an act not committed: the influence of age and suggestibility. *Law and Human Behavior*, **27**, 141–156.

Redlich, A. D., Silverman, M. & Steiner, H. (2003). Factors affecting pre-adjudicative and adjudicative competence in juveniles and young adults. *Behavioral Sciences and the Law*, **21**, 1–17.

Redlich, A. D., Silverman, M., Chen, J. & Steiner, H. (2004). The police interrogation of children and adolescents. In G. D. Lassiter, ed., *Interrogations, Confessions, and Entrapment*. New York: Kluwer Academic/Plenum Publishers, pp. 107–126.

Ruback, R. B. & Vardaman, P. J. (1997). Decision making in delinquency cases: the role of race and juveniles' admission/denial of the crime. *Law and Human Behavior*, **21**, 47–69.

Russano, M. B., Meissner, C. A., Narchet, F. M. & Kassin, S. M. (2005). Investigating true and false confessions within a novel experimental paradigm. *Psychological Science*, **16**, 481–486.

Saywitz, K., Jaenicke, C. & Camparo, L. (1990). Children's knowledge of legal terminology. *Law and Human Behavior*, **14**, 523–535.

Sigurdsson, J. F. & Gudjonsson, G. H. (1996a). The psychological characteristics of false confessors: a study among Icelandic prison inmates and juvenile offenders. *Personality and Individual Differences*, **20**, 321–329.

Sigurdsson, J. F. & Gudjonsson, G. H. (1996b). Illicit drug use among "false confessors": a study among Icelandic prison inmates. *Nordic Journal of Psychiatry*, **50**, 325–328.

Snyder, H. (2004). Juvenile arrests 2002. *Juvenile Justice Bulletin*. Office of Juvenile Justice and Delinquency Prevention, Office of Justice Programs. Washington, DC: U.S. Department of Justice.

Steinberg, L. & Cauffman, E. (2001). Adolescents as adults in court: a developmental perspective on the transfer of juveniles to criminal court. *Social Policy Report*, **XV**, 3–14.

Steiner, H. & Redlich, A. D. (2002). Child psychiatry and the juvenile court. In M. Lewis, ed., *Child and Adolescent Psychiatry: A Comprehensive Textbook*, 3rd edn. Baltimore, MD: Lippincott, Williams, & Wilkins, Inc, pp. 1417–1425.

Tanenhaus, D. S. & Drizin, S. A. (2003). Owing to the extreme youth of the accused: the changing legal response to juvenile homicide. *Journal of Criminal Law & Criminology*, **92**, 641–704.

Teplin, L. A. (1990). The prevalence of severe mental disorder among urban male detainees: comparison with the epidemiologic catchment area program. *American Journal of Public Health*, **80**, 663–669.

Teplin, L. A., Abram, K. M., McClelland, G. M., Dulcan, M. K. & Mericle, A. A. (2002). Psychiatric disorders in youth in juvenile detention. *Archives of General Psychiatry*, **59**, 1133–1143.

Viljoen, J. L., Roesch, R. & Zapf, P. A. (2002). An examination of the relationship between competency to stand trial, competency to waive interrogation rights, and psychopathology. *Law and Human Behavior*, **26**, 481–506.

Viljoen, J. L., Klaver, J. & Roesch, R. (2005). Legal decisions of preadolescent and adolescent defendants: predictors of confessions, pleas, communication with attorneys, and appeals. *Law and Human Behavior*, **29**, 253–277.

Wellborn, J. (1999). Responding to individuals with mental illness. *FBI Law Enforcement Bulletin*, **68**, 6–8.

White, W. S. (2003). *Miranda's Waning Protections: Police Interrogation Practices after Dickerson.* Ann Arbor: University of Michigan Press.

Wilgoren, J. (2002). Confession had his signature; DNA did not. *New York Times*, August 26, p. A1.

Zimbardo, P. G. & Leippe, M. R. (1991). *The Psychology of Attitude Change and Social Influence.* New York, NY: McGraw-Hill Book Company.

5

Assessing children's competence to stand trial and to waive Miranda rights: new directions for legal and medical decision-making in juvenile courts

Thomas F. Geraghty, Louis J. Kraus, and Peter Fink

Introduction

This chapter discusses the distinct but related issues of a child's competence to stand trial, to understand and to waive Miranda rights, and to make a knowing and voluntary statement when interrogated by police and prosecutors.

We begin this chapter with a brief overview of the history of the law relevant to the issues of a child's competence to stand trial. We then discuss the legal and medical frameworks for assessing a child's competence to stand trial.

We go on to present and to analyze the legal and medical frameworks and methodologies for assessing a child's competence to waive Miranda rights. We then turn to the methods by which lawyers and medical personnel evaluate a child's competence in these areas. These assessments play a central role in determining the admissibility into evidence of children's statements to law enforcement.

Finally, we include a section on the interactions and relationships between the judges, lawyers, and medical experts who participate in the assessment process and in the process of adjudicating competence to stand trial and children's capacity to make a knowing, intelligent waiver of Miranda warnings. It is important for all involved in the assessment and adjudicative process to understand the role of each actor in the process, and the dynamics of relationships that can affect the quality of the judge's decision as to admissibility of a child's statement to law enforcement.

The issues discussed in this chapter are of central importance to the juvenile court's adjudicative process. Accurate determinations regarding the competence of juveniles to stand trial and to waive Miranda rights are essential to ensuring the right to a fair trial. Ensuring that a child is competent to stand trial maximizes the

The Mental Health Needs of Young Offenders: Forging Paths toward Reintegration and Rehabilitation, eds. Carol L. Kessler and Louis J. Kraus. Published by Cambridge University Press. © Cambridge University Press 2007.

possibility that there will be meaningful communication between the child, the child's attorney, and the child's parents or guardians. A child's capacity to understand the nature and consequences of the interrogation process, including comprehending the meaning of Miranda rights, furthers the goal of minimizing the possibility of coercion and maximizing reliability of statements taken from children.

Historical background: juvenile courts and due process

Before the Supreme Court of the United States decided *In re Gault*, 387 U.S. 1 (1967), legal formalities were absent in juvenile courts. The founders of the juvenile court movement created a model of investigation and adjudication for children that did not rely upon the adversarial proceedings that characterized the criminal trials of adults. The founders of the juvenile court in Chicago in 1899 were more concerned about the incarceration of children with adults than with the appropriate model for juvenile court adjudications. "By the early 1890s, a number of judges and the city's jailor publicly voiced their concerns about incarcerating young children with adults. On numerous occasions, for example, Judge Kersten told police officers not to bring children under 12 years of age to his court" (Tanenhaus, 2004, p. 8). Lucy Flower and Julia Lathrop, shocked at the conditions to which children were subjected in Chicago's jails, campaigned for legislation that created the Cook County Juvenile Court in 1899 (Tanenhaus, 2004, pp. 11–22).

Before *Gault*, the child's mental status, both at the time of the offense (the basis for what now would be a diminished capacity or insanity defense) or at the time of trial, were not relevant until after the court made a finding of delinquency. (Even today, states differ on their approaches to the relevance and effect of a child's criminal capacity.) This was because the juvenile court's inquiry as far as guilt or innocence were concerned was whether the child was factually guilty or innocent. Mental status was relevant only to the dispositional phase of the proceedings. This approach was based on the notion that juvenile courts acted as parens partriae and that their dispositional orders constituted "treatment" rather than "punishment."

The following is a description of a Chicago juvenile courtroom in 1929: Hearings in the court are informal. In delinquency cases, they are merely an attempt to learn facts both concerning the circumstances of the specific acts complained of and concerning the habits, circumstances of life, and general character of the child. The purpose of the hearing is not to establish guilt or innocence, but to secure facts which will form the basis for intelligently recommending corrective treatment for the child. Hearings before the referees are held in their offices, and nobody is present except those immediately concerned with the case. Hearings before the judge are in a small room, and may be said to be public, though very few people are admitted, and the attempt is made to limit attendance in the court room to persons who have specific business in the court. (Wigmore, 1929)

In 1968, the United States Supreme Court in *In re Gault* required that children in juvenile court proceedings receive basic due process protections including the right to adequate notice, the right to a hearing, and the right to counsel. The Supreme Court ruled that children needed these due process protections in order to protect them from the oft-times arbitrary decision-making of juvenile court judges. The facts that gave rise to the Supreme Court's decision in *Gault* illustrate this phenomenon. In *Gault*, a juvenile was committed to a state reformatory for an indeterminate period of time for allegedly making an obscene phone call. He was not given notice of the charges; the complaining witness was never called to testify. Gault had no lawyer. The State of Arizona defended the procedure that resulted in Gault's incarceration on the basis that juvenile court proceedings were an informal inquiry designed to protect the child and not to punish. The Supreme Court rejected this view, stating *In re Gault*, 387 U.S. 1, 18 (1967) "that juvenile court history has again demonstrated that unbridled discretion, however benevolently motivated, is frequently a poor substitute for principle and procedure."

Beginning in 1968, therefore, juvenile courts were required to provide notice, opportunity to be heard, and the right to counsel. Following *Gault*, the Supreme Court also held that the beyond a reasonable doubt standard of proof, required in criminal cases, applied to juvenile court adjudication (see *In Re Winship*, 397 U.S. 358 (1970)). But the Supreme Court stopped short of requiring juvenile courts to apply the full panoply of rights available to adults when it held that children tried in juvenile court were not entitled to jury trials, *McKeiver v. Pennsylvania*, 403 U.S. 528 (1971). In *McKeiver v. Pennsylvania*, the case in which the Supreme Court held that jury trials are not required in juvenile court proceedings, the Court attempted to strike a balance between advancing and preserving the due process model and maintaining the "informal" nature of juvenile court proceedings.

The Court in *McKeiver* stated,

[t]he imposition of the jury trial on the juvenile court system would not strengthen greatly, if at all, the fact-finding function, and would contrarily, provide an attrition of the juvenile court's assumed ability to function in a unique manner. It would not remedy the defects of the system. Meager as has been the hoped-for advance in the juvenile field, the alternative would be regressive, would lose what has been gained, and would tend once again to place the juvenile squarely in the routine of the criminal process. (McKeiver v. Pennsylvania, 403 U.S. 547 (1971))

Subsequently, the Supreme Court held that the Double Jeopardy Clause of the Fifth Amendment to the Constitution of the United States applies to proceedings in juvenile court, *Breed v. Jones*, 421 U.S. 519 (1975). More recently, the Supreme Court reaffirmed the notion that juvenile court proceedings are not entirely punitive in nature when it upheld the pre-trial detention of children without bail, based upon a lesser standard of proof than is applicable to persons charged in criminal court. *See, Schall v. Martin*, 467 U.S. 253 (1984). Pre-trial detention is "regulatory" rather than "punitive": "Preventive detention under the [New York Family Court Act] serves the legitimate state objective, held in common with every state in the country, of protecting both the juvenile and society from the hazards of pretrial crime." *See, Schall v. Martin*, 467 U.S. 274 (1984). The Fourth Amendment protections available to children in school are also less stringent than those applied to adults, *New Jersey v. T.L.O.*, 469 U.S. 325 (1985).

The Supreme Court, in its recent decision in *Roper v. Simmons*, 543 U.S. 511 (2005) – the juvenile death penalty case – has reaffirmed its view that children are a distinct group for purposes of sentencing and justice policy. The Court in *Roper*, stated that, "once the diminished capacity of juveniles is recognized, it is evident that the penological justifications for the death penalty apply to them with lesser force." (*Roper v. Simmons*, 543 U.S. 1196 [2005]) The Court went on to observe that:

If trained psychiatrists with the advantage of clinical testing and observation refrain, despite diagnostic expertise, from assessing any juvenile under the age of 18 as having antisocial personality disorder, we conclude that States should refrain from asking jurors to issue a far graver condemnation – that a juvenile merits the death penalty. When a juvenile offender commits a heinous crime, the State can exact forfeiture of some of the most basic liberties, but the State cannot extinguish his life and his potential to attain a mature understanding of his own humanity. (*Roper v. Simmonds*, 543 U.S. 1197 (2005))

This statement by the Supreme Court of the United States underscores the fact that courts remain sensitive to the differences between children and adults, and that they incorporate research and findings by medical experts into their decisions. The incorporation of the research of psychiatrists, psychologists, and other experts into the still developing field of children's law underscores the importance of cooperation between legal and medical professionals involved in delinquency proceedings.

Competence to stand trial

The ability of juveniles to understand the adjudicative processes has been the focus of much study and debate. Ordinarily, claims of incompetence are based upon a child's age, cognitive ability, and mental health status. More recently, psychiatrists and psychologists have focused on immaturity as a factor to be considered when evaluating children's competence to stand trial. Dr. Thomas Grisso and his colleagues have found that many children, not identified as unfit because of low intelligence, lack of cognitive skills, or mental disability may, in fact, still be incompetent to stand trial because of immaturity:

. . . juveniles aged 15 years and younger are significantly more likely than older adolescents and young adults to be impaired in ways that compromise their ability to serve as competent defendants in a criminal proceeding. On the basis of criteria established in studies of mentally ill offenders (Otto *et al.*, 1998; Poythress *et al.*, 1999), approximately one-third of all 11–13 year-olds, and approximately one-fifth of 14–15 year-olds are as impaired in capacities relevant to adjudicative competence as are seriously mentally ill adults who would likely be considered incompetent to stand trial by clinicians who perform evaluations for courts. Our results also indicate that the competence-relevant capacities of 16- and 17-year-olds as a group do not differ significantly from those of young adults … Not surprisingly; juveniles of below-average intelligence are more likely than juveniles of average intelligence to be impaired in abilities relevant for competence to stand trial. Because a greater proportion of youths in the juvenile justice system than in the community are of below-average intelligence, the risk for incompetence to stand trial is therefore even greater among adolescents who are in the justice system than it is among adolescents in the community. (Grisso *et al.*, 2003, 333)

The findings of Dr. Grisso and his colleagues suggest that a substantial percentage of children who are tried in juvenile court may not be competent to stand trial according to the competency standards applied to adults. Most of these children, however, are not, under present practice, evaluated to determine whether they are, in fact, competent.

If a substantial proportion of children charged in juvenile proceedings would not be found competent to stand trial in an adult criminal proceeding, what implications does this fact have for proceedings in juvenile court? Grisso *et al.* (2003, p. 359) suggest that in the case of children tried in criminal court, special measures be taken to ensure that these children are competent, including automatic competency evaluations for children subject to discretionary transfer and for those in criminal court as the result of automatic transfer statutes. Dr. Grisso *et al.* (2003, 360) argue for a relaxed competence standard "in juvenile court, a standard applicable to juveniles that would hold a child competent to stand trial if the youth 'has a basic understanding of the purpose of the proceedings and can communicate rationally with counsel.'" They base this argument on Supreme Court doctrine which has made it clear that the requirements of due process in delinquency proceedings are not identical to those that regulate criminal trials. (Grisso *et al.* [2003, 359], citing *McKeiver v. Pennsylvania*, 403 U.S. 528 [1971]). Grisso and his colleagues go on to note that "several courts that have considered competence to stand trial in juvenile court assume that the competence demands of a delinquency proceeding are lower than in an adult trial, and that youths who cannot be transferred to adult criminal court because of incompetence can be tried in juvenile court." This standard, Grisso and his colleagues argue, "will promote practices that implement due process without creating an undue burden on the court system." (Grisso *et al.* [2003, 360], citing *In the Matter of W.A.F.*, 573 A. 2d 1264 [D.C. 1990] and *Ohio v. Settles*, 1998 WL 667635 [Ohio App. 3rd Dist 1998])

Dr. Grisso and his colleagues have proposed a reasonable response to the impact of their findings regarding adjudicative competence. However, the Supreme Court's holding in *McKeiver v. Pennsylvania* – that jury trials are not required in juvenile proceedings – can be distinguished on functional grounds from the long-standing constitutional requirement that a defendant be competent to stand trial. The fact-finding mission of a court can proceed, and can conceivably be fair and impartial, without the participation of a jury. "The requirements of notice, counsel, confrontation, cross-examination, and standard of proof naturally flow . . .. But one cannot say that in our legal system the jury is a necessary component of accurate fact finding. There is much to be said for it, to be sure, but we have been content to pursue other ways for determining facts." (Grisso *et al.*, 2003, p. 543). It is somewhat less realistic to expect that a child who lacks the ability fully to understand the nature of the proceedings, and who is unable to form a meaningful relationship with counsel, can be adequately defended. In addition, it is unclear how a more "relaxed" standard of competency would be applied in practice. The body of case law that defines competence to stand trial in criminal cases is well developed and has proved to be workable in the juvenile court setting. The notion that a lesser standard of due process is warranted because juvenile courts operate in the "best interests" of children and do not exact punishment is challenged by the fact that in many states, juvenile court acts have been recently rewritten to stress punishment and deterrence, rather than treatment and rehabilitation as the objectives of a juvenile court proceeding.

The statement of purpose and policy in the Illinois Juvenile Court Act illustrates this shift in policy:

"It is the intent of the General Assembly to promote a juvenile justice system capable of dealing with the problem of juvenile delinquency, a system that will protect the community, impose accountability for violations of law and equip juvenile offenders with competencies to live responsibly and productively. To effectuate this intent, the General Assembly declares the following to be important purposes of this Article:

(a) To protect citizens from juvenile crime.

(b) To hold each juvenile offender directly accountable for his or her acts.

(c) To provide an individualized assessment of each alleged and adjudicated delinquent juvenile, in order to rehabilitate and to prevent further delinquent behavior through the development of competency in the juvenile offender."

(705 ILCS 405/5-101 (West, 2005))

The child's ability to understand the interrogation process and to waive Miranda rights

That a child's statement to the police should be examined for voluntariness and reliability at a pre-trial hearing was also a concept foreign to the original intent and purpose of the first juvenile court. Indeed, pre-trial hearings on the admissibility of statements in criminal cases were not made mandatory until 1964 when the Supreme Court held that when the voluntariness of a defendant's statement is at issue, judges must make a preliminary assessment regarding the admissibility of that statement (see *Jackson v. Denno*, 378 U.S. 368 [1968]). The prosecutor must prove by a preponderance of the evidence that the statement was voluntary and made in accordance with the requirements of Miranda (see *Lego v. Twomey*, 404 U.S. 477 [1972] and *Colorado v. Connelly*, 479 U.S. 157 [1986]). This constitutional requirement ensures that juries do not consider involuntary confessions when reaching their verdicts.

Despite the fact that there are no jury trials in juvenile court, thus obviating the concern about tainting juries with evidence of an inadmissible confession, juvenile courts overwhelmingly follow the practice of deciding pre-trial the admissibility of a child's inculpatory statement to law enforcement officials. The rationale for this practice is that a pre-trial hearing on the admissibility is a more efficient way to proceed than considering the issue of admissibility and guilt/innocence at the same time.

Beginning in 1932 with the notorious case of *Powell v. Alabama*, 287 U.S. 45 (1932), the Supreme Court began to focus on the phenomenon of miscarriages of justice in our nation's criminal justice systems, creating jurisprudence that required assistance of counsel and that condemned abusive and heavy-handed police interrogation techniques. Two of the leading cases in this area involved the interrogation of juveniles. In 1948, the Supreme Court decided *Haley v. Ohio*, 332 U.S. 596 (1948), and in 1962 decided *Gallegos v. Colorado*, 370 U.S. 49 (1962), cases in which the Supreme Court condemned extreme measures used by the police to extract statements from children. In *Haley* and in *Gallegos* the Supreme Court ruled that police must pay special attention to the vulnerabilities of children during the custodial interrogation process.

The language used by the Supreme Court in *Haley* and *Gallegos* is instructive in identifying the issues that have guided the developing jurisprudence on the admissibility of children's confessions. In *Haley*, the defendant was 15 years old. He was held by the police for three days incommunicado and confessed after a five-hour interrogation. There was evidence that Haley had been beaten by the police. Even though Haley acknowledged in his statement that he was told that he had a right not to make a statement, Justice Douglas, writing for the majority, stated:

What transpired would make us pause for careful inquiry if a mature man were involved. And when, as here, a mere child – an easy victim of the law – is before us, special care must be used. Age 15 is a tender and difficult age for a boy of any race. He cannot be judged by the more exacting standards of maturity. That which would leave a man cold and unimpressed can overawe and overwhelm a lad in his early teens. This is the period of great instability which the crisis of adolescence produces." (*Haley v. Ohio*, 332 U.S. 596, 600 (1948))

Responding specifically to the prosecution's assertion that Haley's confession was admissible because he had been advised of his right to remain silent, Justice Douglas wrote:

That assumes, however, that a boy of fifteen, without aid of counsel, would have a full appreciation of that advice and that on the facts of this record he had freedom of choice. We cannot indulge in those assumptions. Moreover, we cannot give any weight to recitals which merely formalize constitutional requirements. (*Haley v. Ohio*, 332 U.S. 596, 600 (1948))

Justice Douglas reiterated these principles in 1962 in *Gallegos v. Colorado*, 370 U.S. 49 (1962). (Confession of a 14-year-old held inadmissible after the child was held for five days and was denied access to his parents during this time.)

The youth of the petitioner, the long detention, the failure to send for his parents, the failure immediately to bring him before the judge of the juvenile court, the failure to see to it that he had the advice of a lawyer or a friend – all these combine to make us conclude that the formal confession on which his conviction may have rested [citation omitted] was obtained in violation of due process. (*Gallegos v. Colorado*, 370 U.S. 52 (1962))

More recently, the United States Court of Appeals for the 7th Circuit relied on *Haley* and *Gallegos* when it held the confession of an 11-year-old inadmissible, observing that:

when [the child] sat, alone, in the police interrogation room, he was not even old enough to be a caddy on a golf course under Illinois law … [He] had no prior experience with the criminal justice system. [The interrogating police officer] continually challenged [the child's] statement and accused him of lying, a technique which could easily lead a young boy to 'confess' to anything. No friendly adult, moreover, was present during the questioning. (*A. M. v. Butler*, 360 F.3d 787, 800 (7 Cir. 2004). See also, *Hardaway v. Young*, 302 F. 3d 757, 759 (a case in which the 7th Circuit held that statement of a 14 year-old admissible, but only with the "gravest misgivings".))

After the Supreme Court's decision in *Miranda v. Arizona*, 384 U.S. 436 (1966), both federal and state courts have held that Miranda warnings are required before statements can be taken from children who are under arrest. Whether there has been a knowing and intelligent waiver of Miranda rights by a juvenile depends on the totality of the circumstances of the interrogation, including "evaluation of the juvenile's age, experience, education, background, and intelligence and … whether he has the capacity to understand the warnings given him, the nature of his Fifth Amendment rights, and the consequences of waiving those rights." (*Fare v. Michael C.*, 442 U.S. 707 [1979])

Competence to stand trial

A requirement of due process

The Supreme Court of the United States has held that the prohibition against trying defendants who are mentally incompetent to stand trial is fundamental to our adversary system of justice:

> It has long been accepted that a person whose mental condition is such that he lacks the capacity to understand the nature and object of the proceedings against him, to consult with counsel, and to assist in preparing his defense may not be subjected to a trial. Thus, Blackstone writes that one who became 'mad' after the commission of an offense should not be arraigned for it 'because he is not able to plead to it with the advice and caution that he ought.' Similarly, if he became 'mad' after pleading, he should not be tried, 'for how can he make his defense?' [citations omitted]. Some have viewed the common-law prohibition 'as a by-product of the ban against trials in absentia; the mentally incompetent defendant, though physically present in the courtroom, is in reality afforded no opportunity to defend himself. (*Drope v. Missouri*, 420 U.S. 162, 171 (1975))

The classic case of incompetence to stand trial was that presented to the Supreme Court in *Jackson v. Indiana*, 406 U.S. 715 (1972), a case in which the defendant was a deaf mute with a mental ability of a pre-school child. The expert witness in *Jackson* testified that "Jackson's almost non-existent communication skill, together with his lack of hearing and his mental deficiency, left him unable to understand the nature of the charges against him or to participate in his defense" (*Jackson v. Indiana*, 406 U.S. 718 [1972]).

Few cases involve defendants with such pervasive disabilities. Most defendants in criminal cases and children subject to delinquency proceedings who may be incompetent have less overwhelming disabilities that affect their ability to understand the nature and purpose of the proceedings and to cooperate with counsel. These characteristics include low intelligence, mental illness, developmental limitations, and physical disabilities that negatively affect cognitive function.

The paradigm presented by the facts in *Jackson* is present in many cases involving children. A child's communication skills are often poorly developed. It may not be possible for the child to understand precisely what it is that he has allegedly done wrong. The child client may also lack the ability to understand the nature of the trial process and the roles of the various actors in the trial process, making his ability to cooperate with counsel non-existent. Moreover, a child may be unable to develop the kind of trust relationship with his lawyer necessary for meaningful cooperation.

The legal test for competence to stand trial

The Supreme Court of the United States articulated the test for competency to stand trial in criminal cases:

... the test must be whether he [the defendant] has sufficient present ability to consult with his lawyer with a reasonable degree of rational understanding – and whether he has a rational as well as factual understanding of the proceedings against him. (*Dusky v. United States*, 362 U.S. 402 (1960) See also *Pate v. Robinson*, 383 U.S. 375 (1966)).

This test has been incorporated into state laws by legislation. The Illinois statute governing the conduct of fitness hearings is typical of such statutes. It contains a list of factors that a judge must apply when deciding whether a defendant is competent to stand trial:

(1) The defendant's knowledge and understanding of the charge, the proceedings, the consequences of the plea, judgment or sentence, and the functions of the participants in the trial process;
(2) The defendant's ability to observe, recollect and relate occurrences, especially those concerning the incidents alleged and to communicate with counsel;
(3) The defendant's social behavior and abilities; orientation as to time and place; recognition of persons, places and things; and performance of motor processes.

(725 ILCS 5/104-16 (b)(1)–(3))

Competence vs. criminal capacity

It is important at the outset to note the distinction between criminal capacity and competence or "fitness" to stand trial. "Criminal capacity" refers to the ability to form the requisite mental state to establish criminal culpability. "Competence to stand trial" refers to the ability of a person to understand the nature and purpose of the proceedings and to cooperate with counsel. The common law presumed a child under the age of 7 not to have the capacity to commit a criminal offense. Between the ages of 7 and 14, there was a rebuttable presumption against criminal capacity. After the age of 14, the child was presumed to possess criminal capacity, see, e.g., *People v. Lang*, 83 N. E. 2d 688 (1949). In Illinois, the age of criminal capacity is governed by statute, prohibiting the criminal prosecution of children under the age of 13. "No person shall be convicted of any offense unless he had attained his 13th birthday at the time the offense was committed." (720 ILCS 5/6-1.) However, this does not mean that a child under the age of 13 cannot be tried for an offense in juvenile court. In fact, in many states there is no limitation on the age at which a child can be tried, making it theoretically possible that a child of any age could face prosecution in juvenile court. However, in states in which there is no limitation regarding the age of capacity, children below a certain age may not be committed to the state's correctional system. If these children are found guilty, they are referred to the state's child welfare agency instead of to the correctional system.

There is a continuing debate about whether criminal capacity should be a requirement in a juvenile proceeding. Illinois courts have held that criminal capacity is not a requirement in a juvenile proceeding. *In re Carson*, 295 N.E. 2d 740 (Ill. App. Ct., 3rd Dist. 1973); *In Interest of G.T.*, 409 Pa. Super. 15(1991) (finding of delinquency is not the same as a conviction of a crime, so it is not necessary to prove that the juvenile had criminal capacity); but see, e.g., *State v. T.E.H.*, 91 Wash. App. 908 (Div. 1 1998) (statutory presumption of incapacity to commit crimes for children 8–12 applies to juvenile proceedings); *People v. Lewis*, 26 Cal. 4th 334, 378 (2001) (prosecution must rebut the presumption that children under 14 lack criminal capacity). The question of criminal capacity or the ability to possess criminal intent, is a question that defense lawyers, prosecutors, social workers, psychiatrists, and psychologists may be called to address in jurisdiction in which lack of criminal capacity is a bar to delinquency proceedings. Other states have taken a contrary position. At present there is variability from jurisdiction to jurisdiction, and at times from judge to judge (AACAP, 2005).

The requirement of competence to stand trial applies to delinquency proceedings

Although the Supreme Court has not specifically addressed the question of whether the standards applicable to the fitness of adults to stand trial in criminal court are applicable to juvenile court proceedings, state courts have held that competence to stand trial is a requirement in juvenile court. See, Richard E. Redding and Lynda E. Frost, *Adjudicative Competence in the Modern Juvenile Court*, 9 Va. J. Soc. Pol'y & L. 352, 354 (2001); *In re T.D.W.*, 441 N.E.2d 155 (Ill. App. Ct. 1982); *In the Matter of W.A.F.*, 573 A.2d 1264 (D.C. 1990); *In Interest of S.H.*, 469 S.E.2d 810 (Ga. Ct. App. 1996); *In re Welfare of D.D.N.*, 582 N.W.2d 278 (Minn. Ct. App. 1998); and *In re J.M.*, 769 A.2d 656 (Vt. 2001). State courts have reached this result based upon the conclusion that the same due process rules that require notice, opportunity to be heard, and counsel, also require that a child be competent in order to be tried in a delinquency proceeding. See, e.g., *In re E.V.*, 549 N.E. 2d 521 (Ill. App. Ct., 3rd Dist., 1989) and *In re T.D.* 441 N.E. 2d 155 (Ill. App. Ct., 4th Dist., 1982) (holding that despite the fact that there was no provision in Illinois' Juvenile Court Act for a hearing on competence to stand trial, the "right not to be tried or convicted while incompetent" applies to juvenile proceedings).

The procedure followed to determine whether a child is competent to stand trial

The inquiry into the question of whether a child is competent to stand trial focuses on the child's understanding of the nature of the charges, of juvenile court proceedings, and the child's ability to cooperate with counsel. The ability to cooperate with counsel involves an assessment of a child's ability to convey and comprehend information about the charge, about the nature of the proceedings, and about the choices to be made during the course of the proceedings. Every state has a statute governing the procedures to be followed when competence is raised in criminal proceedings, see, e.g., Fla. R. Crim. P. 3.210 to 212; Fla. Code § 15-16-20 to -23; W. Va. Code § 27-6A-1 (1980); and Wis. Stat. Ann. § 971.13(1) (West 1985). Some states have statutes which are specifically applicable to proceedings in juvenile court, see, e.g., Ariz Rev. Stat. §§ 8-291 to 291.11; La. Child Code Art. 832 to 838; VA ST § 16.1-356 to 16.1-361. Under most statutory schemes, the first question to be answered is whether the defendant understands the nature and purpose of the proceedings. The second inquiry is whether the defendant is able to cooperate with counsel. (The Illinois fitness statute provides: "A defendant is presumed to be fit to stand trial or to plead, and be sentenced. A defendant is unfit if, because of his mental or physical condition, he is unable to understand the nature and purpose of the proceedings against him or to assist in his defense." 725 ILCS 5/ 104-10.) State statutes and/or case law set forth the procedure to be followed for raising the issue of competence in court and the burden of proof to be applied at a hearing on the issue of competence to stand trial. Statutory provisions and case law also govern the procedure to be followed for the appointment of experts to examine the defendant (see, *Ake v. Oklahoma*, 470 U.S. 68, 105 S.Ct. 1087 [1985] and cases following *Ake* that discuss an indigent criminal defendant's right to appointment of expert witnesses), and the procedures to be followed if the defendant is found to be not competent to stand trial. (The Illinois statute governing the procedure for inquiring into fitness provides that the issue may be raised by the defense, by the prosecution, or by the judge. When a bona fide doubt exists as to competence, the defendant must be found fit by a preponderance of the evidence and the burden is on the state to go forward with the evidence. The defendant has a right to a jury trial to determine competence to stand trial. See, 725 ILCS 5/104-11, 5/104-12.)

When the issue of the possible incompetence of a child to stand trial is raised, the judge must conduct an inquiry to determine whether a "bona fide doubt" exists as to the child's competence to stand trial (see, e.g., 725 ILCS 5/104-11: "When a bona fide doubt of the defendant's unfitness is raised, the court shall order a determination of the issue before proceeding further.") The inquiry as to whether a "bona fide doubt" exists is ordinarily triggered by a statement or motion by defense counsel, but can be initiated by a judge or a prosecutor who observes that the child is particularly young or is behaving in a way that suggests lack of ability to understand the proceedings or to cooperate with counsel. At this stage, experts may be retained to determine whether a bona fide doubt as to competence exists. If the court-ordered inquiry reveals no bona fide doubt, a hearing to determine competence is not required. If there is a bona fide doubt as to fitness, most jurisdictions require that a hearing be held to resolve the issue of whether the child is competent to stand trial, (see, e.g., *People v. Smith*, 353 Ill.App.3d 236 [2nd Dist. 2004]).

Courts differ on the question of whether the ordering of a fitness examination raises a "bona fide doubt" as to competence. Most courts hold that the mere ordering of a fitness examination does not raise a bona fide doubt.

If the judge decides, after reviewing the experts' assessments, that a bona fide doubt continues to exist, the judge must hold a hearing to determine whether the child is competent. The burden of going forward with the evidence, and the burden of proving the child incompetent to stand trial by a preponderance of the evidence is usually on the defense. (See *Medina v. California*, 505 U.S. 437, 452. But in some states the burden to prove competency is placed on the prosecution by statute. See, e.g., 725 ILCS 5/104-11(c): "When a bona fide doubt of the defendant's fitness has been raised, the burden of proving that the defendant is fit by a preponderance of the evidence and the burden of going forward with the evidence are on the State.")

In some jurisdictions, the content of expert reports is regulated by statute. Some statutes require that the experts state a diagnosis of the child, describe how that diagnosis was reached, and make a judgment about the severity of the disability, (see, e.g., 725 ILCS 5/104-15). In addition, experts are required to give an opinion as to how long the state of incompetence to stand trial is expected to last and what, if any, treatment will enable the child to become competent to stand trial, (see, e.g., 725 ILCS 5/104-15). State statutes also provide that statements regarding the alleged criminal act to examining experts by a child during the course of a fitness examination may not be revealed.

... no statement made by the defendant [in the course of an examination for competence to stand trial] which relates to the crime charged or to other criminal acts shall be disclosed by persons conducting the examination or the treatment, except to members of the examining or treating team without the informed written consent of the defendant, who is competent at the time of giving such consent. (725 ILCS 5/104-14 (b))

Ordinarily, the first inquiry into competence will be conducted by a court-appointed expert or team consisting of a psychiatrist and a psychologist. Although defense counsel may also retain its own expert(s) to conduct a parallel investigation, the procedure for obtaining experts varies from jurisdiction to jurisdiction and from case to case. Some juvenile courts have assessment or clinical services divisions that are available to all children. In those jurisdictions, the judge will refer the question of competence to professionals working in that department. (An example of such an office is the Juvenile Court Clinic of the Juvenile Court of Cook County. See website at http://www.cookcountycourt.org/about/non-judicial.html.) In other jurisdictions, the juvenile court judge will appoint an expert or a team of experts at public expense. Defense counsel may seek an "independent" assessment when the quality or independence of the court-appointed team is in doubt, or when the defense seeks to consult with its own expert or team of experts. Payment for an additional team of experts may often be an issue, given the fact that very few children tried in juvenile court have funds to retain an expert. In such cases, defense counsel must apply to the court for funding. This is most often done when defense counsel fear that a court-appointed expert will not be impartial or when defense counsel questions the competence of court-connected experts to conduct an independent, state-of-the-art examination. Should there be a disagreement between court-appointed and defense-retained experts regarding the child's fitness, a hearing must be held during which the conflicting evidence regarding the child's fitness will be presented.

At this hearing, the expert or experts who have examined the child may be called to testify. They are permitted to testify in accordance with local rules of evidence governing the testimony of expert witnesses. Most states have adopted Federal Rule of Evidence 702, which provides:

> If scientific, technical, or other specialized knowledge will assist the trier of fact to understand the evidence or to determine a fact in issue, a witness qualified as an expert by knowledge, skill, experience, training, or education, may testify thereto in the form of an opinion or otherwise, if (1) the testimony is based upon sufficient facts or data, (2) the testimony is the product of reliable principles and methods, and (3) the witness has applied the principles and methods reliably to the facts of the case. (Fed. Rules of Evidence Rule 702 (3d ed.), Rule 702)

After hearing all of the evidence, the judge issues a ruling, which, in most jurisdictions, must be supported by findings of fact and conclusions of law. A decision finding a child fit to stand trial is not appealable by the defense until after a finding of delinquency and disposition. A decision finding a defendant unfit to stand trial is not appealable by the state. (See, *Alexander v. State*, 107 P. 2d 811 [Okla. 1940]. But some states do allow a defendant to appeal a decision that he is incompetent to stand trial. See, *State v. Guatney*, 299 N.W. 2d 538, 543 [Neb. 1980]; *People v. Fields*, 399 P. 2d 369 (Cal. 1965); *Jolley v. State*, 384 A2d 91 [Md. 1978]; *U.S. v. Gold*, 790 F2d 235 [2nd Cir. 1986]; and *U.S. v. Friedman*, 366 F.3d 975 [9th Cir. 2004].)

If a child is found unfit to stand trial, the court must determine whether the child can be made competent to stand trial, through education about the nature of the charges, about the the trial process, and about the role of the lawyer. Restoration to competence may also include treatment of the disabilities, if any, that caused the incompetence (see, e.g., 725 ILCS 5/104-16[d]). If it appears that the child may be made competent to stand trial through instruction or medication, the judge may order the education and/or treatment necessary, including commitment to a mental health facility and/or to an outpatient facility (Elizabeth S. Scott and Thomas Grisso, *Developmental Incompetence, Due Process, and Juvenile Justice*

Policy, 83 N.C.L. Rev. 793, 829 n.125 [but the authors note that these practices, while helpful in adult cases, are not necessarily appropriate for juveniles]). If it appears, after a period of further evaluation and treatment, that the child cannot be made competent to stand trial, most states provide for a procedure that results in the termination of proceedings against the child (see e.g., La. Child Code Art. 837), or that provides for civil commitment for mental illness, if commitment criteria are met (see e.g., Ariz. Rev Stat 8-291.03 and Kan. Stat Ann 38-1638), or that allows the judge to continue to require efforts to make the child competent, provided there is a showing made by the state that the child would not be acquitted of the charge if the case were to be tried (see, e.g., 725 ILCS 5/104-25). A child may not be held indefinitely pending efforts to make the child competent. Some states require that if the child cannot be made fit within a year, the prosecution must be terminated (*In re Charles B.*, 978 P.2d 659 [Ariz. Ct. App. 1998] [six months with the possibility of a two month extension]; *Department of Children and Families v. Clem*, 903 So.2d 1011 [Fla.App. 2005] [six months]; and Tex. Fam. Code Ann. §55.33 [a][1][A] [Vernon 2002] [90 days].).

The standards to be applied in deciding if a child is competent to stand trial

As noted above, once a bona fide doubt of competence is raised, the burden is usually on the defendant to prove by a preponderance of the evidence that the child is incompetent to stand trial. (See, *Cooper v. Oklahoma*, 517 U.S. 348, 368-69 [1996] [striking down an Oklahoma statute, that required a defendant to prove in competence by clear and convincing evidence. The Court held that a defendant's burden in such case should be the "preponderance of the evidence" standard].) This standard gives judges considerable discretion in deciding whether a child is fit to stand trial. Appellate courts seldom reverse trial courts' findings that a child is competent to stand trial. Most cases in which such findings are reversed involve children who are very young and/or children who test particularly low on IQ tests. (See, *In re Williams*, 116 Ohio App. 3d 237 [2d Dist 1997]. See also, *In re E.V.*, 190 I.. App. 3d 1079 [1st Dist. 1989] [holding that the trial court erred in determining that a juvenile was competent to stand trial without the benefit of any medical testimony or clinical evaluation when there was substantial evidence that the child had suffered brain damage].) There is little appellate case law on this issue, resulting primarily from the fact that most delinquency cases are resolved quickly and few children have the resources to pursue an appeal. Moreover, if a child has been placed on probation and returns home, the incentive to appeal is reduced. Even if sentenced to time in a correctional center, the juvenile will most likely have completed serving his sentence long before an appeal process could be complete.

Ability to understand the nature of the charge and the potential consequences

In order to enter a plea to a charge, and in order to assist in defense of a charge, a child must understand as well as appreciate the nature of the charge. As noted earlier, this aspect of the requirement of fitness is rooted in the notion that a defendant's absolute right to be present during his trial cannot be effectively implemented if, in effect, he is absent by reason of mental incapacity. In addition, a child must be able to understand both the possible consequences of pleading guilty or not guilty and be able to realistically weigh the likely outcomes.

Ability to understand the nature and process of the proceeding

This inquiry focuses on the child's ability to understand the process of the adjudication, including the significance of the various stages of the proceeding and the ability to understand what goes on in the courtroom. The inquiry centers around the question of whether the child understands, or can be educated to understand, the process that will lead to a finding of guilt or innocence and a possible sentence.

There are two parts to this inquiry. First, does the child understand the nature of the proceedings? This question is generally interpreted to focus on the question of whether the child understands that the purpose of the proceeding is to determine whether he committed the offense and, if so, what an appropriate sentence might be (Grisso, 2000).

The second area of inquiry under this category is whether the child understands the mechanics of the proceedings (Grisso, 2000). For example, does the child understand that there could be/will be appearances before the judge for status, for pre-trial hearings, and eventually for a trial? Does the child understand that a trial consists of the calling of witnesses and the introduction of evidence? Does the child understand the concepts of burden of proof, and proof beyond a reasonable doubt? Does the child understand the various roles of the actors during trial? Does he know what the role of the judge will be? Does he understand the role of the prosecutor? Does he understand that evidence will be presented through the testimony of witnesses and the submission of documentary and physical evidence? Does he understand that witnesses will be examined and cross-examined?

Ability to cooperate with counsel

This inquiry focuses on the child's ability to communicate with his lawyer and to assess the advice given to him by his lawyer. This inquiry, of course, is affected by the "role" that defense counsel adopts when defending a delinquency case. Some lawyers and scholars argue that the role of a lawyer in a delinquency case should be no different than that in a criminal case involving an adult (Guggenheim, 1998, 2003, 1996; Shepherd, 1996). The lawyer representing the child should give almost complete autonomy to the child to make decisions regarding the conduct of the case (Guggenheim, 1998, 2003, 1996; Shepherd, 1996). The lawyer for the child should act in accordance with the client's instructions regarding the objectives of the representation even if the lawyer believes that the child's best interests will not be served by the client's choices (Shepherd & England, 1996; Matthews, 1996; Peters, 1996; Edwards & Sagatun, 1995; Davis, 1994). Others argue that the lawyer who represents a child in a delinquency proceeding should play the roles of attorney and guardian, sometimes stepping in to protect the perceived best interests of the child even when the child's position is in conflict with the lawyer's (Luban, 1981). Under both models of representation, a child must have the ability to make a relationship with his lawyer that will foster the child's understanding of the nature of the case, the nature of the proceedings, and appreciation of the role of defense counsel.

Perhaps the most crucial aspect of a child's competence as it relates to the client–lawyer relationship is the child's ability to provide information about either his lack of involvement or his involvement in the case. Some children are either so young or so impaired that they are not able give coherent narratives. Some children may be so intimidated by the lawyer and by the judicial process that they are unable to communicate (Grisso, 2000). Other children may suffer from cognitive shortcomings and emotional problems that make it impossible for the child to construct a coherent narrative of what occurred.

In addition to these factors, the child must also be able to reason about available options without any significant distortion. He must also be able to monitor the events of the trial and realistically challenge the witnesses that the prosecution calls. Courtroom behavior is also a consideration regarding the child's ability to control his behavior in the courtroom as well as to testify if necessary.

The competence inquiry: the roles of defense lawyer, prosecutor, and judge
The role of the defense lawyer

As noted above, a defendant has an absolute constitutional right not to be tried while incompetent. (See, *Pate v. Robinson*, 383 U.S. 375 [1966]; see also, *Brown v. Sternes*, 304 F.3d 677 [2002] [7th Cir].) An incompetent defendant cannot "waive" or give up his right to be tried while incompetent because he is incapable of making reasoned decisions regarding the court proceedings, including waiver of rights. This situation presents a number of difficult legal and ethical challenges for lawyers and for judges. If a child's lawyer suspects or believes that his client is incompetent to stand trial, how should decision-making authority be allocated between client and lawyer regarding whether the issue should be raised? This is a crucial issue because raising the issue of incompetence can have severe negative effects upon the client, including long-term institutionalization during the "restoration" process, and labeling of the client as mentally deficient or mentally ill.

If an allegedly incompetent client objects to the issue being raised, must the lawyer follow the client's direction and decline to bring the issue to the attention of the court? The cases and the American Bar Association Criminal Defense Standards create an obligation on the part of defense counsel to both abide by the client's decisions regarding the objectives of the representation and to seek the appointment of a guardian if, because of mental or physical disability, the client is unable to maintain the lawyer–client relationship (Lafitte, 2004; Drews & Halprin, 2002; Uphoff, 1988). No specific guidance is given for exercising this discretion. The difficulty inherent in this situation is compounded by the fact that failure to raise the issue of incompetence can be a ground for a post-conviction claim of ineffective assistance of counsel.

The question of whether a lawyer should raise the issue of a child client's incompetence presents an additional set of problems. The first is that it is even more unlikely that a child, as compared to an adult, will understand the consequences of raising, or failing to raise, the issue of incompetence. The role of the child's family in this decision-making is an additional complicating factor. What role should a child's parents or guardians play in the decision whether to raise the issue of incompetence? Must the lawyer consult with the child's parents when making this decision? What should the lawyer do if she is convinced that the child is incompetent to stand trial, but the child and the child's parents do not want this issue to be raised?

There are no easy answers to the questions raised above. Even the American Bar Association Juvenile Justice Standards provide little guidance. These Standards provide that the lawyer should maintain an ordinary lawyer–client relationship with the child to the greatest extent possible, allowing the client as much of a role in decision-making as is appropriate under the circumstances.

The role of the prosecutor

Prosecutors in juvenile courts play a somewhat different role than in criminal prosecutions. Their role is influenced by the purpose of juvenile court acts and the nature and purpose of juvenile court proceedings. Although many juvenile court acts have been revised in recent years to implement a more punitive approach to juvenile justice, the objective of most juvenile court prosecutions remains to balance the best interests of the child with the need to protect society. Many juvenile court acts also endorse the notion of balanced and restorative justice that emphasizes the need for children to take responsibility for their actions and then to be reintegrated into family, school, and society. Prosecutors are part of this process and play a key role in supporting efforts, when possible, to minimize the effects of being involved in a juvenile court proceeding on a child's future.

Thus, when confronted with the prospect that a child may not be competent to stand trial, prosecutors in juvenile courts will carefully consider a number of issues when deciding whether to contest the finding. First, prosecutors will carefully examine the findings of the experts to determine whether the finding is well founded. The interests of the victim, the community, and of society often dictate that a case proceed to adjudication. Prosecutors may be unwilling to accede to a claim of unfitness because such a finding can effectively preclude prosecution. Even if a child can be made competent through education and increasing maturity, the delay involved makes cases difficult to prosecute. Thus a finding of incompetence, in the view of a prosecutor, may frustrate the ability to prosecute a young person who should be held accountable for his actions.

If the evidence of incompetence is weak or closely balanced, the prosecutor may conclude that the best way of reaching a credible decision regarding fitness is to contest the claim at a full-blown hearing, relying on the evaluations of prosecution witnesses or cross-examination of the experts called by the defense to expose flaws in the opinions reached by those experts. This process will allow the judge to make the ultimate, and an informed, decision.

The role of the judge

The Supreme Court of the United States has held that judges must initiate the inquiry into possible incompetence of a defendant when there are "alerting circumstances" even when defense counsel and the defendant fail to raise the issue. (See *Pate v. Robinson*, 383 U.S. 375 [1966]; *Drope v. Missouri*, 420 U.S. 162 [1975]; and *Brown v. Sternes*, 304 F.3d 677 [2002].) Making the fitness inquiry before or during trial is essential to the process because of the legal requirement that a child be competent to stand trial and because of the difficulties involved in making post hoc evaluations of fitness when the issue of fitness only comes to light after the child has been adjudicated delinquent. (See *Pate*, 383 U.S. 375 [1966]; *U.S. v. Williams*, 113 F.3d 1155 [10th Cir. 1997]; *People v. Solorzano*, 126 Cal. App. 4th 1063 [2005].) A judge's failure to initiate an inquiry into competence can result in a reversal of a conviction where the record shows that the inquiry should have been made. (See *Pate*, 383 U.S. 375 [1966]; *Brown*, 304 F.3d 677 [2002]; In re *E.V.*, 190 Ill. App. 3d 1079 [1st Dist. 1989].) "Alerting circumstances" include a wide variety of behaviors of the defendant and of information that comes to the attention of the judge. (*Chenault v. Stynchcombe*, 546 F.2d 1191, 1192-93 [1977]; *Pate v. Robinson*, 383 U.S. 375 [1966].) These include the behavior of the client in the courtroom, observable conflicts between the child and his lawyer, information including report of history of mental illness, and information from family members about the past behavior and mental health history of the defendant. (*Green v. State*, 14 S.W. 489 (Tenn. 1890); *Tillery v. Eyman*, 492 F.2d 1056 (9th Cir. 1974); *Odle v. Woodford*, 238 F.3d 1084, 1089 (9th Cir. 2001); *Johnson v. Norton*, 249 F.3d 20 (1st Cir. 2001); *U.S. v. Williams*, 113 F.3d 1155 (10th Cir. 1997).)

Judges are understandably and rightly concerned about injecting themselves into the proceedings when it appears that there may be a fitness issue that counsel has not raised. A judge must presume that a child's lawyer is representing her client effectively. Intruding upon the lawyer–client relationship is only appropriate under compelling circumstances. However, case law gives the judge little choice about whether to require a hearing when alerting circumstances are presented.

Factors that courts take into account when assessing competence to stand trial

The factors that judges take into account in assessing a child's competence to stand trial have been generated by the lawyers, medical professionals, and scholars who have grappled with the question of what capacities children must possess in order to comprehend the charges, to understand the proceedings, and to cooperate with counsel. Most lawyers, judges, and medical professionals agree that the following characteristics of a child should be considered: age, intelligence, mental illness or mental disability, and physical disability. These factors are usually considered together to form a comprehensive assessment of a child's competence.

Age

It is to be expected that the younger the child, the more likely it is that lawyers and judges will question the child's ability to understand the charges, the nature of the proceedings, and the ability of the child to cooperate with counsel. It is also to be expected that lawyers and judges will have more confidence in older children's competence. Thus, age serves as a "trigger" for further inquiry, but is not, by itself, a determinative factor. However, the less mature a child, the more likely it is that the child may not be competent (Grisso, 2005a).

Intelligence

There is no bright line test that, for example, ties competence to stand trial to the results of IQ testing. However, courts do consider the results of intelligence testing to be a high salient factor in assessing competence. The results of IQ testing are often taken into consideration with other factors such as a child's basic under-standing of the process, the child's experience with the process, and reports of professionals who have experience in dealing with the child. Often, these reports are given more weight than the results of tests, particularly because of the cultural biases written into such tests. (The issue of cultural bias in standardized testing procedures is beyond the scope of this chapter. Standardized tests are both confusing and helpful to courts. Psychologists excel in helping the courts under-stand the strengths and limitations of these instruments. Psychiatrists familiar with the strengths and weaknesses of instruments through long-term collaboration with psychologists and the application of psychological test data may also be able to address this issue. It is important to distinguish that just because a test measures what it is designed to measure in a scientifically valid way, does not mean that a particular test finding provides a cause and effect explanation for any particular behavior by a defendant that is logically connected to the skill measured.)

As children age, general intelligence stabilizes and IQ test results show slight decreases in intelligence as children age. However, their ability for abstract reasoning and their maturity relative to their intelligence progresses with age.

Grisso described competency to stand trial as being contextual in nature. Children's cases vary with respect to how much cognitive ability is required so that a child will be deemed competent (Grisso, 2005b).

Mental illness, disability

"Mental illness" and "disability" are used in their legal context. Mental health professionals by convention label mental difficulties as disorders or traits, a convention of the classificatory system in force at the time. The current standard is the *Diagnostic and Statistical Manual*, 4th edition, (APA, 2000). A child who suffers from a mental illness or disability may have symptoms, cognitive or emotional, that impair the child's skills or abilities to understand the nature of the proceedings and/or to cooperate with counsel. The most common such mental illnesses or disabilities that can result in incompetence to stand trial are psychoses and depression. Children who engage in antisocial behavior may be unable to focus on the nature and purpose of the proceedings and may have substantial problems in communicating with their lawyers.

Mental illness, per se does not make someone inherently incompetent. This is true of both adults as well as children. Significant mental disabilities that can affect competency to stand trial include: schizophrenia, schizoaffective disorder, bipolar disorder, and depression. An evaluator may identify a mental disability. If a mental disability is identified, the evaluator then proceeds to determine how that disability could affect competence. One cannot simply state a diagnosis and use this for the purpose of rendering an opinion regarding competency. Neither mental illness, mental retardation, nor amnesia automatically constitutes incompetence. These may be circumstances under which competency should be assessed. It is critically important to assess prior treatment records for children with diagnoses of mental illness, and prior educational records for those children with potential learning disabilities. Prior pertinent psychological testing should also be reviewed.

Immaturity

Developmentally immature children whose IQ test performance scores are in the normal range may be incompetent to stand trial. While some courts may consider immaturity as a basis for finding a child incompetent to stand trial, other jurisdictions do not recognize it. Developmental immaturity refers to the relatively delayed appearance of adult-like reasoning capacities and occurs most often in those in between ages of 14–16, most often in those children who enter puberty later than their peers. Developmental immaturity is not a bright line concept. Instead, clinicians use the concept of developmental immaturity to describe those children and adolescents who for their age, physical development, cognitive capacities, and life experiences demonstrate functional skills and interests more typical of a younger individual. Measures of reasoning found on psychological testing should be correlated with the clinical interview and collateral data about the life experience of the adolescent. In some cases adolescents who demonstrate scores on tests of reasoning (problem-solving and cognitive flexibility), may have yet failed to apply these skills consistently and in their day-to-day lives. Adolescents may fail to consider long-term consequences of their actions, a trait that can put them at a distinct disadvantage during the legal process (Bonnie & Grisso, 2000).

Physical disabilities and impairments

The ability to hear, to speak, to see, and to process sensory input and thought are essential elements of the ability to understand and to communicate. Those individuals with acquired or congenital sensory loss, as well as those suffering from various kinds of congenital or acquired organic brain damage, demonstrate impairments that may render them incompetent to participate in the legal process. Although these disabilities can be overcome through the employment of various means of communication appropriate to the disabled client in social or educational settings, it is not at all clear that they can be overcome in the courtroom. Courtroom proceedings place a premium on an individual's ability to react in a reasonable period of time to the oral and visual testimony, the statements of judges and attorneys, and the ability to read and comprehend the information contained in documents. The skills and abilities described become the elements of understanding and participation in the legal process.

Conducting a fitness evaluation

It is important to remember that competency to stand trial refers to the child's *present* mental functioning, not what the child's mental capacity was at the time of the offense. The evaluation process consists of clinical interviewing, and mental status examination, with or without a screening neurological, performed by the psychiatrist. The psychologist performs a clinical interview and standardized testing. Psychologists apply their knowledge of the applicability of standardized testing instruments that include instruments that examine cognitive and emotional functioning. In addition, psychologists may administer specialized forensic tests, such as the MacArthur instruments for Miranda rights and adjudicative competency assessment where the tests are designed to look at mental skills related to particular legal functional requirements.

The interview, whether done by a psychiatrist and/or psychologist, should focus on both the mental health data typically relied upon by mental health professionals for making diagnoses, as well as the competency issues in question. Typical areas include obtaining the following relevant background information concerning the child and their family.

1. What the child knows about his developmental history such as important milestones, setbacks, traumas.
2. What the child knows about his family history in terms of family relationships, medical and social problems, criminal history, and mental health history.
3. What the child knows of his medical, social, and mental health history.
4. What the child knows of his important family or non-family relationships.
5. Obtaining from the child a description of his interests and his means of deriving enjoyment from those interests.
6. What the child knows about his adaptive strengths and weaknesses.
7. The child's work history, or in lieu of work history any commitment and/or experience the alleged offender has with having a duty to perform, a task, such as household chores, or child care.
8. What the child knows or is willing to tell about his history of chemical use, abuse, or dependency. (If the interviewer learned that the child habitually used drugs or alcohol in association with activities that led to police scrutiny, then a history of substance use and abuse might have some bearing on the alleged offender's state at the time of interrogation. A website, www.ProjectCork.org, provides resources for evaluating substance abuse in adolescents.)
9. The information the child is willing or able to provide concerning his past contact with the police or the juvenile justice system.
10. The identification of potential sources of collateral data, such as the names of schools, treating professionals, or institutions where the child received treatment. If possible, individuals who have knowledge about the alleged offender's skills, abilities, and deficits should be interviewed.
11. If the child was interrogated by the police, obtain the child's account of what transpired before, during, and after the interrogation. This portion of the evaluation should attempt to obtain specifics of the child's report of his recollections of the events leading to his alleged comprehension of Miranda rights at the time he reportedly waived those rights. In this portion of the evaluation, attention to post-waiver contacts and experiences that could influence the recollection process, e.g., experiences whether from reading, fellow detainees, attorneys, or other sources should be considered (Oberlander *et al.*, 2003).

12. Obtain, through the interview process, an evaluation of the child's knowledge of the ajudicative process. In addition, the evaluator(s) should evaluate the juvenile's capacity for narrative recall of their actions and behaviors during the time of the alleged offense. The evaluator(s) should evaluate the juvenile's ability to communicate what he knows to his attorney. As this may be potentially incriminating material, the evaluator needs to pose questions carefully and should remind the juvenile that he needs to answer questions carefully. (Because there is no evaluator equivalent of attorney–client privilege, the juvenile may reveal incriminating information about the alleged offense. While some states make such data by statute non-discoverable, others do not.) For example, when interviewing the child regarding the offense, the evaluator should frame the questions in terms of the child's understanding of the charges as opposed to what the child has actually done.

13. If possible, the evaluator should attempt to evaluate the child's ability to understand the testimony of both peers and adults. Evaluation of these skills requires the evaluator to have some measure of the juvenile's ability to listen to spoken speech, comprehend, paraphrase, and comment on what they have heard.

14. An assessment of the child's ability to understand choices inherent in making a plea or agreeing to a plea bargain.

15. If the evaluator is a physician, and notes during the evaluation data that suggest difficulty with nervous system functioning, then the physician evaluator may perform a screening neurological within the limits of their training and experience. Evaluation information obtained may suggest that further neurological evaluation is required.

16. If possible, family members should be interviewed about their relationship with the child, and for verification of the child's account of his life history and present functioning.

In many cases, a psychiatrist will conduct the first competency assessment. Depending on the case, the psychiatrist may ask a clinical psychologist to investigate and/or confirm concerns identified by the psychiatrist. The psychologist typically uses standardized instruments and measures to examine cognitive skills, attention, judgment, and problem-solving. Typically child psychologists with neuropsychological training and forensic experience have the widest range of instruments and interpretive experience. As part of his evaluation protocol, the psychologist does a clinical interview providing another content oriented interaction with the child.

Psychiatric assessment, beyond the waiver of confidentiality issue, involves getting a sense from the alleged offender of their knowledge of their development. Attention is focused on the course of development of motor, language, other cognitive skills, impulse control, judgment, problem-solving, and relevant life experiences. What the alleged offender lacks in information should ideally be supplemented from collateral interview of the child's parent or guardian. The child's and the parents' narration and understanding of the alleged offender's education, medical, social, and family (social, medical, and mental health) history, and mental health history is part of the assessment. Collateral descriptions may deviate from what was expected based on the conversation with the juvenile. Consequently, examples from the interviewed collateral sources typically clarify the evaluator's understanding.

The psychiatric assessment also includes a "mental state examination." The mental state examination includes, but may not be limited to, standard clinical cognitive assessment tools associated with the term "mental state examination." "Mental state examination" is a term of art that reflects a clinical method used to assess cognitive and emotional function.

Although psychiatrists typically do not conduct physical examinations when conducting a competence evaluation, it is important to inquire or even ask to look for tattoos, marks, or scars that could indicate abuse or a history of fighting or attempts at self-injury. Inquiring about sexual experience and/or molestation is also useful in understanding a juvenile's experience and maturity.

Competence of children to knowingly waive Miranda rights and to make voluntary and accurate statements during the interrogation process

As noted above, the Supreme Court of the United States has long been concerned about the reliability of confessions obtained from children. In *Gallegos v. Colorado*, 370 U.S. 49 (1962) and in *Haley v. Ohio*, 332 U.S. 596 (1948), the Court announced a doctrine that requires that "special care" be taken when interrogating children. The concern expressed by the Supreme Court reflects our society's condemnation of the "third degree," and our belief that coerced confessions are highly likely to be unreliable. Both of these concerns resonate strongly when children are the subject of police interrogation.

In an effort to provide a means of ensuring the voluntariness of confessions, the Supreme Court of the United States in *Miranda v. Arizona*, 384 U.S. 436 (1966) required that in order for a defendant's statement to be admissible in court, the defendant must be advised of his right to remain silent, of the fact that any statement made may be used against him, and of his right to counsel. ("[U]nless other fully effective means are devised to inform accused persons of their right of silence and to assure a continuous opportunity to exercise it, the following measures are required. Prior to any questioning, the person must be warned that he has a right to remain silent, that any statement he does make may be used as evidence against him, and that he has a right to the presence of an attorney, either retained or appointed. The defendant may waive effectuation of these rights, provided the waiver is made voluntarily, knowingly and intelligently.") Failure to give these warnings prior to the taking of a statement, the Court ruled, could result in exclusion of the statement from evidence. Even if the Miranda warnings are given, Supreme Court jurisprudence requires that the statement be made voluntarily. The giving of Miranda warnings is only one part of the totality of the circumstances that courts must take into account in determining whether the statement was the product of undue coercion.

The Supreme Court's decision in Miranda has generated an extensive jurisprudence, which is well beyond the scope of this chapter. (There are several leading criminal procedure texts containing detailed descriptions of this jurisprudence. See, e.g., Kamisar *et al.*, 2005.) We focus here on a basic outline of the law with respect to the admissibility of confessions made by children to police during the custodial interrogation process, and the framework utilized by psychologists and psychiatrists to evaluate the ability of children to understand and to waive Miranda rights, and to make knowing and accurate statements during a custodial interrogation.

Courts utilize a totality of the circumstances test when ruling on the admissibility of a statement made by a child during a custodial interrogation. The totality of the circumstances includes considering the age, background, and intellectual ability of the child, the presence of a parent or friendly adult to provide the child with advice, the conduct of the police in conducting the interrogation, including the manner in which Miranda rights are read to the child, the timing of the interrogation (at night, during the day), the length of the interrogation, the conditions under which the child was held for interrogation, whether the child was fed while in custody, as well as other factors relevant to the particular interrogation under review.

Courts pay special attention to all of the above factors when considering the admissibility of a very young child, especially those between the ages of 7–13. (See, e.g., *A.M. v. Butler*, 360 F.3d 787 [2004] [7th Cir.].) It is in these cases that lawyers and judges are most likely to consult with experts to determine whether the child actually understood the Miranda warnings and whether the child made the statement knowingly and voluntarily. (See e.g., *In re JW*, 346 Ill. App. 3d [2004]; *In re Wesley B.*, 764 A.2d 888 [NH 2000]; and *TSD v. State*, 743 So 2d 536 [Fla App. 1999].) Thus expert witnesses are called to assess the questions of whether the child was capable of understanding the concept of the right to remain silent, whether the child understood the concept of self-incrimination, and whether the child understood the implications of his right not to proceed with questioning without a lawyer being present.

Given the vulnerability of children and the special attention that is needed to ensure that a child's statement is voluntary, several states have been experimenting with other ways of ensuring that a statement by a child is not a product of coercion. One such method is the use of "per se" rules to ensure voluntariness. These rules are either statutory or court created, and generally require the presence of an "interested adult" for a child's rights' waiver to be held valid. (See e.g., *People v. Saiz*, 620 P.2d 15 [Colo.

1980]; *Commonwealth v. Smith*, 372 A.2d 797 [1977].) This person can be a parent or an attorney. This approach provides that any statement that was obtained without the presence of this "interested adult" will be held inadmissible. There are several variants of this approach, such as requiring both the child and the adult to consent to the waiver of Miranda rights (see, *Whipple v. State*, 523 N.E.2d 1363 [Ind. 1988]); others require that the "interested adult" be present for the entire interrogation (*In re Robert M.*, 576 A.2d 549 [Conn. App. 1990]; *In re E.T.C.*, 449 A.2d 937, 940 [Vt. 1982]; *Commonwealth v. A Juvenile*, 449 N.E.2d 654, 657 [Mass. 1983]; *State v. Presha*, 748 A.2d 1108 [N.J. 2000]). The most protective of these statutes requires that under a certain age the child must have an attorney present during the custodial interrogation (see, 705 ILCS 405/5-170 [West 2005]).

Medical and social science: research on children's ability to understand and waive Miranda rights

Over the past three decades, Dr. Thomas Grisso has undertaken several studies to assess juvenile's abilities to waive their Miranda rights. Dr. Grisso found that 90 percent of juveniles waived their Miranda rights (Grisso & Pomicter, 1977). In a 1981 study, he found that for juveniles who were part of the 1977 study under the age of 15, virtually all of them waived their right to remain silent (Grisso, 1981). In that same study, juveniles under the age of 14 scored low on comprehension of Miranda rights. Fifteen- and sixteen-year-olds varied widely in their ability to comprehend their rights. Those with an IQ score under 80 did not understand their rights any better than the younger children; those with average or above IQs fared closer to adults (Grisso, 1981).

Later studies have demonstrated that about one third of juveniles studied did not understand the nature of the attorney–client relationship and did not understand why an attorney would want their client to tell them the truth. A significant number of juveniles also misinterpreted the right to silence, perceiving that the judge could waive that right. They also felt that the warning "anything you say can and will be used against you in court" referred to using profane language or criticizing the judge (Grisso, 1981, 2006).

Neuroimaging studies have now been able to show that there is a linear decrease in cortical gray matter and an increase in white matter across ages through to the early 20s. Adolescents are a group of risk takers. Youth can understand right from wrong, but often cannot foresee the long-term ramifications of their behavior. This may have a direct impact on an adolescent's understanding of Miranda, in particular during stressful situations such as police interrogations.

Neuroimaging research has primarily focused on the development of the adolescent's frontal lobe and neuroconnections (Giedd *et al.*, 1999). The frontal lobe controls such issues as concentration, orientation, language, attention, judgment, affect, and motor functioning. For the most part, it controls the executive functions of our brain and helps in controlling one's behavior in a way that offers a protective mechanism. The limbic system on a more primitive level of function is related to the flight or fight response. The limbic system's firing is related to a behavior; as we grow appropriate pruning occurs where the myelination and neurological tracts are placed. The frontal lobe then has better control over the midbrain. The younger a teenager is, the more impulsive he will be, and the more apt he will be to waive his Miranda rights.

Protocol for conducting an examination regarding competence to waive Miranda rights

An evaluation of rights' waiver is a complex process that asks whether the child has an adequate conceptualization of risk, safety, self-protection, and empowerment. This is usually called for in cases where the child is at an intermediate age, such as 12–15, because there are more variable outcomes than with very young or older juveniles. When an evaluation is ordered, the psychiatrist should first review the warnings and assess the alleged offender's current understanding of those warnings. Retrospective memory is often colored by motives of the present. Furthermore, memory is not the same as videotape, DVD, or recorded conversations. Recollections of, or failure to recollect, conversations, information, or events are not uncommon. Furthermore, individuals can subjectively believe they remember something as true that did not occur or happen.

The literature on childhood recollections of sexual abuse suggests that the concept of recovered, influenced, suggested, and false information, incorporated into memory, is not uncommon. (While this topic of memory is beyond the scope of this chapter, there are many sources in the literature regarding age related aspects of memory.) Therefore it is important to compare what the child says about past statements, contacts with authorities, and other measures of understanding, knowing, and remembering information. For example, it is not unusual for some children who suffer from attention-deficit/hyperactivity disorder (ADHD) to remember in the moment and fail to remember or respond to information given five minutes later as if they had never received the information in the first place. Relative deficiencies of working memory and retaining information in sequence, if a consistent finding, is most likely not faked but a reality of that person's working memory and problem-solving skills.

To the extent that the child can recall, it is useful to ask about what the child remembers concerning his level of energy or fatigue, whether he experienced coercion, and any implied or directly promised reward for his waiver offered by the officers. Police may tell a juvenile that if he just gives them certain information, then he can go home. A juvenile who is suggestible or naïve, or is used to giving authority figures what they want (state wards, children with long experience in child protective services or foster care) is especially vulnerable to complying with direction from adults rather than asserting his rights.

If the juvenile demonstrates the ability to provide recitation in his own words that he understood that he was a target of investigation, that as a target he was in danger, and that because of what he said he might not go home and/or could go to jail, then that child has demonstrated important elements of knowing, voluntary, and intelligent waiver. The challenge is then accuracy and validity of post hoc assessment of abilities. In other words, is what the child is telling the evaluator a valid representation of his mental state at the time of the interrogation or has it been colored by post-event experience? Teasing these issues out is often quite difficult. Nevertheless the methods and findings of the evaluator(s) adds to the data considered by the court under the "totality of the circumstances" standard.

Table 5.1 shows some possible examples of responses that may be given during an evaluation of competency to waive Miranda rights.

Table 5.2 provides some examples of indicators for the capacity for knowing, voluntary, and intelligent waiver.

Referrals to psychiatrists, psychologists, educational consultants, and social workers

Lawyers and judges confronted with the necessity of referring a child for a competency evaluation, benefit if they have the necessary training and information to make appropriate referrals. Should the referral be made to a psychiatrist with the expectation that the psychiatrist will associate with a psychologist? If educational deficits are identified, will a specialist in special education need to be retained? If a physical disability is the cause of the perceived incompetence, will a physician who specializes in the impact of disabilities be made part of the team? From this it is apparent that the choice of experts is crucial to an adequate investigation of the child's competence.

Lawyers and judges are not experts in the appropriate protocols to be employed in the evaluation. However, it is crucial that lawyers and judges have enough knowledge to assess the processes to be employed by the experts. This can most effectively be done by developing on-going relationships with experts that will provide the required overview of the most up-to-date professional standards. Lawyers and judges should also keep abreast of developments through reading and attending seminars on adolescent forensic psychiatry and psychology. (The following organizations publish and hold conferences on this subject: International Society for Adolescent Psychiatry and Psychology, American Academy of Child and Adolescent Psychiatry, American Society for Adolescent Psychiatry, American Academy of Psychiatry and the Law.)

Table 5.1. Competency to waive Miranda rights

Prong	Miranda warning	Response that does not meet the Miranda standard	Response that could meet the Miranda standard
1	You have the right to remain silent.	I shouldn't ask any questions.	I don't have to talk if I don't want to.
2	Anything you say can and will be used against you in a court of law.	What I say now can come up in court	If I talk to you now, you can use what I say and put me in jail. In jail I can't see my friends, go to my home, school, or be with my family, until you let me out.
3	You have a right to have an attorney present at the time of questioning.	I can have an attorney here.	I can have a lawyer, because this is tricky. I probably need someone to protect me from things I don't know about.
4	If you cannot afford an attorney then one will be provided for you.	You will pay for a lawyer.	Having a lawyer is important enough that you'll give me one for free. Having a lawyer is important for me.
5	At any time, if you do not want to talk to us, then you can stop. At any time, you can stop and ask to talk to an attorney.	I can stop and rest but I have to continue to answer questions if you want me to. When I rest I can have a conference with a lawyer.	I can stop when I want for any reason even if I started talking to you. Especially if I am worried, scared, or tired. I can stop and if I stop, I can still ask for a lawyer even though I did not ask for a lawyer before. Lawyers are for my protection.

Table 5.2. Knowing, voluntary, and intelligent waiver of Miranda rights

Category	Could meet the criteria	Could fail to meet the criteria
Knowing	If by course of dealing with authorities the alleged offender has experience with the choice to provide or not provide information, for example if they have been targets before and a confession led to a consequence.	First time alleged offender with no previous practical experience with the legal system.
Voluntary	Reviewed the choices with a trusted adult or attorney.	Is tired, frightened, and/or has a pattern of deferring to authority when confronted with alleged misdeeds.
Intelligent	Tested IQ > 70 where pragmatic expressive language and demeanor indicate understanding.	IQ < 70 where none of the factors in the previous column are met.

The lawyers and judges who make referrals to forensic experts must also have the knowledge necessary to refer cases to knowledgeable and experienced experts. Experts who examine children for competence to stand trial should be licensed psychiatrists and psychologists. For children and adolescents, less than age 18, they should be specialists in child and adolescent psychiatry or psychology. They should have experience working in legal settings, and ideally be familiar with the most recent studies concerning competence of juveniles to stand trial. Finally, the experts chosen should have the necessary education, training, and experience to be allowed to testify as an expert, known as qualifying as an expert. In this area of inquiry, it is highly relevant, although not determinative, that courts in the relevant jurisdiction or elsewhere have accepted the expert witness as a qualified expert.

Making sure that the evaluation team has all relevant records

It is both the responsibility of the lawyers and the competence assessment team, to collect all available records involving the child's educational, medical, mental health, legal, and social history. For an individual or a team to undertake a thorough evaluation without such records, especially if available, is a flawed evaluation that most likely will fail to provide the information required for competency determination (see, *Brown v. Sternes*, 304 F.3d 677 [2002]). In cases where there are no locatable pre-event records, minimal records, or incomplete records, the competency assessment team does the best job it can. In those cases, the competency evaluators construct the evaluation process to answer as many questions as possible. In these types of cases, the evaluators' formulation of their findings should highlight the relevance of the missing information. In particular the evaluators should discuss how missing data could affect their confidence in the findings and their relevance to the competency issue in question.

Frequently requested records

Medical records

These records inform the evaluator whether the alleged offender has ever suffered from traumatic brain injury, or other neurological conditions, for example epilepsy, Tourette's disorder, or pre-natal starvation. Could the individual have suffered a stroke due to, say, sickle cell disease or a toxic encephalopathy such as those due to lead intoxication, West Nile virus, or AIDS?

Mental health treatment records

Individual juveniles may have had emotional, behavioral, or conduct difficulties that led their caretakers to seek mental health evaluation and/or treatment. Mental health diagnostic evaluations, with or without treatment records, provide the evaluating and/or treating professionals insight about the the juvenile's impulse control, judgment, and suggestibility versus independence. These clinical records provide data for comparison with that acquired by the forensic evaluator. If the juvenile had received treatment that helped, then the continuation versus discontinuation of treatment may be a relevant factor in the juvenile's compentency at the time in question. Juveniles involved with child protective agencies often have protective services evaluations and follow-ups that can include data helpful to the compentency evaluator. Clearly, diagnoses that indicate developmental disabilities, such as retardation, autism spectrum difficulties, ADHD, psychotic disorders, and mood disorders, or severe anxiety disorders, such as obsessive compulsive disorder, may have relevance. However, more than diagnoses, descriptions of the functional capacity of the juvenile, their ability to relate and work with evaluating and treating professionals provide descriptive material for competency evaluators.

Educational records

School records provide the competency evaluator with the alleged offender's academic achievement and effort, speech and language skills, behavioral patterns, special education participation, standardized testing assessments for either special education or to assess district or state educational expectations. These records provide a mix of subjective and objective data regarding cognitive functioning, growth, the ability to learn from and work with others, as well as the juvenile's ability to sustain their interest and effort in a learning process. Educational records often contain information about behavioral regulation difficulties in the form of suspensions, expulsions, or other administrative actions. Behavior reports may highlight possible gang involvement. Special education evaluation and services may indicate relevant cognitive issues to the competency evaluator, for example, an auditory processing disorder, separate from effort and motivation.

Police records

These records, concerning the investigation and questioning of the alleged offender, have self-evident value in that they are proximate to the time of legal competence in question. If the interviews were videotaped or tape recorded they provide further understanding of the individual's behavior around the time when waiver reportedly took place. Collateral interviews of witnesses at times may provide additional insight into juvenile functioning either contrasting with or tending to corroborate the observations of others.

Previous police contacts provide a review of the individual's police contacts that rose to the level of formal reporting. Often these records contain adjudication results that may or may not have involved an adjudication procedure and/or a past evaluation of Miranda competency. These records would allow the attorney to track down adjudicatory records from previous incidents to determine if court-ordered competency or mental health evaluations were performed, and, if so, to obtain those evaluations. In addition, these records may identify collateral sources potentially available for interview.

Juvenile detention records

Juveniles in detention may have had evaluations initiated by their attorney, or come to the attention of detention health screeners who may have ordered evaluations including psychological testing. Review of detention school records, detention notes, or detention-related evaluations or treatment is another source of data proximate to waiver issues and for assessment of competency to proceed to adjudication.

Court records

There may have been hearings or filings by the attorneys that contain data relevant to competency skills. These are often determined by the context of a given case and evaluation.

The other side's psychiatric and psychological evaluations

Information from forensic evaluations performed by the "other side" from the one the mental health professional is assisting, provide that professional's evaluation of the competency issue in question. Review of the "other side's" data as well as the formal report may indicate issues, and collateral sources that you, as the current evaluator, did not know. Additionally, review of other's evaluations of the juvenile regarding the forensic issues may indicate inadequate or partial evaluations such that the basis for the opinions stated rest on a defective foundation.

Data from sources that examine an individual's functioning but do not directly attempt to assess the specific competency issues in question must be weighed regarding the relevant issues. For example, a history of conduct problems at school, head injury, previous abuse and neglect may or may not have specific bearing on questioned competency issues unless the reviewer of this data can relate the information in a meaningful manner to the competency required. The weight each element is given requires judgment on its merits after looking at the individual piece of data in the context of all the data available.

Disclosure of data, notes, and reports

Discovery rules applicable to delinquency proceedings require that the data, notes, and reports of testifying experts be preserved and disclosed. (We distinguish between "consulting" and "testifying" experts. Generally, a lawyer may consult with an expert who is not expected to testify. That expert becomes a part of the attorney's "team" for purposes of the lawyer–client privilege.) Thus, when an expert is appointed by the court or retained by the defense or by the prosecution, the expert can expect to be asked to produce the data he relied upon, the notes taken during the interview with the child, and any reports that he has written (*Karn v. Ingersoll Rand*, 168 F.R.D. 633, 639 [N.D. In. 1996]; *Fid. Nat'l Title Ins. Co. v. Intercounty Nat'l Title Ins. Co.*, 412 F.3d 745, 751 [7th Cir. 2005]). An expert may also be asked to produce the drafts that were the basis for the final report submitted. The fact that data, notes, and drafts are discoverable should dictate that these documents be preserved by the expert and that the lawyers who retain the experts instruct the witnesses concerning document retention. Destruction of documents relating to the evaluation undermines the credibility of the expert and may violate discovery rules, perhaps resulting in a ruling prohibiting the expert from testifying.

Due to the fact that this information is discoverable, it is essential that the child understand the nature, purpose, and non-confidential nature of the interview as well. Informed consent, commonly known as "waiver of confidentiality," should be obtained before proceeding with any forensic evaluation. Typically, the juveniles are interviewed in a detention setting without either an attorney or a parent immediately available. To obtain the informed consent, the evaluator(s) need to explain to the defendant their discipline, their agency (defense or prosecution), and the explicit purpose of the interview, i.e., to assess the alleged offender regarding the competency issue(s) in question. The alleged offender should be told that talking to the evaluator(s) is a choice they are making, and is not mandatory unless court ordered.

When the evaluation is court ordered, then the juvenile's preferences or comprehension of confidentiality may have no bearing because the presence of a court order indicates that they were represented by their attorney in the process that resulted in the court-ordered evaluation. Before proceeding with the evaluation interview(s) or testing, the alleged offender should have consulted with their attorney regarding the evaluation. If the juvenile has not consulted with their attorney, as happens on occasion, then it is advisable to contact the attorney who requested your evaluation for instructions on how to proceed. If your attorney is not available for instructions, then it is best to stop at this point until the evaluator can be assured that the juvenile has had the benefit of his attorney's advice and counsel.

Interaction between judges, lawyers, and expert witnesses

The assessment team receives its referral from the judge or from the lawyers involved in the case. Thus, the issues to be examined by the assessment team are framed by the judge and/or the lawyers. The expert should ensure that she understands the nature of the question presented, together with the specifics of the issues that require investigation. The judge and/or the lawyers should provide the expert with all relevant information concerning the child's background and perceived disabilities. This information, while not determinative of the expert's investigation and findings, should be taken into account as deemed appropriate by the expert.

While the assessment is ongoing, the expert and the lawyers should feel free to communicate with each other. However, it is important that during this process, the expert take steps to preserve her independence, especially if she is retained by one of the parties. The expert should explain at the outset the boundaries of communication necessary to preserve the appearance and reality of independence. Once the examination is completed, the court-appointed expert submits her report to the court. The court then distributes the report to the parties.

When the expert is retained by the prosecution or defense, there is usually discussion between the lawyers and the expert regarding the expert's findings. At this stage, the expert may still fall within the definition of a "consulting expert." However, because the children being examined are sometimes in custody, an examination sought by the defense will be known to the prosecution. Likewise, an examination sought by the prosecution will always be known to the defense. Discussions between lawyers and retained experts are sensitive discussions, given the fact that there is inevitably tension between the expert's desire to provide an objective assessment and the lawyers' role as advocates. The bottom line is that while lawyer and expert may discuss the expert's findings and the conclusions to be reached in a report, the lawyer may not tell the expert what to say. If the expert's examination of the child results in a conclusion adverse to the party by whom she has been retained, the referring lawyers may decide not to ask the expert to write a report.

Organization of expert witness report on fitness to stand trial

While there are no specific guidelines for writing a forensic report there are general guidelines that can be followed. Overall, the report should proceed logically. The key is to be thorough yet succinct. Reports that contain too much information may overwhelm the fact finder, while those with too little tend to be strictly conclusory in nature. To ensure that the reader has a clear picture of what you are expressing avoid the use of jargon, and if you must use a technical term, be sure to define it so a lay person can understand. The sections generally used are as follows:

1. Circumstances of the referral – State the referral source and any prior legal history and the current legal situation.
2. Purpose of the evaluation – Describe the legal issues involved in the case.
3. Informed consent – This section is used, when appropriate, to ensure that the person understands that the purpose of the evaluation is legal, not therapeutic, in nature and that they understand the limits of confidentiality.
4. Date and nature of the clinical contacts – Here the evaluator lists the dates and duration of contacts with the person or others related to the evaluation, such as family members. Also included should be the nature of the contact, whether it be an interview, testing, etc.
5. Data sources – In this section the evaluator would list the documents reviewed, such as academic or medical records. In addition it should identify the sources of interviews conducted and list all tests conducted.
6. Relevant history – This section should include information that is relevant and sufficient to support your opinions regarding competency. Information here may include among other things history of past mental difficulties, history of substance abuse, and history, or lack of a history, of involvement in the criminal justice system.
7. Clinical findings – This is where the evaluator summarizes his observations as well as results determined from documents, interviews, or testing. Observations about present mental functioning as well as any diagnoses would also be included in this section. It may be helpful to use direct quotes at times, if it helps to make your point clearer.

8. Summary and recommendations – This section states what the evaluator feels he can say with "reasonable certainty." The evaluator would also use the information reported in the previous sections to address the possible relevance of that data to the legal issue at hand.

Preparing the expert witness to testify

Neither experts nor lawyers should expect testimony to be understandable and complete without preparing for the courtroom presentation. Testimony should be presented in a way that effectively conveys the expert's opinion and the bases for the opinion. The first step in expert witness preparation is to identify the precise issue that will be the subject of the witness' testimony. If the issue to be addressed is competence to stand trial, the general issue is fairly straightforward. However, the expert may be called upon to give her opinion regarding subsidiary issues, such as how a particular characteristic of the child impedes or does not impede competence to stand trial. These questions must be formulated with precision. The next question is whether the expert possesses the requisite expertise to give the necessary opinions. For example, does the psychiatrist who leads the assessment team have the qualifications necessary to diagnose an educational deficit? If not, should the psychologist member of the team offer this opinion, or may the psychiatrist rely on the psychologist's conclusions as data reasonably relied upon by experts in his field (see, *Fed. R. Evid.* 702 et. seq.).

Once these basic issues are resolved, the lawyer calling the witness must gain an understanding of the procedures followed by the team in reaching its conclusions. This inquiry includes learning what procedures were followed in the investigation of competency, what investigation was conducted by the evaluation team, and how the facts gathered were applied to the governing legal standards. It is important, during this part of the preparation session, for the lawyer to determine whether the protocol followed by the assessment team meets the standards of those within the profession who conduct competency evaluations of children to stand trial. It is also crucial that the lawyer establish that the experts applied the proper legal standards to the analysis of the information gathered about the child.

Case vignettes

Case example 1

John is a 12-year-old male currently in the fifth grade, who was taken into custody and charged with aggravated battery. John was picked up by the police because he matched the description given by the store clerk who had been hit with a baseball bat.

John had never been taken into custody by the police before. He was taken to the station when both of his parents were out shopping.

At the police station, his parents were contacted and said that they would be coming down shortly. The detectives after briefly interrogating John called the state's attorney, who arrived at the station prior to the parents being there. At this time, John was read Miranda rights. Regarding each part, John's actual response to the Miranda warning was "Yes, I understand that" at which point the state's attorney repeated "Yes, you understand you have the right to . . ." and John agreed. The detective wrote down this information stating that John had an understanding of Miranda warnings. The state's attorney then asked a variety of questions about the incident. These were leading questions. During the questioning John began to cry, and he was told that it would be okay if he would simply tell them that he committed the crime. He could go home with his parents if he confessed.

When John's parents arrived at the police station, they were told that John had admitted to hitting the store clerk with a baseball bat because he had been caught shoplifting from the store.

John's parents were in shock because John had no prior juvenile offenses. They were told that the state's attorney had just finished writing down John's confession and he was going to sign it. The parents stood there unsure of what to do while John signed the confession.

Six weeks later, as John's defense attorney had been collecting collateral information, he learned that John had failed the third grade, had a verbal IQ of 84, and a performance IQ of 63. At this point, his attorney hired a child and adolescent psychiatrist to assess John, and to collect available collateral information to render an opinion regarding John's competency to understand Miranda warnings.

The opinion of the expert was that John was not competent to understand Miranda warnings. He based this on John's inability to comprehend the ramifications of the Miranda warnings. In addition, it was his opinion that John's level of anxiety without his parents being there, in association with his young age and lack of abstract reasoning ability, even further impacted his competency to understand Miranda warnings.

Case example 2

Adam is a 16-year-old male who is charged with kidnapping a 4-year-old child. Adam has been in special education classes since the fourth grade. He is emotionally and educationally disabled. His full scale IQ is 94.

His defense attorney questioned whether he is competent to stand trial. The lawyer questioned Adam's inability to work with him, and his inability to understand the potential repercussions that could occur in court.

All of the collateral educational information and mental health history was reviewed. Adam also has a diagnosis of ADHD. He is currently taking methyl-phenidate. According to his psychiatrist's notes, Adam's attention has been stabilized on this medication.

Adam's parents were interviewed. They reported that Adam was picked up by the police on several prior occasions. The issue of competency to stand trial had never been previously raised. The parents reported that at home, Adam sometimes has to be reminded several times to do household chores but does his chores when reminded to do so. They reported that Adam is capable of taking care of his activities in daily living, such as washing, cleaning his room, and even washing his own clothes.

When initially interviewing Adam, the psychiatrist asked Adam if he knew who his attorney was. He stated that he did not. He had no idea what a court was, who a judge was, or what a trial was. He was half smiling when answering this. Adam was then asked what his favorite sports team was in Chicago. He reported that it was the White Sox. He knew the starting line-up for the past three years and was able to describe the last two games, inning by inning. Adam had no severely defined mental health issues other than his ADHD and a mild oppositional-defiant disorder. He had a learning disability in reading, where he was approximately two-and-a-half years behind age level. There were no other significant educational issues.

Adam's mother was asked to come into the room. It was explained to her that Adam stated that he had no idea who his attorney was, what a court was, and what a trial was. At this point, his mother looked at him and said, "Stop wasting the examiner's time and tell him." Adam than recited the name of his attorney, how many times he had seen her, and what they spoke about in their last meeting. Adam understood what the charges were against him. He understood the role of his attorney, the state's attorney, and the judge.

He did not initially understand some of the complexities of the court such as plea bargaining. He reported that nobody ever discussed this with him. As such, he did not understand what it meant. As the general concepts of plea bargaining were explained to him, Adam responded "So, if I agree to a lesser charge maybe I won't have to go to juvenile, but I'll still have some type of record." He was unable to answer "Who will make that decision?"

Adam was competent to stand trial. This case is noteworthy as it helps to explain that many times, a youth's initial presentation will be guarded, with the hope of having a positive finding.

Case example 3

Jennifer is 14 years old. She is charged with criminal sexual assault. The alleged event occurred while she was baby-sitting her six-year-old nephew. Jennifer was brought to the police station by her uncle, the police station in which her uncle (the father of the victim) works. He was not involved with the interview process. Jennifer's uncle stood up during the interrogation of Jennifer and told her that she needed to tell the police the truth. Jennifer stated that she hadn't done anything. Jennifer's parents were called but were not available. Jennifer spent the next eight hours at the police station. She was quite anxious and even though offered food couldn't eat. At the end of that time, her uncle said "Just tell them what they want to hear, you are not going to get in trouble, at the most you may have to have some therapy." At this point, it was 12:30 am and Jennifer was exhausted. Specific allegations were described to her. Jennifer responded "Yeah." The state's attorney asked if that meant "Yes," which she acknowledged. The state's attorney then took a four-page statement from Jennifer.

During the time that Jennifer was at the police station, the victim was being evaluated through a victim-sensitive interview at a university based pediatric emergency room for signs of sexual assault. The victim had no signs of trauma or sexual assault.

Jennifer had signed her admission and was then told that she could not return home and would have to stay at the pre-trial detention facility.

The public defender questioned Jennifer's competency to understand Miranda warnings secondary to the level of exhaustion and the undue influence from her uncle.

It was determined by the initial expert that Jennifer was not able to understand Miranda warnings secondary to the undue influence and her exhaustion. Without undue influence or exhaustion, she had the cognitive ability to understand the basic concepts of Miranda.

The state's attorney then retained an expert whose opinion differed. This expert believed that although the uncle did bring her to the police station, that he was not part of the interview process and as such did not unduly influence his niece to make a statement. The expert also relied upon the fact that Jennifer typically stayed up in the summer months until 1:00 or 2:00 am. Typically she slept until 11:00 am.

As time progressed, the six-year-old child told his father that he had not been honest about what had happened. He reported that his cousin had never touched him in any way. He stated that night he was watching a show on cable television and repeated what he had seen on the cable movie. The comments that the six-year-old made were basically consistent with the victim-sensitive interview and physical assessment. This additional information was given to the state's attorney and the charges were dropped.

There are many concerning questions regarding this vignette. The issues of undue influence, not being able to reach the parents, and having a very superficial amount of initial information to even have charges, are danger signs. Lastly, there was little or no concern about the impact of leading questions on this child, and what the result of the short- and-long term sequela could be on this child based on the false allegations and lengthy interrogation.

Conclusion

As this chapter has demonstrated, defense lawyers, prosecutors, judges, and medical professionals play significant roles in the assessment and adjudication of children's competence to stand trial and to participate knowingly and intelligently in the police interrogation process. In order for all involved to make the best decisions on behalf of the child, on behalf of the public, and on behalf of the justice system, each professional involved must understand the legal rules, the procedural constraints, and the medical research and evaluation techniques that impact the way in which the important decisions regarding competency to stand trial and ability to understand the interrogation process are made.

All too often, important decisions are made by defense lawyers and prosecutors without knowledge or full understanding of the latest medical research. It is also often the case that a full picture of a child's overall functioning may not be presented in court because of medical professionals' lack of knowledge concerning the questions that are of most concern to the legal professionals involved. Finally, decisions regarding competence to stand trial and ability to understand the interrogation process may be sub-optimal because of the way in which evidence is presented in court. Lawyers and medical professionals must focus on the best way in which to accurately and effectively communicate complex information, some of which is counter-intuitive.

With the expansion of knowledge regarding the capacity of children to understand complex transactions and to make important decisions, juvenile courts will be forced to adapt. Do juvenile courts do enough to provide children with understandable information about the procedures to which they will be subjected, and to identify those children who are incapable of understanding the proceedings and cooperating with counsel? If not, should we be concerned about a child's lack of understanding given the treatment-oriented approaches of many juvenile court judges? Are Miranda warnings essentially meaningless to a child who is being interrogated? If so, should we re-evaluate the way in which we approach determining the admissibility of children's admissions to police investigators?

The answers to these questions are beyond the scope of this chapter. However, we can predict with some certainty that the impact of scientific research will lay the foundation for changes in the operation of juvenile courts in much the same way that research on the actual functioning of juvenile courts paved the way for the "due process revolution" initiated by the Supreme Court of the United States in *In re Gault*, 387 U.S. 1 (1967).

References

AACAP (2005). *Recommendations for Juvenile Justice Reform*, 2nd edn. Committee on Juvenile Justice Reform. Available at http://www.aacap.org/galleries/LegislativeAction/JJmonograph1005.pdf.

APA (2000). *Diagnostic and Statistical Manual*, 4th edn., text revision (DSM-IV-TR). Washington, DC: American Psychiatric Association.

Bonnie, R. J. & Grisso, T. (2000). Adjudicative competence and youthful offenders. In T. Grisso and R. G. Schwartz, eds., *Youth on Trial: A Developmental Perspective on Juvenile Justice*. Chicago, IL: University of Chicago Press.

Davis, S. M. (1994). The role of the attorney in child advocacy. *Journal of Family Law*, **32**, 817–831.

Drews, M. D. & Halprin, P. (2002). Determining the effective representation of children in our legal system. *Family Court Review*, **40**, 383–386.

Edwards, L. P. & Sagatun, I. J. (1995). Who speaks for the child? *University of Chicago Law School Roundtable*, **2**(1), 67–94.

Giedd, J. N., Blumenthal, J., Jeffries, N. O. *et al.* (1999). Brain development during childhood and adolescence: a longitudinal MRI study. *Nature Neuroscience*, **2**(10), 861–863.

Grisso, T. (1981). *Juveniles' Waiver of Rights*. New York, NY, Plenum Press, p. 191.

Grisso, T. (2000). What we know about youths' capacities as trial defendants. In T. Grisso and R. G. Schwartz, eds., *Youth on Trial: A Developmental Perspective on Juvenile Justice*. Chicago, IL: University of Chicago Press.

Grisso, T. (2005a). *Clinical Evaluations for Juveniles' Competence to Stand Trial: A Guide for Legal Professionals*. Professional Resource Press, pp. 13–14.

Grisso, T. (2005b). *Evaluating Juveniles' Adjudicative Competence: A Guide for Clinical Practice*. Professional Resource Press, p. 12.

Grisso, T. (2006). Adolescents' decision making: a developmental perspective on constitutional provisions in delinquency cases. *New England Journal of Criminal and Civil Confinement*, **32**, 3–14.

Grisso, T. & Pomicter, C. (1977). Interrogation of juveniles. *Law and Human Behavior*, **1**, 321.

Grisso, T., Steinberg, L., Cauffman, E. *et al.* (2003). Juveniles' competence to stand trial: a comparison of adolescents' and adults' capacities as trial defendants. *Law and Human Behavior*, **27**, 333–363.

Guggenheim, M. (1996). A paradigm for determining the role of counsel for children. *Fordham Law Review*, **64**, 1399–1424.

Guggenheim, M. (1998). Reconsidering the need for counsel for children in custody, visitation and child protection proceedings. *Loyola University of Chicago Law Journal*, **29**, 229–352.

Guggenheim, M. (2003). Ethical considerations in child welfare cases: the law guardian's perspective. *PLI-CRIM*, **192**, 455–459.

Kamisar, Y., Letave, W. R., Israel, J. H. & King, N. J. (2005). *Modern Criminal Procedure: Cases, Comments, and Questions*, 11th edn. West.

Laffitte, E. (2004). Model Rule 1.14: the well-intended rule still leaves some questions unanswered. *Georgetown Journal of Legal Ethics*, **17**, 313–317.

Luban, D. (1981). Paternalism and the legal profession. *Wisconsin Law Review*, **3**, 454–493.

Matthews, M. (1996). Ten thousand tiny cheats: the ethical duty of representation in children's class-action cases. *Fordham Law Review*, **64**, 1435–1458.

Oberlander, L. B., Goldstein, N. E. & Goldstein, A. M. (2003). In I. Weiner and A. M. Goldstein, eds., *Handbook of Psychology, Volume II, Forensic Psychology*, pp. 335–357.

Peters, J. K. (1996). The roles and content of best interests in client-directed lawyering for children in child protective proceedings. *Fordham Law Review*, **64**, 1519–1565.

Shepherd, R. E., Jr. (1996). *Juvenile Justice Standards, Annotated*. IJA-ABA.

Shepherd, R. E., Jr. & England, S. S. (1996). I know the child is my client, but who am I? *Fordham Law Review*, **64**, 1917–1942.

Tanenhaus, D. (2004). *Juvenile Justice in the Making*. New York, NY: Oxford University Press.

Uphoff, R. (1988). The role of the criminal defense lawyer in representing the mentally impaired defendant: zealous advocate or officer of the court? *Wisconsin Law Review*, **65**.

Wigmore, J. D., ed. (1929). *The Illinois Crime Survey*. Chicago, IL: Illinois Association for Criminal Justice, p. 681.

6

The etiology of antisocial behavior: biopsychosocial risk factors across development

Kayla Pope and Christopher R. Thomas

The criminal character was first described in 1812 by Benjamin Rush, after he consulted on a series of cases with young people who exhibited a "total perversion of moral faculties." He speculated that in all of these cases of "innate, preternatural moral depravity, there is probably an original defective organization in those parts of the body which are occupied by the moral faculties of the mind." For the remainder of the nineteenth century, scientific thought was devoted to understanding the inherent traits or physical defects that characterized the criminal character. At the beginning of the twentieth century, this focus of inquiry gave way to considerations of environmental influences on the development of criminal character among those working with juvenile offenders. Recognition of the importance of environmental factors was captured in the thoughts of W. Douglas Morrison (1898) who wrote that, "Unless a man has acquired criminal habits in early life it is comparatively seldom that he degenerates into an habitual criminal . . . Juvenile crime arises out of the adverse individual or social conditions of the juvenile offender, or out of both sets of conditions acting in combination." The changing view of antisocial behavior in youth served as the basis for establishing the first juvenile court in Chicago in 1899, emphasizing rehabilitation instead of punishment. This directly led in 1909 to the creation of the Juvenile Psychopathic Institute, later renamed the Institute for Juvenile Research, under the direction of William Healy. He argued that interventions with delinquents must be based on a scientific understanding of the causes and context of antisocial behaviors (Healy, 1917). This shift from inherent factors to environmental influences was reinforced by psychoanalytic theory and the work of August Aichorn, who in the 1930s began to describe disruptive behavior as the unregulated expression of primitive instinctual satisfaction without regard for the surrounding world. Environmental factors continued to be the mainstay of scientific inquiry until the ground-breaking work of Thomas and Chess in the 1950s (Chess & Thomas, 1984), and their studies on temperament. Understanding criminal behavior as a biological or physiological

The Mental Health Needs of Young Offenders: Forging Paths toward Reintegration and Rehabilitation, eds. Carol L. Kessler and Louis J. Kraus. Published by Cambridge University Press. © Cambridge University Press 2007.

phenomenon has continued in its ascendancy by advances made in the fields of genetics and neuroscience in understanding behavior.

From this long history of inquiry, the picture that has emerged is that criminal behavior can best be understood as an intricate dance between nurture and nature, and it is the culmination of biological and social influences that are determinant. Criminal behavior is thus a developmental phenomenon that does not suddenly appear in adolescence or early adulthood, but rather, begins early in life and evolves as the child passes through subsequent developmental stages (Aber, Brown & Jones, 2003; Broidy *et al.*, 2003; Frick *et al.*, 2003; Shaw *et al.*, 2003; Dionne *et al.*, 2003). The development of criminal behavior is also a biopsychosocial phenomenon, and factors that influence its development derive from multiple sources, ranging from genetic heritability to gang participation. Further, risk factors associated with the development of criminal behavior can be found for each developmental phase, with the most significant risk factors for each developmental period being those that influence the achievement of developmental milestones. Thus, during infancy, factors that interfere with the formation of a secure attachment appear to be most detrimental while during adolescence, risks associated with peer relationships are most critical. The remainder of this chapter will be devoted to exploring these biological and environmental risk factors, and their effect on behavior across development.

Biological factors

Risk factors influencing the developing brain

Advances made in the fields of genetics and the neurosciences have greatly enriched our understanding of the neurological mechanisms that regulate the experience and expression of human emotions. In the most fundamental sense, criminal behavior can be understood as a dysregulation of the experience and expression of anger resulting in aggressive behavior. The areas of the brain that are responsible for anger regulation comprise the limbic system, and during the prenatal period these areas are rapidly developing and are thus vulnerable to toxic influences. Most critical in early development is the amygdala, which has been referred to by LeDoux (1993) as the "central emotional processor of the brain." This area plays a vital role in associating emotion to experience, and is online at birth and is responsible for early processing of emotions, including anger. This region of the brain also alters the way the body will experience threats from the environment, and will influence physiological responses including heart rate and blood pressure, thus playing a key role in the internal state experienced by the infant in response to threats in its environment. Damage to this area has been associated with deficits in the interpretation of social cues and in the ability to suppress negative emotion (Davidson *et al.*, 2000). Later in development, the frontal lobe becomes more central to regulating behavior. Decreased functioning or damage to this area has been associated with violence and impulsive aggression (Pliszka, 1999; Raine *et al.*, 1998; Volkow *et al.*, 1995; Brower & Price, 2001). There is some evidence to suggest that damage to different lobes will result in different types of aggression, with impairment to the frontal lobe resulting in patterned aggressive responses, and damage to the temporal lobes resulting in more reactive forms of aggression without provocation or premeditation (Golden *et al.*, 1996).

The effect of genetic loading, exposure to environmental toxins, or both, can lead to the development of a predisposition for poor regulation of aggression. The precise mechanism through which these insults are translated into aggressive behavior is unknown, but likely involves a disruption of the neural circuitry responsible for regulating aggression described above. What is supported by research is that several behavioral deficits, thought to result from prenatal insults, have been observed in adolescents who engage in aggressive behavior including: poor impulse control and attention deficits (Hinshaw, 1994; Fowles, 2001; Simonoff *et al.*, 2004); both increased and decreased responsiveness to stressful stimuli (Lorber, 2004; Scarpa & Raine, 2000); and difficult temperament (Bates *et al.*, 1991).

Genetics

The importance of genetics as a contributory factor in the development of anti-social behavior finds support in a growing body of research. Although specific genes may have a special relevance for certain behaviors, antisocial behavior is likely a polygenetic phenomenon, resulting from different genes being expressed at different times (Rutter *et al.*, 1997; Torgerson, 1997). If viewed on a behavioral level, there appears to be a moderate degree of heritability for aggression, delinquency, and antisocial behavior from childhood to adulthood (Eley, Lichenstein & Stevenson, 1999; Taylor, Iacono & McGue, 2000). Behavioral genetics research has shown that there are genetic factors that help to explain differences in behaviors that are thought to play a role in conduct problems in middle childhood, including impulsivity, temperament, and attention deficits (Cadoret *et al.*, 1995; Miles & Carey, 1997). Twin studies also show that genetic factors account for moderate amounts of variance associated with externalizing problems in childhood (Eley *et al.*, 1999), and in self-reports of adolescent delinquent behavior (Rowe, 1985).

More recent research has focused on the heritability of physical aggression. This line of inquiry may prove to be particularly fruitful given that physical aggression during childhood has been shown to be one of the best predictors of aggression in adolescence (Broidy *et al.*, 2003; Nagin & Tremblay, 1999). Physical aggression is also a useful marker given that children begin to display physical aggression during infancy with significant variability among infants (Hay, Castle & Davies, 2000; Tremblay, 2000). Further, the display of physical aggression has been shown to be quite stable across development, from pre-school to elementary school (Cummings, Iannotti & Zahn-Waxler, 1989; Hay *et al.*, 2000) and into adolescence (Broidy *et al.*, 2003). A recent study by Dionne *et al.* (2003) utilized this approach, and examined the heritability of physical aggression in 562 19-month-old twins. The majority of the children were found to exhibit low levels of aggression, but 5 percent of the sample showed significantly higher levels of aggression. Overall, heritability was found to account for 58 percent of the variance in aggressive behavior.

Environmental toxins

In addition to genetic endowment, fetal exposure to a number of toxins has been shown to predispose children to aggressive behavior later in development. Of the environmental toxins, lead has received the most attention, and has been shown to be related to conduct problems later in development (Needleman *et al.*, 1996). With respect to drug toxicity, fetal exposure to opiates and methadone has been shown to increase the risk for conduct problems in 10- to 13-year-olds (de Cubas & Field, 1993). Similarly, fetal exposure to alcohol, marijuana, and cigarette by-products has been shown to increase the risk for later aggressive behavior (Day *et al.*, 2000; Goldschmidt, Day & Richardson, 2000; Olson, Brookstein & Theide, 1997).

Maternal smoking as a risk factor in the development of conduct problems has received a fair amount of attention. In multiple studies, smoking has been associated with an increased risk for the development of conduct disorder and delinquency in male offspring (see Wakschlag *et al.*, 2002 for a review). The interpretation of these studies has been confounded by the fact that many of these children also exhibited symptoms of hyperactivity, and it wasn't clear until a recent study by Wakschlag *et al.* (2006) whether an independent relationship could be established between smoking and conduct problems. In the Wakschlag study, boys exposed to pre-natal smoking were found to be more likely to develop oppositional-defiant disorder (ODD) or co-morbid ODD and attention-deficit/hyperactivity disorder (ADHD), but not more likely to develop ADHD alone. Further, these children were more likely to have an earlier onset of delinquent behavior than boys not exposed to prenatal smoking.

Neurotransmitters and neurochemicals

Investigation of the role of neurotransmitters and neurochemicals has yielded some promising results in furthering our understanding of how aggression is regulated. Serotonin has been the most studied of the neurotransmitters, and has been repeatedly shown to be predictive of aggressive behavior. Low levels of serotonin in cerebro-spinal fluid (CSF) have been linked to concurrent and future levels of aggression in children, and low levels of 5-HIAA (a serotonin metabolite) have been found in conduct disordered children (Kruesi et al., 1990; 1992). High blood levels of serotonin have been correlated with childhood onset conduct disorder (CD) and adolescent violence (Unis et al., 1997). The hormone cortisol has also been demonstrated to be predictive of aggression, with low levels of salivary cortisol being associated with early onset and persistence of aggression in boys (McBurnett et al., 2000) with ODD (van Goozen et al., 1998), and being predictive of boys who progressed from CD to antisocial personality disorder (APD) (Vanyukow et al., 1993). High testosterone levels have also been associated with aggressive behavior including the early onset of aggression (Pliszka, 1999).

The role of neurochemistry in regulating aggression is likely a complicated one, a point borne out in a study evaluating the role of the enzyme monoamine oxidase A (MAOA) (Caspi et al., 2002). This study investigated the role of MAOA in determining whether children who were maltreated would grow up to develop antisocial behavior. What the study found was that maltreated children who inherited a polymorphism of the gene that resulted in high levels of expression of MAOA were less likely to develop conduct problems.

Autonomic nervous system

It has been theorized that individuals with a propensity toward violence have lower levels of autonomic arousal at baseline and in response to stressful stimuli either due to deficient fear conditioning (Lykken, 1957) or deficiencies in orienting to threatening stimuli (Hare, 1968). A significant amount of research has been conducted to test the relationship between antisocial behavior and autonomic arousal, and to identify physiological markers that could be used to identify individuals with a propensity toward violence.

The most promising measurements of autonomic arousal have been skin conductance and heart rate. Skin conductance, or electrodermal response (EDR) to arousing stimuli, has been shown to be inversely correlated in children with CD and comorbid CD and ADHD (Herpertz et al., 2003). However, in a meta-analysis of studies evaluating EDR, no significant relationship was found between EDR and children who exhibited aggressive behavior or CD. In contrast, an inverse relationship between EDR and psychopathy/sociopathy in adults was found. Heart rate (HR) been more consistently shown to be a marker for aggressive behavior in children. A low resting heart rate at age 3 years has been shown to be predictive of aggression at age 11 (Raine et al., 1997), has been associated with adolescent antisocial behavior (Mezzacappa et al., 1997), and is predictive of later criminal behavior (Raine et al., 1990).

Whether HR or EDR can be used to distinguish different forms of aggressive behavior in children was addressed in a meta-analysis by Lorber (2004). What they found was that aggressive and sociopathy/antisocial behavior could be distinguished in adults by low HR in the former group and low EDR in the latter. In children and adolescents, however, both aggressive and conduct disordered children and adolescents demonstrated low HR at rest and in response to stimulus, with conduct disordered children also demonstrating low EDR at rest. Thus, conduct disordered children exhibit the autonomic profile of both adult aggressors and psychopaths/sociopaths, suggesting that their developmental trajectory may as yet be undecided.

Psychological factors

Attachment

The most significant developmental milestone of the first two years of life is the formation of a secure attachment with a caregiver (Bowlby, 1969). Evidence of the importance of attachment has been demonstrated in studies that have shown that infants with secure attachments show more effective emotion regulation, higher sociability, and higher compliance with parental requests (Bretherton, 1985; Richters & Water, 1991). Children who are insecurely attached have been shown to have more problems with peers and less self-control during preschool years (Carlson & Sroufe, 1995; Thompson, 1999); they are more likely to be referred to mental health clinics (Greenberg, 1999), and have higher rates of behavior problems as reported by preschool teachers (Egeland *et al.*, 1990).

The inability to regulate emotion is a key component of externalizing disorders. Learning to regulate emotions begins with early parent–child interactions, where the child relies on the proximity of an available and responsive caregiver to manage emotionally arousing experiences in her environment. By referencing the parent's response, the child learns how to regulate feelings of anxiety, fear, and distress. When the caregiver is appropriately responsive to the infant's emotional state, it enhances the infant's ability to tolerate and regulate affect, and the child learns to respond in socially appropriate ways. These repeated patterns of interaction between the parent and the child are thought to have an impact on emotion regulation via neural organization and conditioning processes (Schore, 2003).

In cases of insecure attachment, infants are deprived of the opportunity to experience emotions in a safe and secure manner and to learn mastery over their emotional experiences. Three general patterns of insecure attachment have been defined: avoidant, anxious/resistant, and disorganized, with each pattern resulting in behaviors that place the child at risk for later externalizing behaviors. The avoidant attachment pattern is observed in children whose caretaker is observed to be rejecting in response to the infant's expressions of distress. In response to rejection, these infants will minimize their distress in order to maintain proximity to the caregiver. Children with an avoidant attachment style have been found to be more overtly angry later in development, are more apt to displace frustration and anger to other people (Goldberg *et al.*, 1995), and have been found to be more aggressive, hostile, and impulsive in school settings (Greenberg, 1999). Infants who are anxious/resistant in their attachment style have caregivers who are inconsistent in their response to expressions of distress. These infants tend to exhibit exaggerated dependence on the caregiver and, it is thought, fail to relax and be soothed for fear of loosing contact with the caregiver. Children with this attachment pattern have also been found to be more overtly angry and cry more frequently. They are also more likely to exhibit passive withdrawal and to become scapegoats or victims of children with avoidant attachment patterns (Suess *et al.*, 1992; Troy & Sroufe, 1987). The third insecure attachment pattern has been labeled disorganized/disoriented. These children have been shown to exhibit controlling behavior, bossiness, and parentification (Main & Cassidy, 1988).

Attachment style is also thought to affect cognitions about relationships, and an insecure attachment can bias a child's perception of self and others in subsequent relationships. Experiencing a secure attachment enables the child to develop a perception of self as valued and competent. In contrast, insecure attachments may "... play a role in the development of representations characterized by mistrust, anger, anxiety, and/or fear ..." that may lead to hostile attributional biases and the potential for reactive aggression. (Guttmann-Steinmetz & Crowell, 2006; Pettit *et al.*, 2001).

Temperament

Temperament is regarded as characteristics of an individual that are observable very early in development, and appear to be biologically based. While the constructs of temperament have been variably defined, one approach has been to classify children in terms of behavioral activation versus behavioral inhibition. Behavioral activation is characterized by novelty and sensation seeking, impulsivity, hyperactivity, and predatory aggression. In contrast, behavioral inhibition is characterized by fearfulness, anxiety, timidity, and shyness (Thomas & Chess, 1968). Studies have shown that early signs of behavioral activation are predictive of externalizing behavior by middle childhood (Prior *et al.*, 1999), and that high levels of daring behavior at ages 8–10 are predictive of convictions and self-reported delinquency before age 21 (Farrington, 1998). A more recent study by Caspi (2000) found that temperament classification at age three was predictive of adult social functioning. Using data gathered from the Dunedin Study, children classified as "undercontrolled" at age three were found to be unreliable, antisocial, and to have more conflicts at age 21 than were children who were classified as inhibited, who were more likely to be unassertive and depressed.

Temperament, when difficult or dysregulated, can also become a risk factor by evoking maladaptive parenting. (Lytton, 1991). Thus, the relationship between parenting style and temperament appears to be bidirectional, and the negative effects of difficult temperament and maladaptive parenting appear to have an additive risk in the development of externalizing behavior (Calkins *et al.*, 1999; Cummings *et al.*, 2000).

Intelligence and academic performance

Failure to demonstrate competence in the academic environment has been shown to be significantly related to conduct problems, though it is unclear whether the behavior is the cause of poor school performance or whether failure at school precipitates the development of the behavior. Research has established that children who exhibit conduct problems have higher levels of learning disabilities, which helps to set the stage for failure in the school setting. It has also been shown that children's early experiences with failure are predictive of later conduct problems in adolescence (Moffitt *et al.*, 1981), and that poor self-concept with respect to academic performance at age seven is predictive of antisocial behavior in adolescence (Pisecco *et al.*, 2001). Early school failure appears to be more strongly correlated to adolescent behavior problems than is low intelligence (Hinshaw, 1992). And while retention in earlier grades may help to ameliorate academic difficulties, being held back is negatively perceived by peers, which may exacerbate the development of antisocial behaviors.

The relationship between intelligence and antisocial behavior is far from clear. While it was long considered to be true that children with externalizing behavior had lower intelligence quotients (IQs), a meta-analysis conducted by Hogan (1999) found that controlling for ADHD showed there to be no relationship between CD and low intelligence. However, a more recent study again showed that low intelligence was significantly correlated with conduct problems and adult antisocial behavior (Simonoff *et al.*, 2004). Interestingly, boys with psychopathic characteristics and conduct problems were found to have IQs equal to controls, and higher than boys with conduct problems without psychopathic traits (Christian *et al.*, 1997).

With respect to verbal IQ, there does appear to be a relationship between verbal IQ and antisocial behavior, with several studies showing delinquent juveniles having a lower verbal than non-verbal IQ (Moffitt *et al.*, 1993), and high verbal IQs being related to a decrease in CD symptoms (Lahey *et al.*, 1995). Similarly, reading disorders appear to be more common among children with CD. It is hypothesized that this reflects a language processing deficit in the left temporal lobe (Pine *et al.*, 1997) which may be apparent very early in development (Hinshaw, 1992; Sanson *et al.*, 1996).

Social cognitive functioning

It has been theorized that children who engage in antisocial behavior have deficits in social cognition that impair their ability to attend to and to accurately perceive social cues. Research to date, supports both of these tenets. Work by Dodge *et al.* has demonstrated that children with social skills impairment fail to attend to social cues (1995), and that aggressive children demonstrate a bias to attribute hostile intentions to others (Dodge, 1993). This has also been shown to be true of incarcerated delinquent boys (Wong & Cornell, 1999). Further, it appears that they are also more apt to select aggressive responses to problems (Matthys *et al.*, 1999).

A second area of research has been in the development of empathy and its role in regulating the expression of aggression. Empathy has been shown to mitigate aggressive behavior (Kaukiainen *et al.*, 1999). It has also been demonstrated that children with CD have lower levels of empathy and less ability to identify interpersonal cues (Cohen & Strayer, 1996).

Social factors

Parenting

Maladaptive parenting serves as a risk factor across development. Several aspects of parenting have been implicated in promoting the development of antisocial behavior during the toddler stage, including disciplinary style, the display of nurturing behaviors, and the skills and ability of the parent to teach socially appropriate behavior. With respect to disciplinary styles, inconsistent and harsh discipline has been shown to be a major risk factor in the later development of antisocial behavior (Glueck & Glueck, 1950). The importance of inconsistent discipline has been highlighted by Patterson's work. He has argued that parental response to antisocial behavior in early childhood lays down the behavioral response to demands later in life. He has found that children of parents who make demands of their children, then capitulate when the child aversively responds, have children with higher levels of chronic conduct problems (Patterson, 1995). The harshness of parental discipline has also been implicated in the later development of behavior problems, especially when the discipline crosses the boundary into physical abuse (Deater-Deckard & Dodge, 1997; Rutter *et al.*, 1998).

In addition to disciplinary styles, the warmth and nurturance of parents has been shown to influence the development of antisocial behavior. The lack of warmth between parent and child has been shown to contribute to antisocial outcomes (McFayden-Ketchum *et al.*, 1996; Pettit, Bates & Dodge, 1993). Further, the presence of maternal warmth has been shown to lead to positive social outcomes for children.

A third component of parenting that appears to play an important role during the toddler stage is the teaching behaviors of parents. This is especially true in the modeling of prosocial behaviors. Social coaching and advice giving appear to be important in young children's initial social encounters with peers, as well as with other children in the family. (Ladd & Pettit, 2002). Parent's proactive teaching of social skills in early childhood years has been shown to predict lower levels of behavioral problems in middle childhood and early adolescence (Pettit, Bates & Dodge, 1997).

In addition to parenting, there is evidence that early out-of-home care also plays a role in the development of antisocial behavior. One study showed that high rates of out-of-home placement during the first five years of life was related to display of aggressive behavior in kindergarten (Bates *et al.*, 1994). This remains controversial, however, as it is not clear whether it is the amount of out-of-home care that is important, or whether it is the quality of care received in the out-of-home place-ment or the quality of the care being provided at home (Colwell *et al.*, 2001; NICHD Early Child Care Research Network, 2002). However, both the quality and amount of out-of-home care have been shown to be important factors in school-aged children (Flannery, Williams & Vazsonyi, 1999; Posner & Vandell, 1999; Vandell & Posner, 1999). Further, it has been shown that children who spend large amounts of time in unsupervised after-school care in the early elementary grades are at elevated risk for behavior problems in adolescence (Pettit *et al.*, 1997).

Parental influence continues to be a significant factor in predicting delinquency during adolescence. The importance of parenting at this stage is its ability to serve as a mechanism to limit exposure to antisocial peers (Poole & Regoli, 1979). Unfortunately, however, even the effects of good parenting have been shown to be fully mediated by gang participation (Henry *et al.*, 2000) and that poor parenting leads to a greater interest in and susceptibility to antisocial peer groups and subsequently to antisocial behavior (Dishion *et al.*, 1995).

Thus, the aspects of parenting that appear to be most critical during adolescence is the parent's monitoring of the adolescent's activities as well as their ability to communicate with their children to determine how they are spending their time. In one study, Dishion and McMahon (1998) found that parental monitoring and supervision served a critical function in limiting adolescents' exposure to deviant peers groups. Further, the importance of parental monitoring in pre-dicting delinquency and violent behaviors appears to be significant regardless of income status, education, and ethnicity (Capaldi & Patterson, 1996; Florsheim,

Tolan & Gorman-Smith, 1996; McCord, 1980). In contrast, however, for adolescents raised in urban neighborhoods with high crime and poverty, both too much and too little parental monitoring has been associated with juvenile delinquency (Patterson *et al.*, 1992). It appears that the importance of parental monitoring may be due to the knowledge it accords parents of their children's activities. Thus, parents who did minimal monitoring were shown to have a limited understanding of their children's activities, and were found to have children that were significantly more likely to be engaged in deviant behavior, even after controlling for behavior problems earlier in development (Laird *et al.*, 2003; Pettit *et al.*, 1999). This finding was confirmed in a later study by Pettit *et al.* (2001).

In addition to parental monitoring and knowledge of adolescent activity, the manner of communication and bonding between parent and adolescent also appears to be important in predicting delinquent behavior. Parents who seek information from adolescents in an accusatory or uninterested manner were significantly more likely to have adolescents engaged in delinquent behavior (Hawkins & Lishner, 1987). Similarly, mothers of antisocial adolescents were found to be more hostile in their efforts to obtain information from their children (Dishion & McMahon, 1995).

Child abuse and family violence

The effects of child maltreatment and family violence on the development of antisocial behavior has been the subject of a considerable amount of research. It has been estimated that 20 percent of children who are abused will become delinquent before reaching adulthood (Lewis, Mallouh & Webb, 1989). Physical and sexual abuse have been shown to significantly increase the risk of CD in children (Fergusson *et al.*, 1996), and to be predictive of later antisocial personality disorder (APD) (Luntz & Winom, 1994) as well as the development of psychopathy (Weiler & Widom, 1996). Different forms of maltreatment have been evaluated in terms of their effects on later displays of antisocial behavior. Physical abuse has been shown to alter children's social processing skills, making them more likely to exhibit hostile attributional biases and positive evaluations of aggression (Deater-Deckard & Dodge, 1997; Dodge *et al.*, 1995). There appears to be no protective factor that can fully ameliorate the effect of physical abuse on the later development of conduct problems. Sexual abuse has also been shown to increase the risk of later development of conduct problems and externalizing behaviors (Trickett & Putnam, 1998).

The witnessing of violence in the home has also proven to increase the risk of later antisocial behavior, a significant concern given that an estimated 3.3 million children witness physical or verbal abuse annually (Jaffe Wolfe & Wilson, 1990). The risk appears to be greatest for boys and younger children (Reid & Crisafulli,

1990). Violence between parents also increases the risk of child maltreatment (McKibben, De Vos & Newberger, 1989), and the effects of witnessing violence and being the victim of child abuse are additive in increasing the risk for later antisocial behavior (Hughes, Parkinson & Vargo, 1989).

Peer relationships

With respect to peer relationships, the school setting can be the first exposure to aggressive peers, a factor which has been shown to be a risk factor for the development of aggressive behavior (Sinclair *et al.*, 1994). The failure to be liked and accepted by peers at this stage can also place the child at risk for developing aggressive behavior (Rubin, Bukowski & Parker, 1998). The duration of peer rejection also plays a role. In one study, children shown to be rejected by peers over a two-year period were shown to be more aggressive in their social interactions than were children who were only rejected during their first year of school (Pettit *et al.*, 1996). In follow-up studies, children who were rejected for two or three years by the second year of grade school were found to have a 50 percent chance of displaying clinically significant conduct problems later in adolescence, in contrast with children who avoided peer rejection, who had a 9 percent chance of demonstrating significant behavior problems (Dodge *et al.*, 2003).

As children approach adolescence, peer associations take on greater importance as a source of risk for the development of delinquent behavior. Peer influences are important at earlier stages of development with respect to feelings of self-worth and the need for acceptance and affiliation. However, as children reach adolescence, simple association with delinquent peers becomes significantly related to delinquent behavior (Coie, Terry & Lochman, 1995; Thornberry *et al.*, 1993). Studies have repeatedly found that association with deviant peers is the most significant factor with respect to onset of delinquency and escalation of violence (Dishion, Andrews & Crosby, 1995; Henry, Tolan & Gorman-Smith, 2001). The importance of peer associations is reflected in Aultman's finding that two-thirds of all delinquent acts were committed by adolescents in groups of twos or threes (1980). It is also reflected in the fact that the presence of a delinquent adolescent in a peer group can have a significant influence over the activity of the entire group resulting in delinquent behavior, even if the other members have a limited history of conduct problems (Patterson *et al.*, 1992).

Gang participation has also been shown to promote delinquent behavior. The influence of gangs on violent behavior in adolescence is greater than that from associating with antisocial peers (Battin *et al.*, 1998; Thomas *et al.*, 2003). A longitudinal study indicates that it is active participation in a gang that exacerbates delinquency and aggression, rather than gangs recruiting more violent individuals (Thornberry *et al.*, 1993). This study also found that the effect is not permanent and if a youth quits a gang, his violent behavior usually decreases. Conversely, association with peers involved in prosocial activities including community centers, athletic activities, and extracurricular school activities has been shown to have a protective effect against delinquent behavior (Hawkins & Lishner, 1987).

Larger social forces: role of communities and the media

During adolescence, the larger community/social context takes on increasing importance in predicting adolescent delinquent behavior. In a study by Sampson (1997), neighborhood social processes were significantly correlated with levels of crime. The most important factors appeared to be the degree of connectedness within the community as well as the amount of informal control, which included monitoring of behavior, supervision of children, and maintaining public order. Other neighborhood factors increasing the risk of antisocial behavior in adolescence include community disorganization, availability of drugs, and adults involved in crime (Herrenkohl et al., 2000). Community disorganization appears to influence antisocial behavior independently of factors such as single parent homes or poverty (Peeples & Loeber, 1994). Tolan and Gorman-Smith (1997) found that while strong parenting might provide only limited protection in the face of neighborhood problems and poor social processes, these neighborhood characteristics did not add to the risk posed by poor parenting. Poor neighborhood attachment and frequent residential moves may also contribute to increased risk of delinquency by disrupting the influence of social networks and bonds, although this effect may be short term (Herrenkohl et al., 2000).

The influence of media as a contributory factor in the development of antisocial behavior is the subject of a growing body of research. Violent television programs and films have received the most attention, and there is a considerable body of evidence to suggest that there are both short-term and long-term effects of viewing violence on aggressive and violent behavior in children (Huesmann & Miller, 1994; Bushman & Huesmann, 2006). While viewing violent material is not felt to be a sufficient risk factor for the development of antisocial behavior, in the presence of other risk factors, viewing violent material has been shown to have a short-term effect of "priming" an individual for violent acts (Huesmann, 1998). Viewing violent material is also thought to have long-term effects on the cognitions surrounding violent behavior (Berkowitz, 1993; Huesmann, 1998), serving to normalize it, or to desensitize the observer. Further, the long-term effect of viewing violence appears to carry over from childhood to adulthood. In a recent study by Huesmann et al. (2003), viewing TV violence between the ages of six and ten was found to be predictive of violent and aggressive behavior fifteen years later in adulthood. Further, this relationship held true even after controlling for other known risk factors, including socioeconomic status, intellectual ability, and parenting practices.

More current research has begun to examine the impact of other media sources, including computers and video games, on aggressive and violent behavior. Results indicate that violence viewed in this format appears to have a similar effect on increasing aggressive behavior (Villani, 2001).

Implications for future policy and research

Current research demonstrates that myriad factors influence the development of antisocial behavior, with individual risk factors having variable impact depending on the timing and duration of exposure. It is also clear that no one factor can be identified as the sole reason or even leading cause for antisocial behavior in general. Certain factors appear to be associated with specific stages of development, such as exposure to environmental toxins, or influence of peers. While certain factors may precede others in the sequence of effect on any given individual, it is their sum total that is important in the course of development of antisocial behavior. Epidemiological research has found that the presence of a single risk factor has little influence on the appearance of a disorder, but rates increase dramatically with exposure to multiple risks (Rutter *et al.*, 1975). Studies also indicate that there may be special configurations of multiple risks. Research with school-age children found a specific and cumulative contribution of risks by individual, parenting, peer, and social–cultural domains (Deater-Deckard *et al.*, 1998). Cluster analysis identified differing configurations in risks that strongly predicted later antisocial behavior with differing pathways.

Similar research has been carried out with adolescents, exploring cumulative risk of exposure to multiple risk factors (Herrenkohl *et al.*, 2000). In this prospective study, psychological and social risk factors were evaluated in youths at ages 10, 14, and 16 years of age, for their predictive value of violence at age 18. What they found was that many of the risk factors increased the likelihood of later violence, and that youths with exposure to 5 or more risk factors at age 10 were 7 times more likely to commit violent acts at age 18, with the odds increasing to 10 times more likely at age 14, and 11 times more likely at age16. These and other longitudinal studies support models describing different pathways in the development of antisocial behaviors, and in understanding and organizing the influence and interaction of multiple contributing factors (Loeber & Hay, 1994).

Research is now beginning to consider that various risk factors must interact to exert their effect on individuals. The Dunedin Multidisciplinary Health and Development Study (Caspi *et al.*, 2002) considered the interaction between genes and environment. Building on previous research (Brunner *et al.*, 1993) that found a relationship between aggression and deficiencies in monoamine oxidase inhibitor (MAOA), this study found that boys with a variant allele resulting in decreased MAOA activity were at greater risk than boys with normal MAOA activity for becoming physically violent in later life only if they were physically abused as children.

Further research is necessary to determine the relative importance of each of these individual risk factors, and the precise interactive and additive effect of exposure to multiple risk factors. In light of the developmental nature of antisocial behavior and the complexity of its etiological determinants, future research must evaluate risk longitudinally as well as assess the interaction of risk factors across biological, psychological, and social domains. Given the individual and societal costs associated with antisocial behavior, the benefits of such an investment seem clear.

References

Aber, J. L., Brown, J. L. & Jones, S. M. (2003). Developmental trajectories toward violence in middle childhood: course, demographic differences, and response to school-based intervention. *Developmental Psychology*, **39**(2), 324–348.

Aultman, M. (1980). Group involvement in delinquent acts: a study of offense type and male–female participation. *Criminal Justice and Behavior*, **7**, 185–192.

Bates, J. E., Bayles, K., Bennett D. S., Ridge, B. & Brown, M. M. (1991). Origins of externalizing behavior problems at eight years of age. In D. J. Pepler and K. H. Rubin, eds., *The Development and Treatment of Childhood Aggression*. Hillsdale, NJ: Erlbaum, pp. 93–120.

Bates, J. E., Marvinney, D., Kelly, T. *et al.* (1994). Child-care history and kindergarten adjustment. *Developmental Psychology*, **30**, 690–700.

Battin S., Hill K., Abbott R., Catalano R. & Hawkins, J. (1998). The contribution of gang membership to delinquency beyond delinquent friends. *Criminology*, **36**(1), 93–115.

Berkowitz, L. (1993). *Aggression: Its Causes, Consequences, and Control.* New York: McGraw-Hill.

Bowlby, J. (1969). *Attachment and Loss.* Vol. 1. *Attachment.* New York: Basic Books.

Bretherton, I. (1985). Attachment theory: retrospect and prospect. *Monographs of the Society for Research in Child Development*, **50**, 3–25.

Broidy, L. M., Tremblay, R. E., Brame, B. *et al.* (2003). Developmental trajectories of childhood disruptive behaviors and adolescent delinquency: a six-site, cross-national study. *Developmental Psychology*, **39**(2), 222–245.

Brower, M. C. & Price, B. H. (2001). Neuropsychiatry of frontal lobe dysfunction in violent and criminal behavior: a critical review. *Journal of Neurology, Neurosurgery and Psychiatry*, **71**, 720–726.

Brunner, H. G., Nelen, M., Breakefield, X. O., Ropers, H. H. & van Oost, B. A. (1993). Abnormal-behavior associated with a point mutation in the structural gene for monoamine oxidase-A. *Science*, **262**, 578–580.

Bushman, B. H. & Huesmann, L. R. (2006). Short-term and long-term effects of violent media on aggression in children and adults. *Archives of Pediatric and Adolescent Medicine*, **160**(4), 348–352.

Cadoret, R. J., Yates, W. R., Troughton, E., Woodworth, G. & Stewart, M. A. (1995). Genetic-environment interaction in the genesis of aggressivity and conduct disorders. *Archives of General Psychiatry*, **52**, 916–924.

Calkins S., Gill K., Johnson M. & Smith, C. (1999). Emotional reactivity and emotion regulation strategies as predictors of social behavior with peers in toddlerhood. *Social Development*, **8**, 310–341.

Capaldi, D. M. & Patterson, G. R. (1994). Interrelated influences of contextual factors on antisocial behavior in childhood and adolescence for males. *Progress in Experimental Personality and Psychopathology Research Review*, 165–198.

Carlson, E. & Sroufe, L. (1995). Contribution of attachment theory to developmental psycho-pathology. In D. Cicchetti and D. Cohen, eds., *Developmental Psychopathology, Vol. 1 Theory and Methods*. New York: Wiley, pp. 581–617.

Caspi, A. (2000) The child is father of the man: personality continuities from childhood to adulthood. *Journal of Personality and Social Psychology*, **78**(1), 158–172.

Caspi, A., McClay, J., Moffitt, T. E. *et al.* (2002). Role of genotype in the cycle of violence in maltreated children. *Science*, **297**, 851–854.

Chess, S. & Thomas, A. (1984). *Origins and Evolution of Behavior Disorders: From Infancy to Early Adult Life*. New York, NY: Brunner Mazel.

Cohen, D. & Strayer, J. (1996). Empathy in conduct disordered and comparison youth. *Developmental Psychology*, **32**, 988–998.

Coie, J. D., Terry, R. & Lochman, J. E. (1995). *Changing social networks and their impact on juvenile delinquency*. Paper presented at the annual meeting of the American Society of Criminology, Phoenix, AZ.

Colwell, M. J., Pettit, G. S., Meece, D., Bates, J. E. & Dodge, K. A. (2001). Cumulative risk and continuity in nonparental care from infancy to early adolescence. *Merrill-Palmer Quarterly*, **47**, 207–234.

Christian, R. E., Frick, P. J., Hill, N. J., Tyler, L. & Frazer, D. R. (1997). Psychopathy and conduct problems in children: II. Implications for subtyping children with conduct problems. *Journal of the American Academy of Child and Adolescent Psychiatry*, **36**(2), 233–241.

Cummings, E. M., Iannotti, J. J. & Zahn-Waxler, C. (1989). Aggression between peers in early childhood: individual continuity and developmental change. *Child Development*, **69**, 887–895.

Cummings, E., Davies, P. & Campbell, S. (2000). *Developmental Psychopathology and Family Process: Theory, Research and Clinical Implications*. New York: The Guilford Press.

Davidson, R. J., Putnam, K. M. & Larson, C. L. (2000). Dysfunction in the neural circuitry of emotion regulation: a possible prelude to violence. *Science*, **289**, 591–594.

Day, N. L., Richardson, G. A., Goldschmidt, L. & Cornelius, M. D. (2000). Effects of prenatal tobacco exposure on preschoolers' behavior. *Journal of Developmental and Behavioral Pediatrics*, **21**, 180–188.

de Cubas, M. M. & Field, T. (1993). Children of methadone-dependent women: developmental outcomes. *American Journal of Orthopsychiatry*, **63**, 266–276.

Deater-Deckard, K. & Dodge, K. A. (1997). Externalizing behavior problems and discipline revisited: nonlinear effects and variation by culture, context and gender. *Psychological Inquiry*, **8**, 161–175.

Deater-Deckard, K., Dodge, K. A., Bates, J. E. & Pettit, G. S. (1998) Multiple risk factors in the development of externalizing behavior problems: group and individual differences. *Development and Psychopathology*, **10**, 469–493.

Dionne, G., Boivin, M., Tremblay, R., Laplante, D. & Perusse, D. (2003). Physical aggression and expressive vocabulary in 19-month-old twins. *Developmental Psychology*, **39**(2), 261–273.

Dishion, T. J. & McMahon, R. J. (1998). Parental monitoring and the prevention of child and adolescent problem behavior: a conceptual and empirical formulation. *Clinical Child and Family Psychology Review*, **1**(1), 61–75.

Dishion, T. J., Andrews, D. W. & Crosby, L. (1995). Antisocial boys and their friends in early adolescence: relationship characteristics, quality, and interactional processes. *Child Development*, **66**, 139–151.

Dodge, K. A. (1993). Social-cognitive mechanisms in the development of conduct disorder and depression. *Annual Review of Psychology*, **44**, 559–584.

Dodge, K. A., Petit, G. S., Bates, J. E. & Valente, E. (1995). Social information processing patterns partially mediate the effects of early physical abuse on later conduct problems. *Journal of Abnormal Psychology*, **104**, 632–643.

Dodge, K. A., Lansford, J. E., Burks, V. S. *et al.* (2003). Peer rejection and social information-processing factors in the development of aggressive behavior problems in children. *Child Development*, **74**(2), 374–393.

Egeland, B., Kalkoska, M., Gottesman, N. & Erickson, M. (1990). Preschool behavior problems: stability and factors accounting for change. *Journal of Child Psychology and Psychiatry*, **31**, 891–909.

Eley, T. C., Lichenstein, P. & Stevenson, J. (1999). Sex differences in the etiology of aggressive and nonaggressive antisocial behavior: results for two twin studies. *Child Development*, **70**, 155–168.

Farrington, D. P. (1998). Predictors, causes and correlates of male youth violence. In M. Tonry and M. H. Moore, eds., *Youth Violence*, Vol. 24. Chicago, IL: University of Chicago Press, pp. 421–447.

Fergusson, D. M., Horwood, L. J. & Lynsky, M. T. (1996). Childhood sexual abuse and psychiatric disorders in young adulthood, II: psychiatric outcomes of childhood sexual abuse. *Journal of the American Academy of Child and Adolescent Psychiatry*, **35**, 1365–1374.

Flannery, D. J., Williams, L. L. & Vazsonyi, A. T. (1999). Who are they with and what are they doing? Delinquent behavior, substance abuse, and early adolescents' after-school time. *American Journal of Orthopsychiatry*, **69**(2), 247–253.

Florsheim, P., Tolan, P. H. & Gorman-Smith, D. (1996). Family Processes and risk for externalizing behavior problems among African American and Hispanic boys. *Journal of Consulting and Clinical Psychology*, **64**(6), 1222–1230.

Fowles, D. C. (2001). Biological variables in psychopathology: a psychobiological perspective. In P. B. Sutker and H. E. Adams, eds., *Comprehensive Handbook of Psychopathology*, 3rd edn. New York: Kluwer Academic/Plenum Press, pp. 85–104.

Frick, P. J., Cornell, A. H., Bodin, S. D. *et al.* (2003). Callous-unemotional traits and developmental pathways to severe conduct problems. *Developmental Psychology*, **39**(2), 246–260.

Glueck, S. & Glueck, E. (1950). *Unraveling Juvenile Delinquency*. Cambridge, MA: Harvard University Press.

Goldberg, S., Gotowweic, A. & Simmons, R. (1995), Infant–mother attachment and behavior problems in healthy and clinically ill preschoolers. *Developmental Psychopathology*, **7**, 267–282.

Golden, C. J., Jackson, M. L., Peterson-Rohne, A. & Gotkovsky, S. T. (1996). Neuropsychological correlates of violence and aggression: a review of the clinical literature. *Aggressive Violent Behavior*, **1**, 2–25.

Goldschmidt, L., Day, N. L. & Richardson, G. A. (2000). Effects of prenatal marijuana exposure on child behavior problems at age 10. *Neurotoxicology and Teratology*, **22**, 325–336.

Greenberg, M. (1999). Attachment and psychopathology in childhood. In J. Cassidy and P. Shaver, eds., *Handbook of Attachment: Theory, Research and Clinical Implications*. New York: The Guilford Press, pp. 469–496.

Guttmann-Steinmetz, S. & Crowell, J. (2006). Attachment and externalizing disorders: a developmental psychopathology approach. *Journal of the American Academy of Child and Adolescent Psychiatry*, **45**, 440–451.

Hare, R. D. (1968). Psychopathy, autonomic functioning and the orienting response. *Journal of Abnormal Psychology*, **73**, 1–24.

Hawkins, J. D. & Lishner, D. M. (1987). The social development model: an integrated approach to delinquency prevention. *Journal of Primary Prevention*, **6**, 73–95.

Hay, D. F., Castle, J. & Davies, L. (2000). Toddlers use of force against familiar peers: a precursor of serious aggression? *Child Development*, **71**, 457–467.

Healy, W. (1917). *The Individual Delinquent*. Boston, MA: Little, Brown & Co.

Henry, D., Guerra, N. G. Huesmann, L. R. *et al.* (2000). Normative influences on aggression in urban elementary class rooms. *American Journal of Community Psychology*, **28**(1), 59–81.

Henry, D. B., Tolan, P. H. & Gorman-Smith, D. (2001). Longitudinal family and peer group effects on violence and nonviolent delinquency. *Journal of Clinical Child Psychology*, **30**(2), 172–186.

Herpertz, S. C., Wenning, B., Mueller, B. *et al.* (2003). Psychophysiologic responses in ADHD boys with and without conduct disorder: implications for adult antisocial behavior. *Journal of the American Academy of Child and Adolescent Psychiatry*, **40**, 1222–1230.

Herrenkohl, T. I., Maguin, E., Hill, K. G. *et al.* (2000). Developmental risk factors for youth violence. *Journal of Adolescent Health*, **26**(3), 176–186.

Hinshaw, S. P. (1992). Externalizing behavior problems and academic underacheivement in childhood and adolescence: casual relationships and underlying mechanisms. *Psychological Bulletin*, **111**, 127–155.

Hinshaw, S. P. (1994). Conduct disorder in childhood: conceptualization, diagnosis, comorbidity, and risk status for antisocial functioning in adulthood. In D. C. Fowles, P. Sutker and S. H. Goodman, eds., *Progress in Experimental Personality and Psychopathology Research 1994: Special Focus on Psychopathy and Antisocial Personality: A Developmental Perspective*. New York: Springer-Verlag, pp. 3–44.

Huesmann, L. R. (1998). The role of social information processing and cognitive schemas in the acquisition and maintenance of habitual aggressive behavior. In R. G. Green and

E. Donnerstein, eds., *Human Aggression: Theories, Research and Implications for Policy.* New York: Academic Press, pp. 73–109.

Huesmann, L. R. & Miller, L. S. (1994). Long-term effects of repeated exposure to media violence in childhood. In L. R. Huesmann, ed., *Aggressive Behavior: Current Perspectives.* New York: Plenum Press, pp. 153–186.

Huesmann, L., Moise-Titus, J., Podolski, C. L. & Eron, L. D. (2003). Longitudinal relations between children's exposure to TV violence and their aggressive and violent behavior in young adulthood: 1977–1992. *Developmental Psychology*, **39**(2), 201–221.

Hughes, H. M., Parkinson, D. & Vargo, M. (1989). Witnessing spouse abuse and experiencing physical abuse: a double whammy? *Journal of Family Violence*, **4**, 197–209.

Jaffe, P., Wolfe, D. & Wilson, S. K. (1990). *Children of Battered Women.* Newbury Park, CA: Sage Publications, Inc.

Kaukiainen, A., Bjorkqvist, K., Lagerspertz, K. *et al.* (1999). The relationships between social intelligence, empathy and the three types of aggression. *Aggressive Behavior*, **25**, 81–89.

Kruesi, M. J. P., Rapoport, J. L., Hamburger, S. *et al.* (1990). Cerebrospinal fluid monoamine metabolites, aggression, and impulsivity in disruptive behavior of children and adolescents. *Archives of General Psychiatry*, **47**, 419–426.

Kruesi, M. J., Hibbs, E. D., Zahn, T. P. *et al.* (1992). A 2-year prospective follow-up study of children and adolescents with disruptive behavior disorders. Prediction by cerebrospinal fluid 5-hydroxyindolacetic acid, homovanillic acid, and autonomic measures? *Archives of General Psychiatry*, **49**(6), 429–435.

Ladd, G. W. & Pettit, G. S. (2002). Parenting and the development of children's peer relations in the context of family and neighborhood factors. *Child Development*, **66**, 360–375.

Lahey, B. B., Loerber, R., Hart, E. L. *et al.* (1995). Four year longitudinal study of conduct disorder in boys: patterns and predictors of persistence. *Journal of Abnormal Psychology*, **104**, 83–89.

Laird, R. D., Pettit, G. S., Bates, J. E. & Dodge, K. A. (2003). Parents' monitoring-relevant knowledge and adolescents' behavior: evidence of correlated developmental changes and reciprocal influences. *Child Development*, **74**(3), 752–768.

LeDoux, J. E. (1993). Emotional networks in the brain. In M. Lewis and J. M. Haviland, eds., *Handbook of Emotions.* New York: Guilford Press, pp. 109–118.

Lewis, D. O., Mallouh, C. & Webb, J. (1989). Child abuse, delinquency and violent criminality. In D. Chicchetti and V. Carlson, eds., *Child Maltreatment: Theory and Research on the Causes and Consequences of Child Abuse and Neglect.* New York: Cambridge University Press.

Loeber, R. & Hay, D. F. (1994). Developmental approaches to aggression and conduct problems. In M. Rutter and D. F. Hay eds., *Development Through Life: A Handbook for Clinicians.* Oxford: Blackwell Scientific, pp. 488–515.

Lorber, M. F. (2004). Psychophysiology of aggression, psychopathy and conduct problems: a meta-analysis. *Psychological Bulletin*, **130**(4), 131–152.

Luntz, B. K. & Widom C. S. (1994). Antisocial personality disorder in abused and neglected children grown up. *American Journal of Psychiatry*, **151**, 670–674.

Lykken, D. T. (1957). A study of anxiety in sociopathic personality. *Journal of Abnormal and Social Psychiatry*, **55**, 6–10.

Lytton, H. (1991). Parents' different socialization of boys and girls: a meta-analysis. *Psychological Bulletin*, **109**, 267–296.

Main, M. & Cassidy, J. (1988). Categories of response to reunion with parent at age 6: predictable from infant attachment classification and stable over a one month period. *Developmental Psychology*, **50**, 66–106.

Matthys, W., Cuperus, J. M. & Van Engeland, H. (1999). Deficient social problem solving in boys with ODD/CD, with ADHD, and with both disorders. *Journal of the American Academy of Child and Adolescent Psychiatry*, **38**, 311–321.

McBurnett, K., Lahey, B. B., Rathouz, P. J. & Loeber, R. (2000). Low salivary cortisol and persistent aggression in boys referred for disruptive behavior. *Archives of General Psychiatry*, **57**, 38–43.

McCord, J. (1979). Some child-rearing antecedents of criminal behavior in adult men. *Journal of Personality and Social Psychology*, **37**(9), 1477–1486.

McFayden-Ketchum, S. A., Bates, J. E., Dodge, K. A. & Pettit, G. S. (1996). Patterns of change in early child aggressive-disruptive behavior: gender differences in predictors from early coercive and affectionate mother–child interactions. *Child Development*, **67**, 2417–2433.

McKibben, L., De Vos, E. & Newberger, E. (1989). Victimization of mothers of abused children: a controlled study. *Pediatrics*, **84**, 531–535.

Mezzacappa, E., Tremblay, R. E., Kindlon, D. *et al.* (1996). Relationship of aggression and anxiety to autonomic regulation of heart rate variability in adolescent males. *Annals of the New York Academy of Sciences*, **794**, 376–379.

Miles, D. R. & Carey, G. (1997). Genetic and environmental architecture of human aggression. *Journal of Personality and Social Psychology*, **72**, 207–217.

Moffitt, T. E., Gabrielli, W. F., Mednick, S. A. & Schulsinger, F. (1981). Socioeconomic status, IQ, and delinquency. *Journal of Abnormal Psychology*, **90**, 152–156.

Moffitt, T. E., Caspi, A., Harkness, A. R. & Silva, P. A. (1993). The natural history of change in intellectual performance: Who changes? How much? Is it meaningful? *Journal of Child Psychology and Psychiatry*, **34**(4), 455–506.

Morrison, W. D. (1898). *Juvenile Offenders*. New York, NY: D. Appleton and Co.

Nagin, D. S. & Tremblay, R. E. (1999). Trajectories of boys' physical aggression, opposition, and hyperactivity on the path to physically violent and nonviolent juvenile delinquency. *Child Development*, **70**, 1181–1196.

Needleman, H. L., Reiss, J. A., Tobin, M. J., Biesecker, G. E. & Greenhouse, J. B. (1996). Bone lead levels and delinquent behavior. *Journal of the American Medical Association*, **275**(5), 363–369.

NICHD Early Child Care Research Network (2002). Parenting and family influences when children are in child care: Results from the NICHD Study of Early Child Care. In J. G. Borkowski, S. L. Ramey and M. Bristol-Powers, eds., *Parenting and the Child's World: Influences on Academic, Intellectual, and Social-Emotional Development*. Monographs in Parenting Series. New York: College Entrance Exam Board, pp. 59–89.

Olson, S., Bookstein, F. L. & Theide, K. (1997). Association of prenatal alcohol exposure with behavioral and learning problems in early adolescence. *Journal of the American Academy of Child and Adolescent Psychiatry*, **36**, 1187–1194.

Patterson, G. R. (1995). Coercion – a basis for early age onset for arrest. In J. McCord, ed., *Coercion and Punishment in Long-Term Perspective*. New York: Cambridge University Press, pp. 81–105.

Patterson, G. R., Reid, J. B. & Dishion, T. J. (1992). *A Social Learning Approach: Volume 4. Antisocial Boys*. Eugene, OR: Castalia.

Peeples, F. & Loeber, R. (1994). Do individual factors and neighborhood context explain ethnic differences in juvenile delinquency? *Journal of Quantitative Criminology*, **10**(2), 141–157.

Pettit, G. S., Bates, J. E. & Dodge, K. A. (1993). Family interaction patterns and children's conduct problems at home and at school: a longitudinal perspective. *School Psychology Review*, **22**, 401–418.

Pettit, G. S., Clawson, M., Dodge, K. A. & Bates, J. E. (1996). Stability and change in children's peer rejected status: the role of child behavior, parent–child relations, and family ecology. *Merrill-Palmer Quarterly*, **42**, 91–118.

Pettit, G. S., Bates, J. E. & Dodge, K. A. (1997). Supportive parenting, ecological context and children's adjustment. *Child Development*, **68**, 908–923; *Developmental Psychology*, **23**, 267–275.

Pettit, G. S., Bates, J. E., Dodge, K. A. & Meece, D. W. (1999). The impact of after-school peer contact on early adolescent externalizing problems is moderated by parental monitoring, perceived neighborhood safety, and prior adjustment. *Child Development*, **70**(3) 768–778.

Pettit, G. S., Laird, R. D., Dodge, K. A., Bates, J. E. & Criss, M. M. (2001). Antecendents and behavior-problem outcomes of parental monitoring and psychological control in early adolescence. *Child Development*, **72**(2), 583–598.

Pine, D. S., Bruder, G. E., Wasserman, G. A. *et al.* (1997). Verbal dichotic listening in boys at risk for behavioral disorders. *Journal of the American Academy of Child and Adolescent Psychiatry*, **36**, 1465–1473.

Pisecco, S., Wristers, K., Swank, P., Silva, P. A. & Baker, D. B. (2001). The effect of academic self-concept on ADHD and antisocial behaviors in early adolescence. *Journal of Learning Disabilities*, **34**(5), 450–461.

Pliszka, S. R. (1999). The psychobiology of oppositional defiant disorder and conduct disorder. In H. C. Quay and A. E. Hogan, eds., *Handbook of Disruptive Behavior Disorders*. New York: Kluwer Academic/Plenum, pp. 371–395.

Poole, E. & Regoli, R. (1979). Parental support, delinquent friends, and delinquency: a test of interaction effects. *Journal of Criminal Law and Criminology*, **70**(2), 188–193.

Posner, J. K. & Vandell, D. L. (1999). After-school activities and the development of low-income urban children. A longitudinal study. *Developmental Psychology*, **35**, 868–879.

Prior, M., Smart, D., Sanson, A. & Oberklaid, F. (2001). Longitudinal predictors of behavioural adjustment in pre-adolescent children. *The Australian and New Zealand Journal of Psychiatry*, **35**(3), 297–307.

Raine, A., Venables, P. H. & Williams, M. (1990). Relationships between central and autonomic measures of arousal at age 15 years and criminality at age 24 years. *Archives of General Psychiatry*, **47**(11), 1003–1007.

Raine, A., Venables, P. H. & Williams, M. (1997). Low resting heart rate at age 3 predisposes to aggression at age 11 years: evidence from Mauritius Child Health Project. *Journal of the American Academy of Child and Adolescent Psychiatry*, **36**, 1457–1464.

Raine, A., Stoddard, J., Bihrle, S. & Buschbaum, M. (1998). Prefrontal glucose deficits in murderers lacking psychosocial deprivation. *Neuropsychiatry, Neuropsychology and Behavioral Neurology*, **11**, 1–17.

Reid, W. J. & Crisafulli, A. (1990). Marital discord and child behavioral problems: a meta-analysis. *Journal of Abnormal Child Psychology*, **18**, 105–117.

Richters, J. & Waters E. (1991). Attachment and socialization: the positive side of social influence. In M. Lewis and S. Feinman, eds., *Social Influences and Socialization in Infancy*. New York: Plenum Press, pp. 185–213.

Rowe, D. C. (1985). Sibling interaction and self-reported delinquent behavior: a study of 265 twin pairs. *Criminology*, **23**, 223–240.

Rubin, K. H., Bukowski, W. & Parker, J. G. (1998). Peer interactions, relationships, and groups. In W. Damon (series ed.) and N. Eisenberg (vol. ed.), *Handbook of Child Psychology: Vol. 3. Social, Emotional, and Personality Development*, 5th edn. New York: Wiley, pp. 619–700.

Rush, B. (1812). *Medical Inquiries and Observations upon the Diseases of the Mind*. Philadelphia, PA: Kimber & Richardson.

Rutter, M., Yule, B., Quinton, D. *et al.* (1975). Attainment and adjustment in two geographical areas: III. Some factors accounting for area differences. *British Journal Psychiatry*, **126**, 520–533.

Rutter, M., Dunn, J., Plomin, R. & Simonoff, E. (1997). Integrating nurture and nature: Implications of person–environment correlations and interactions for developmental psychopathology. *Development and Psychopathology*, **9**, 335–364.

Rutter, M., Giller, H. & Hagell, A. (1998). *Antisocial Behavior by Young People*. New York: Cambridge University Press.

Sampson, R. J. (1997). The embeddedness of child and adolescent development: a community-level perspective on urban violence. In J. McCord, ed., *Violence and Childhood in the Inner City*. Cambridge, England: Cambridge University Press, pp. 31–77.

Sanson, A., Prior, M. & Smart, D. (1996). Reading disabilities with and without behavior problems at 7–8 years: prediction from longitudinal data from infancy to 6 years. *Journal of Child Psychology and Psychiatry*, **37**, 529–541.

Scarpa, A. & Raine, A. (2000). Violence associated with anger and impulsivity. In J. C. Borod, ed., *The Neuropsychology of Emotion*. Series in Affective Science. New York: Oxford University Press, pp. 320–339.

Schore, A. (2003). *Affect Dysregulation and Disorders of the Self*. New York: NY, WW Norton & Company.

Shaw, D. S., Gilliom, M., Ingoldsby, E. M. & Nagin, D. S. (2003). Trajectories leading to school-age conduct problems. *Developmental Psychology*, **39**(2), 189–200.

Simonoff, E., Elander, J., Holmshaw, J. *et al.* (2004). Predictors of antisocial personality: continuities from childhood to adult life. *British Journal of Psychiatry*, **184**, 118–127.

Sinclair, J. J., Pettit, G. S., Harrist, A. W., Dodge, K. A. & Bates, J. E. (1994). Encounters with aggressive peers in early childhood: frequency, age differences and correlates of risk for behavior problems. *International Journal of Behavioral Development*, **17**, 675–696.

Suess, G., Grossman, K. E. & Sroufe, L. A. (1992). Effects of infant attachment to mother and father on quality of adaptation in preschool: from dyadic to individual organization of self. *International Journal of Behavioral Development*, **15**, 43–65.

Taylor, J., Iacono, W. G. & McGue, M. (2000). Evidence for a genetic etiology of early-onset delinquency. *Journal of Abnormal Psychology*, **109**, 634–643.

Thomas, A. & Chess, S. (1968). *Temperament and Behavior Disorders in Childhood*. New York, NY: New York University Press.

Thomas, C., Holzer, C. & Wall, J. (2003). Serious delinquency and gang membership. *Adolescent Psychiatry*, **27**, 61–81.

Thompson, R. (1999). Early attachment and later development. In J. Cassidy and P. Shaver, eds., *Handbook of Attachment: Theory, Research and Clinical Applications*. New York, NY: The Guilford Press, pp. 265–286.

Thornberry, T. P., Krohn, M., Lizotte, A. J. & Chard-Wierschem, D. (1993). The role of juvenile gangs in facilitating delinquent behavior. *Journal of Research in Crime and Delinquency*, **30**, 55–87.

Tolan, P. H. & Gorman-Smith, D. (1997). Families and development of urban children. In H. J. Walburg, O. Reyes and R. P. Weissberg, eds., *Urban Children and Youth: Interdisciplinary Perspective on Policies and Programs*. Thousand Oaks, CA: Sage, pp. 67–91.

Torgerson, S. (1997). Genetic basis and psychopathology. In S. M. Turner and M. Hersen, eds., *Adult Psychopathology and Diagnosis*, 3rd edn. New York, NY: Wiley, pp. 58–85.

Tremblay, R. E. (2000). The development of aggressive behavior during childhood: what have we learned in the past century? *Journal of Behavioral Development*, **24**, 129–141.

Trickett, P. K. & Putnam, F. W. (1998). Developmental consequences of child sexual abuse. In P. K. Trickett and C. J. Schellenbach, eds., *Violence Against Children in the Family and the Community*. Washington, DC: American Psychological Association, pp. 39–56.

Troy, M. & Sroufe, A. (1987). Victimization among preschoolers: role of attachment relationship history. *Journal of the American Academy of Child and Adolescent Psychiatry*, **26**, 166–172.

Unis, A. S., Cook, E. H., Vincent, J. G. *et al.* (1997). Platelet serotonin measures in adolescents with conduct disorder. *Biological Psychiatry*, **42**, 553–559.

Vandell, D. L. & Posner, J. K. (1999). Conceptualization and measurement of children's after-school environments. In S. L. Friedman and T. D. Wachs, eds., *Measuring Environment Across the Life Span: Emerging Methods and Concepts*. Washington DC: American Psychological Press, pp. 167–196.

Van Goozen, S. H. M., Matthys, W., Cohen-Kettenis, P. T. *et al.* (1998). Salivary cortisol and cardiovascular activity during stress in oppositional defiant disorder boys and normal controls. *Biological Psychiatry*, **43**, 531–539.

Vanyukow, M. M., Moss, H. B., Plial, J. A. *et al.* (1993). Antisocial symptoms in preadolescent boys and in their parents: associations with cortisol. *Psychiatry Research*, **46**, 9–17.

Villani, S. (2001). Impact of media on children and adolescents: a 10-year review of the research. *Journal of the American Academy of Child and Adolescent Psychiatry*, **40**(4), 392–401.

Volkow, N. D., Tancredi, L. R., Grant, C. *et al.* (1995). Brain glucose metabolism in violent psychiatric patients: a preliminary study. *Psychiatry Research*, **61**, 243–253.

Wakschlag, L., Pickett, K., Cook, E., Benowitz, N. & Leventhal, B. (2002). Maternal smoking during pregnancy and severe antisocial behavior in offspring: a review. *American Journal of Public Health*, **92**, 969–974.

Wakschlag, L., Pickett, K., Kasza, K. E. & Loeber, R. (2006). Is prenatal smoking associated with a developmental pattern of conduct problems in young boys? *Journal of the American Academy of Child and Adolescent Psychiatry*, **45**, 461–467.

Weiler, B. L. & Widom, C. S. (1996). Psychopathy and violent behavior in abused and neglected young adults. *Criminal Behaviour and Mental Health*, **6**, 253–271.

Wong, W. & Cornell, D. C. (1999). PIQ>VIQ discrepancy as a correlate of social problem solving and aggression in delinquent adolescent males. *Journal of Psychoeducational Assessment*, **17**, 104–112.

7

Substance abuse in youth offenders

Deborah R. Simkin

Introduction

A Congressional study in 2004 found that two-thirds of juvenile detention facilities hold youth who are waiting for community based mental health care. Part of the lack of services can possibly be related to a shortage of both outpatient community based and inpatient beds. Overall, the number of inpatient psychiatric beds per capita for adults and children in the United States has dropped by 62 percent since 1970. Publicly run facilities (state and county) have had a more dramatic decline of 89 percent inpatient psychiatric beds per capita. Due to the lack of facilities, a 2003 study by the General Accounting Office found that 9000 families relinquished custody of their children to juvenile justice systems for the sole purpose of accessing mental health services they could not find or afford. However, in 2001, only 16 percent of crimes committed by juveniles were violent. So we have a history of decreased mental health services, increased numbers of youth who are housed in juvenile justice systems awaiting treatment, and insufficient resources either in the juvenile justice facilities or in the community to handle the needs of these youth (Koppelman, 2005).

Although adolescents in the juvenile justice system experience much higher rates of psychiatric disorders than adolescents in the general population (Shelton, 2001), what brings them to the attention of the juvenile justice system is an often co-occurring substance abuse disorder.

Prevalence of disorders

Nearly two-thirds of males and three-quarters of females in the juvenile justice system have at least one psychiatric disorder as opposed to 20 percent of all children. Forty-seven percent of females and 51 percent of males had a substance abuse disorder (Teplin, 2002). In order to avoid youth involvement with the juvenile justice system, more emphasis needs to be placed on early detection and intervention.

The Mental Health Needs of Young Offenders: Forging Paths toward Reintegration and Rehabilitation, eds. Carol L. Kessler and Louis J. Kraus. Published by Cambridge University Press. © Cambridge University Press 2007.

In a study involving female juvenile offenders, 80 percent had emotional or substance abuse disorders, and two-thirds of these girls had a history of recidivism. Among female youths who had a history of recidivism, 82 percent had a history of substance abuse and 47 percent had used mental health services in their lifetime.

Cocozza and Skowyra (2000) estimate that about 20 percent of youth in the juvenile justice system have serious mental disorders, sometimes one but usually a combination of disorders (bipolar, ADHD, schizophrenia, disruptive disorders), and that 25–32 percent have been sexually or physically abused (Teplin, 2002).

Although not all adolescents with a substance abuse disorder become involved with the juvenile justice system, use of alcohol and/or drugs is against the law. Whether an adolescent is caught using drugs or not, the use implies that anyone that does could become involved in the juvenile justice system. Therefore, this chapter will first concentrate on all risk factors that increase the risk for substance abuse, including psychiatric disorders.

Prevention

Risk factors

Newcomb (1997) has not only discussed risk factors that can lead to increased risk for substance abuse, he has also divided these risk factors in the developmental stage at which these factors have the most effect. These risk factors are listed below, and are subdivided into several domains:

1. Cultural/societal
    Laws favorable to drug use
    Social norms favorable to drug use
    Availability of drugs
    Extreme economic deprivation
    Neighborhood disorganization
2. Interpersonal
    Childhood interpersonal factors
    Family alcohol and drug behavior and attitudes
    Poor and inconsistent family management practices
    Parent personality and other characteristics
    Family conflicts
    Physical or sexual abuse
    Adolescent interpersonal factors
    General stressful life events (e.g., relocation)

        Peer rejection in school and other contexts

        Association with drug-using peers

3. Psychobehavioral

        Child and adolescent psychobehavioral influences

        Age

        Early and persistent behavior problem (including drug use)

        Academic failure

        Low degree of commitment to school

        Post adolescent psychobehavioral factors

        Occupational satisfaction and success

        Child-rearing demands

        Multiple role obligations

        Achievement of sex role expectations

        Intimate relationship functioning

        Educational/financial attainment and security

4. Psychobehavioral antecedents and consequences throughout life

        Alienation, rebelliousness, or antisocial personality

        Sensation seeking

        Psychopathology (psychiatric disorders)

        Attitudes favorable to drug use

        Cognitive motivations or expectancies for drug use

        Inability to delay gratification

5. Biogenetic

        Inherited susceptibility to drug use

        Psychophysiological vulnerability to drug effects

Recognition and intervention for these risk factors is important to the child and adolescent psychiatrist in order to reduce the risk of future substance abuse. Since protective factors can cushion the effect of risk factors, the psychiatrist should try to convert the risk factors into protective factors as quickly as possible.

Interpersonal risk factors clearly delineate those factors with the most influence during childhood and adolescence. Research examples of interpersonal risk factors that would be expected to demonstrate the most influence during childhood include the effects of parent modeling; parents' belief in the harmlessness of substances; parent monitoring; family abuse; family disruption; negative communication patterns and lack of anger control in families of substance abusers; lack of closeness and involvement with children's activities; maternal passivity; and low academic aspirations (Baumrind, 1983; Bennett & Kempfer, 1994; Duncan, Biglan & Ary, 1998; Kandel, Kessler & Marguiles, 1978).

It seems that protective factors tend to have an extreme influence in the prevention of the development of substance use disorders. In a study of resilience in sons of alcoholic fathers, more good life events and an internal locus of control seem to cushion against the development of a substance use disorder.

Because protective factors tend to cushion risk factors, finding interventions that turn risk factors into protective factors would be useful in treating adolescents and in reducing continued use and progression of substance use disorders. This conversion of risk factors into protective factors is even more important when one considers that an accumulation of risk factors appears to have a more powerful effect than an accumulation of protective factors. Examples of protective factors include a stable environment, a high degree of motivation, a strong parent–child bond, consistent parental supervision and discipline, bonding to pro-social institutions, high religiosity, association with peers who hold conventional attitudes, and consistent, community-wide anti-drug use messages.

Early intervention education programs

Education programs that are research validated can decrease the risk of future substance abuse and address many of the above risk factors that can increase risk for substance abuse. According to Hansen (1996), evidence now exists that certain aspects of program development are essential to provide effective interventions. They are program focus, delivery technique, evaluation, training, and support.

Program focus describes the expected outcome. According to Hansen, there are three periods of program development: institution-driven, theory-driven, and data-driven. Earlier efforts formulated by institution-driven programs allowed researchers to test the programs and learn from their mistakes. One such well-intentioned effort was the Drug Abuse Resistance Education (DARE) program. Results demonstrated that drug use in control schools and those using the DARE program was almost equal. No substantial short-term or long-term effects were documented.

Some programs grew out of research and, hence, were called theory-driven programs. The problem with these programs was that resources needed to evaluate these programs were minimal. Overall, programs that had an informational or affective component had very little effect, whereas those that used social influence approaches, or life skills approaches with social influence approaches were the most effective. Examples of these types of programs include Project SMART, Life Skills Training, and Project STAR.

The third type of program to develop was based on data-driven prevention. Hansen pointed out that data-driven prevention programs used only variables that had strong statistical relationships with drug use, whereas theory-driven programs used all variables.

He performed a meta-analysis on 242 studies, and found 11 major variables in etiological studies. The variables that had a strong statistical relationship included drug use by peers, previous drug use, bonding, commitment to school, and deviance. Variables with average statistical relationships were beliefs about psychological and social consequences of drug use, pressure to use substances, and perceived attitudes about drug use among others. Belief about health consequences was not as strongly correlated. The weakest variables were home factors, psychological traits of parents, parental marital status, parental education, family composition, and socioeconomic status. Parental attentiveness, parenting style, and parental drug use had higher correlation. Just as Newcomb's work has helped to indicate at what crucial developmental stage risk factors for substance abuse have the greatest effect and, therefore, at what stage intervention might be most effective, Hansen's work can help to prioritize which of these risk factors to target initially, due to the stronger statistical relationship to the development of substance abuse.

Of course, for clinicians who are evaluating children and their families, recognizing potential risk factors and addressing them during the treatment process is important to prevent development of substance abuse.

One population that is only beginning to receive attention is that of adolescents in the juvenile justice system. One study by Thomas Dishion et al. (1996) looked at groupings of delinquent boys over a two-year period. It compared pairings of boys composed of a delinquent and a non-delinquent, two delinquents, or two non-delinquents. In the mixed pair and the pair with two non-delinquent youths, the interaction centered on normative talk and laughter. The delinquent pair interaction was typical of interaction that increased self-reported delinquent behavior. Therefore, interventions that pool high-risk youth into homogeneous groups should be avoided.

A description of education programs can be found in a newly revised booklet produced at the National Institute for Drug Abuse (NIDA, 2003) called *Preventing Substance Abuse Among Children and Adolescents – A Research-Based Guide.*

Media

The media can have a negative effect as well as a positive effect. It is thought that the anti-marijuana ad campaign launched in 2002 by the Office of National Drug Control Policy, in conjunction with the Partnership for a Drug Free America, was the reason for the 2003 decrease in perceived risk. When perceived risk goes up among adolescents, use usually goes down. Of course, ad campaigns that encourage drug use among adolescents should continue to be reduced through legislative efforts (Johnston, 2005). Since use of prescription drugs increased in 2006, perhaps the next campaign should target these drugs (Johnston, 2006).

Co-morbidity

There is a high rate of co-morbidity in adolescents with substance use disorder. Early intervention and recognition of co-morbid disorders is extremely important to reducing risk for not only substance abuse but, as noted before, risk of entering the juvenile justice system. In a recent literature search (Couwelenbergh *et al.*, 2006), adolescents and young adults with substance use disorders (SUD) and co-morbid psychiatric disorders had a high risk of entering the juvenile justice system. In fact, in a study by Turner *et al.* (2005) incarcerated youth were subtyped according to depressive and anxiety symptoms using the Children's Depression Inventory and the Revised Children's Manifest Anxiety Scales. Cluster analysis confirmed the presence of negative mood in 34 percent of the population. These adolescents reported higher levels of both marijuana and alcohol use to regulate mood states.

However, it should be pointed out that the limited availability of services for mental health and substance abuse issues in the juvenile justice system allows disorders to become more severe with time. Hence, recidivism increases with time. However, in a study of young offenders by Lennings *et al.* (2006), although 40 percent of the sample revealed signigicant substance abuse problems, only 18 percent were offered appointments with juvenile justice drug and alcohol counselors. Therefore, adolescents in the juvenile justice system should be evaluated periodically in order to reassess the change in the severity of the problem, and whether appropriate referrals have been made (Harrington *et al.*, 2005).

E. Jane Costello *et al.* (1999) has looked at the onset of several disorders to determine if they are likely to precede the development of a substance abuse disorder, or are more likely to follow the onset of a substance abuse. All disorders, including ADHD (attention-deficit/hyperactivity disorder), conduct disorder, oppositional-defiant disorder, and anxiety disorder, occurred well before the onset of any substance use. Therefore, early recognition of these disorders and proper interventions may decrease the risk of developing a substance abuse disorder. However, depressive symptoms occurred one year after the onset of alcohol abuse, but two years before the onset of smoking. The latter information may indicate that some untreated psychiatric disorders may be risks for the development of substance abuse, whereas other psychiatric disorders may be more likely to follow the use of substances.

Mood disorders and conduct disorders

Although ADHD, major depression, and conduct disorder may be important components of substance dependence, depression may be the primary variable related to substance use disorder in women (Whitmore *et al.*, 1997).

Although girls are more likely to have internalizing disorders, a study by Couwenbergh *et al.* (2006) has shown that externalizing disorders, especially in boys were consistently linked to SUD in treatment-seeking adolescents. Those with conduct disorders had a higher risk of ending up in a juvenile justice system. However, depression in boys may be linked to earlier onset of conduct disorder. In a study of adolescent deviant boys with conduct disorder and co-morbid substance abuse reported by Riggs and Whitmore (1999), depressed boys were more likely to have ADHD, posttraumatic stress disorder (PTSD), anxiety disorder, and an earlier onset of conduct disorder when compared to non-depressed boys. In this same study, the depressive symptoms did not seem to be relieved after four weeks of abstinence.

Rao *et al.* (2000) identified a unique feature of girls with conduct disorder, substance use disorder (SUD), and depression. These girls had more anxiety disorders and elevated cortisol near sleep onset (when the hypothalamic-pituitary system is expected to be more active) than depressed girls without SUD. It is felt that the use of alcohol and/or stress in these girls may be the reason why cortisol levels are much higher than in girls with conduct disorder and depression alone. The role that this may play in treatment, if any, is unclear at this time.

One study has examined the risk of SUD independent of the diagnosis of conduct disorder in late onset bipolar disorder. Tim Wilens *et al.* (1999) has reported that those with adolescent-onset bipolar disorder had an 8.8 times greater risk of developing SUD than those with childhood-onset bipolar disorder. No other disorder, including conduct disorder, accounted for the risk.

Anxiety disorders

Teachers and clinicians will often not recognize children with social phobia because they do not necessarily present with behavioral problems. However, those who are recognized due to their aggressiveness should also be evaluated for shyness. In one study by Neil Swan (1995), the combination of shyness and aggressiveness in boys was a more valid predictor of future cocaine use than a history of aggressiveness alone.

One study of juvenile justice adolescents noted that 11 percent of juvenile detainees met criteria for PTSD, and that more than half had witnessed violence that precipitated their trauma (Abram, 2004). Two direct relationships have been found between childhood trauma and exposure, and adult criminal behavior in women. Having been in foster care or adopted was positively related to engaging in sex associated with prostitution. However, early experiences of traumatic events (e.g., death of a close relative, serious accidents) were related to engaging in violent crime. For African American as well as Caucasian women offenders, childhood traumatic events were related to the development of adolescent substance abuse (Grella, Stein & Greenwell, 2005).

ADHD

It is well recognized that ADHD with conduct disorder has a much greater risk for developing substance abuse than ADHD alone. In fact, in a twin study done by Elizabeth Disney *et al.* (1997) of 626 pairs of 17-year-old twins, ADHD did not increase the risk for substance abuse unless it was associated with a co-occurring conduct disorder. Wilens *et al.* (1999) has shown that untreated ADHD has more risk for future substance abuse than ADHD that is treated. If an adolescent has ADHD and is not treated, the risk of developing substance use disorder is two times higher than those who have ADHD and were treated with stimulants.

Schizophrenia

In a study by Hambrecht and Hafner (2000), a vulnerability hypothesis was constructed to help explain the frequent use of marijuana in patients with schizophrenia. This vulnerability hypothesis was divided into three groups. Frequent use in Group 1 may have decreased the threshold for the appearance of schizophrenia, since they had used for several years before the onset of the disorder. Group 2 may be made up of a vulnerable group in which the dopaminergic stress factor may precipitate the onset of schizophrenia. This group developed the onset of schizophrenia in the same month they began to use marijuana. Group 3 may use marijuana to self medicate, since they developed the onset of marijuana abuse after the onset of the schizophrenia. This vulnerability hypothesis may explain the effects that other substances of abuse may have on the developing brain and how other psychiatric disorders and/or learning disorders may emerge or interplay with drugs of abuse. More research is needed in regard to this hypothesis.

About one percent of the juvenile justice system has psychosis (Teplin, 2002).

Suicide

David Brent *et al.* (1987) revealed that completed suicide among 10- to 19-year-olds was 4.9 times more likely to have occurred while drinking. Besides active substance use disorder, other risk factors for suicide completers, as shown by Bukstein *et al.* (1993), include co-morbid major depression or affective illness, suicidal ideation within the past week, family history of depression and substance abuse, legal issues, and the presence of a handgun in the home. In a study of suicide risk in juvenile justice youth during intake (Wasserman & MacReynolds, 2006), while more girls reported recent attempts regardless of depression, depressed boys' attempt risk was as high as the girls. Depression contributed to attempt history more than substance abuse disorders did.

Among Australian young offenders, younger admission age to the juvenile justice system, repeat admissions, and drug offences predicted earlier death. The mortality rate was 7.2 deaths per 10 000 person-years of observations (Coffey *et al.*, 2004).

Learning disorders

Academic failure and low commitment to school are other psychobehavioral factors associated with drug use during childhood and adolescence. Beyond early onset of use, poor academic achievement, poor social skills and competence, teaming disorders, and poor self-esteem were found to be related to drug abuse. Hyman Hops *et al.* (1999) found that substance abuse at age 14 or 15 could be predicted by academic and social behavior between the ages of 7 and 9.

In a 2002 report on the California Juvenile Justice system, a pathway was described that denotes how children, beginning in the school system, are identified with risk factors, but fail to receive an appropriate comprehensive evaluation that might prevent entrance into the juvenile justice system (Hartney *et al.*, 2002). First, the child may be identified as having a mental health need at age five by a teacher. A referral is made to special education by age seven. The child may interact with the mental health and child welfare services by age nine, and inpatient hospitalization may occur by age 12. The pathway ends by entrance into the juvenile justice system by age 14. Windows of opportunities for proper evaluation and intervention are missed along the way. For instance, before a referral to special education occurs, an evaluation for psychiatric disorders may not occur or learning difficulties like dyslexia may not be identified. In fact, in a study that looked at young offenders and dyslexia, 50 percent were dyslexic (Kirk & Reid, 2001).

Developmental neurobiological and genetic risks for substance abuse

In order to examine why substance abuse may occur in offenders, it is important to examine what developmental neurobiological and genetic risks can increase the development of substance abuse in anyone. There are two important factors to consider: genetic factors and developmental factors.

Genetic factors and the neurobiology of addiction

Adoptive studies have shown that genetic susceptibility seemed to be a stronger predictor of risk for substance abuse than exposure to adoptive parents using substances. However, both genetic and environmental influences may be correlated to substance initiation, whereas progression to substance abuse and dependence may be more related to genetic factors alone. In adoption studies conducted by Kenneth Kendler (1998a, 1998b), 485 monozygotic and 335 dizygotic female twins demonstrated that cannabis use was influenced by genetic and familial environmental factors, whereas cannabis abuse and dependence were solely related to genetic factors. This was also true for cocaine use versus abuse and dependence. Marc Schuckit (Schuckit 1999; Schuckit et al., 2004) has shown greater tolerance in children of alcoholics. In his study, children of alcoholics had to use greater proportions of alcohol before the reflex response to a stimulus was delayed to the same degree found in responses of children of non-alcoholics. In children of non-alcoholics, reflex response to a stimulus was delayed to the same degree on lower proportions of alcohol. This diminished response to alcohol was also measured by subjective feelings, levels of body sway, electrophysiological functioning, and change in three hormones.

The number of dopamine receptors genetically inherited may play another role in genetic vulnerability. Nora Volkow has noted that an increase in dopamine increases the magnitude of the effect from pleasurable experiences and directs the brain to things that are salient and pleasurable. However, an increase in dopamine can decrease the number of postsynaptic receptors, thereby causing natural reinforcers to no longer be salient. However, during these circumstances, although natural reinforcers may not be salient, drugs are (Volkow et al., 2002c). Volkow has shown that people with increased D2 receptors, when given cocaine, have an aversive reaction to cocaine. When Volkow increased D2 receptors in mice (by using an adenovirus), alcohol consumption by the mice decreased by 70 percent (Volkow et al., 2002b). Therefore, people born with an increase in D2 receptors may be at less risk to develop substance abuse, and those who inherit a decrease in D2 receptors may be more vulnerable.

The role of D2 receptors may also influence compulsion, according to Volkow. When D2 receptors are decreased in the nucleus accumbens, there is a corresponding decrease in metabolism in the orbital frontal gyrus and the cingulate gyrus. The cingulate gyrus initiates the ability to restrain control, and the orbital frontal gyrus shifts attention to what is salient. If the orbital frontal gyrus is destroyed, Volkow believes the drug abuser will continue to use drugs, even if using them is no longer pleasurable. Therefore, if decreased D2 receptors decrease the metabolism in the cingulate gyrus (so it can no longer inhibit the drive to use drugs) and the orbital frontal gyrus (so that it continues to compulsively use drugs even though it is no longer pleasurable to do so), a person who has inherited decreased D2 receptors would be at more risk for developing substance abuse (Volkow et al., 2002a). Couple the decreased D2 receptors with the changes that occur in the motivational circuitry during adolescence and it becomes clear why exposure to substances of abuse during adolescence may increase the risk for developing substance abuse.

The genetic and neurobiological explanations of addiction are, in many ways, early in the stages of research. Much more research is needed (especially in helping clinicians to use preventative and pharmacological interventions) to prevent and treat substance abuse.

Developmental factors

Age of exposure to substances of abuse, age of exposure to stimulants for the treatment of ADHD, age of exposure to interventions for learning disorders, academic failure, temperament, and neurobiological changes that occur during adolescence may all play a role in increasing the risk for substance abuse.

Age of exposure to substances of abuse

Early use is a risk factor likely to influence the onset of substance use during childhood and adolescence. Children and adolescents who began drinking at an early age – 11–12 years of age – had a higher percentage probability of meeting the revised third edition of the Diagnostic and Statistical Manual of Mental Disorders (DSM-III-R) criteria for substance abuse (13.5 percent) and substance dependence (15.9 percent) compared to those who began drinking at age 13 or 14 (13.7 and 9.0 percent, respectively). Those who started to drink at age 19 or 20 had rates of 2 and 1 percent, respectively (DeWitt et al., 2000; Kandel et al., 1992). Importantly, rapid progression of alcohol and drug disorders occurred most often with earlier age of onset and increased frequency, rather than duration of use. Those individuals with earlier onset had a shorter time span from first exposure to dependence than did an adult-onset group (Clark et al., 1998). Age of onset of heavy drinking also predicted alcohol-related problems (Lee & DeClemente, 1985). Early age of onset also predicted higher risks for the abuse of other substances. Adolescent-onset adults had higher lifetime rates of cannabis and hallucinogen use disorders, shorter times between the development of their first and second dependence diagnosis, and higher rates of disruptive behaviors and major depression (Clark et al., 1998).

Early use of substances has been found in juvenile offenders as well. In a study that examined early substance initiation in childhood as reported by juvenile offenders, a majority of males and females reported using at least one substance (other than cigarettes) such as alcohol, marijuana, or inhalants by age 13. Thirty-two percent of males and 39 percent of females reported drinking alcoholic beverages at a frequency of several times per month or higher by age 13 (Prinz & Kerns, 2003).

As noted, Wilens et al. (1999) has shown that treatment with stimulants for ADHD reduces the risk for future substances abuse. Reasons for this may be explained by research done by Castellanos (2002). Castellanos reviewed total cerebral volume of treated and untreated adolescents with ADHD. Total white matter in the unmedicated ADHD adolescents was lower than medicated and normals. It is hypothesized that perhaps the trophic effect on myelination, dendritic branching, and length of spines in the treated ADHD youth was somehow protective. The use of diffusion-tensor magnetic resonance imaging (MRI) has indicated that increases in white matter in the temporal-parietal area (responsible for reading ability) was related to increased reading performance (Beaulieu *et al.*, 2005). Luna (Luna & Sweeney, 2004) has shown that a normal process that occurs during adolescence is an increase in myelination. The effect is an increase in processing speed. Therefore, the lack of myelination may decrease reading performance and/or processing speed, and these effects may increase the risk for substance abuse associated with poor academic success.

Age of exposure to interventions for learning disorders

Given that up to 50 percent of juvenile justice offenders will have some form of dyslexia, early intervention is extremely important. The timing of the intervention may be crucial. Wright (2004) has suggested that processing problems associated with language impairment, dyslexia, and auditory processing problems are developmental delays that if not corrected before age ten, will become permanent during adolescence. Therefore, if these disorders are not detected and intervened upon at the appropriate time, a window of opportunity may be lost.

Dyslexia can be confused with ADD/ADHD and therefore may be undetected unless actively looked for. For instance, phonologic dyslexia is associated with auditory processing problems. Simkin and Graves (2001) tested ADD/ADHD children who had responded well to stimulants in elementary school who began to struggle in Middle or High School. Of those tested, 77 children had ADD/ADHD alone or ADD/ADHD with a co-morbid anxiety and/or depression, which were well controlled for. Of these children, the average intelligence quotient (IQ) was 122. Ninety-two percent were found to have an auditory processing problem, 70 percent had a processing speed problem (on the cognitive battery of the Woodcock Johnson-III), and 87 percent had a disorder of written expression (on the Woodcock Johnson-III). This is extremely important since ADD/ADHD can be confused with processing problems. Tapert *et al.* (2002) found that adolescents with attention difficulties predicted substance abuse and dependency eight years later. This study controlled for substance involvement, education, conduct disorder, family history of substance abuse, and learning disorders. The attention difficulties were not necessarily related to ADD/ADHD. Perhaps the attention problems are related to undetected processing problems. Stimulants may help ADD/ADHD but should learning disorders be detected, accommodations must be made in order to ensure continued success. Early detection of processing problems should occur whenever any child has difficulties with reading in order to prevent the risk of developing substance abuse problems and involvement with the juvenile justice system.

Academic failure

Any academic failure and low commitment to school are other psychobehavioral factors associated with influencing drug use during childhood and adolescence. Beyond early onset of use, poor academic achievement, poor social skills and competence, teaming disorders, and poor self-esteem were found to be related to drug abuse (Scheier *et al.*, 1999; Stacy *et al.*, 1993). Hyman Hops *et al.* (1999) found that substance abuse at age 14 or 15 could be predicted by academic and social behavior between the ages of 7 to 9.

Temperament

Temperament may explain why some adults continue to demonstrate characteristics of dependence. Both C. Robert Cloninger and Thomas Babor identified personality traits consistent with those who have poorer prognoses (Cloniger *et al.*, 1985; Babor *et al.*, 1992). Cloninger's type 2 and Babor's type B alcoholics share common characteristics: early onset of spontaneous alcohol-seeking behavior; diagnosis during adolescence; rapid course of onset; genetic precursors that put them at risk to develop substance abuse; severe symptoms of deviant behavior, including fighting and arrests when drinking; and greater psychological vulnerability. Cloninger's type 2 and Babor's type B alcoholics may be related to youth who are thought to have conduct disorder. The conduct disorder is thought to be related to genetic vulnerability and such negative environmental factors as poverty, parental neglect, marital discord, parental illness, and/or parental alcoholism. The disorder is also believed to be associated with an impairment in frontal lobe activity, which affects the ability to plan, to avoid harm, and to learn from negative consequences – traits often found in type 2 or type B alcoholics.

Adolescent neurobiological changes that increase the risk for substance abuse

J. Andrew Chambers *et al.* (2003) reviewed changes influencing the motivation circuitry in the brain that occurs during adolescence. Three important events occur. First, in simple terms, hormones may influence the motivational circuitry by increasing the sensitivity to experiences that are pleasurable, by impacting dopamine discharge into the nucleus accumbens, or by direct influences on neuronal activity of the accumbens. Hence, pleasurable experiences may become more pleasurable. Second, serotonin receptors are pruned during adolescence, which causes increases in impulsivity. And third, the frontal cortex, which is responsible for inhibiting motivational drives, is immature during adolescence. Taken together, during adolescence, the brain may be more developmentally vulnerable to seek out motivational drives for novel experiences, have less ability to inhibit these motivational drives, and be more likely to impulsively seek out pleasurable and risky behaviors, including experimentation with and abusive use of addictive drugs. Therefore, adolescents may be at more risk for the development of substance abuse, especially those who have had little academic or athletic success. These adolescents may be more at risk to seek out ways to feel empowered, such as experimenting with substances of abuse.

Assessment and treatment

Assessment

The assessment of substance use should include the stage of use in which the adolescent is actively engaged. Knight (1997) has described the stages as follows: primary abstinence (never used); experimentation; regular use; problem use (negative consequences associated with use); abuse (continued use despite harm, preoccupation, and loss of control); dependency (withdrawal and tolerance); and secondary abstinence (recovery and treatment). Physical withdrawal is not as common in adolescents as it is in adults. To add to this, DSM-IV describes abuse as continued use despite negative consequences, and dependency as continued use despite adverse consequences, loss of control, and preoccupation with using substances. Therefore, another way to describe these stages may be as follows:

Primary abstinence – never used

Experimentation – use with peers in a social context usually out of curiosity, due to peer pressure, and/or to "fit in"

Regular use or social use (Nowinski, 1990) – usually in the context of peer acceptance and on a regular basis in social situations

Problem use, misuse, or instrumental use (Nowinski, 1990) – either:

Compensatory use – use to relieve a negative mood, affect or disposition, such as shyness or sadness, or

Hedonistic use – use to discover ways to feel good or to experience something new

Abuse – continued use despite adverse consequences. Whereas with problem use the adolescent may not notice any change in mood when not using different from pre-experimentation, with abuse the adolescent does not feel "normal" when not using. Daily use may begin and the adolescent may change from non-using friends to only those that do use. Tolerance becomes worse and the adolescent cannot imagine being without the drug. A pre-use depression will worsen or a secondary depression may develop wherein the adolescent feels only anhedonia when not using. Girls may have drug dealers as boyfriends in order to obtain drugs more readily, or they may exchange sex for drugs. Boys may sell drugs or steal in order to be able to continue to buy their own drugs (Nowinski, 1990)

Dependence or addiction – continued use despite adverse consequences, loss of control, and compulsion to use.

When discussing drug use in adolescents, one should be aware that the use of rationalization during the problem use stage might be a key to further progression to higher stages. For instance, adolescents who see no direct relationship between the first negative consequences associated with substance use are likely to continue despite adverse consequences, or to move into the stage of abuse. An example of rationalization would be when an adolescent has not eaten all day, drinks, and vomits on his/her friend's carpet. The adolescent rationalizes that he/she vomited due to drinking on an empty stomach, rather than recognizing the direct correlation between drinking and getting sick.

Examples of behavior in adolescents that would signal abuse would be: motor vehicle accidents while driving; declining grades; truancy; deteriorating or poor performance in previous favorite activities such as sports; disapproval of use by non-using friends; engagement in activities that may not have happened had the adolescent not been intoxicated, such as fights or non-consensual or unprotected sex; arrests; running away from home; suspension from school; change to friends who use; and/or change in music or clothes. These behaviors signal abuse, since the adolescent continues to use despite these adverse consequences.

Dependency would involve a compulsion to use, which results in a worsening of the above problems and resorting to any lengths in order to continue to use. Adolescents with substance dependence are preoccupied with only one goal – to continue to use. Dependence would involve tolerance, because this becomes the driving force behind compulsively using more to get the same effects. Of course, for those who do experience withdrawal, the diagnosis of dependency would apply, but withdrawal would not be necessary to fit the criteria of dependency, especially in adolescents.

Knight (1997) has also described an intervention for each of these stages, as follows. For primary abstinence, positive reinforcement and intervention for risk factors that could lead to abuse would be appropriate. For regular use, risk reduction could be used. For problem use, the adolescent can be given the chance to prove there is no problem by agreeing to remain abstinent, or by agreeing to a trial of a controlled use if he/she refuses to abstain. For abuse and dependence, treatment matched interventions should be used. For secondary abstinence, support, reinforcement, and relapse prevention should be used.

Awareness of risks factors and assessment of the adolescent and family through the use of a thorough biopsychosocial evaluation (bio = individual or familial psychiatric or medical risk factors, and level and severity of the disorder; psycho = learning disorders or other impediments to educational success, coping skills, and emotional stability; and social = environmental risk factors, such as family chaos or cohesiveness, peer involvement, family support, abuse or neglect, and financial or environmental stress). Using appropriate evaluation tools, which will be discussed later, these risks factors may be targeted initially and throughout the course of treatment, so that future substance use and relapse might be reduced.

Once the stage of use is determined, the process of determining the stage of readiness to change or motivation for treatment should be examined next. Prochaska and DiClemente (1982) described the stages of change, and Knight (1997) described the interventions for each of these stages as follows:

Precontemplation – In this stage, the task is to intervene by raising doubt and by increasing awareness of risks and problems.

Contemplation – In this stage, the adolescent makes excuses, refuses to quit, and will not consider making a change. The intervention is to work toward the acknowledgement of ambivalence, and to evoke reasons to change by comparing pre-use behaviors with present behaviors that are detrimental to the success of the adolescent.

Determination – In this stage, the adolescent is ambivalent about quitting, but is considering changing. The intervention is to help determine the best course of action.

Action – In this stage, the adolescent is ready for change. The intervention is to provide assistance in moving forward.

Maintenance – In this stage, the adolescent must maintain stability by staying away from activities involving drug use or peers that use. The intervention is to use relapse prevention strategies and positive reinforcement.

Relapse – Here the adolescent may relapse even when motivated to change. The intervention is to avoid demoralization, enhance movement back toward action, and assist in learning what triggered the adolescent to relapse so that the situation or the reaction to the situation can be avoided the next time it occurs.

The technique best used to implement these interventions is known as motivational enhancement therapy (MET) (Miller & Rollnick, 1991; Miller & Sanchez, 1994). This technique will be discussed in the section on treatment. However, this technique is a skill that is advantageous to use during the evaluation process in order to form an alliance with the adolescent; hence, treatment begins during the evaluation. Anyone can learn MET and in doing so will increase the possibility that the adolescent will be responsive to the technique.

Screening tools

Screening tools have been developed by several clinicians. However, none, as of this writing, have shown validity except for the Adolescent Drinking Inventory (ADI) (Harrell & Wirtz, 1989), and the CRAFFT (Knight *et al.*, 1999; 2002). The

ADI has 88 percent sensitivity and 82 percent specificity. A score of two or higher on the CRAFFT was optimal for identifying any problem use (sensitivity, 0.76; specificity, 0.94), any disorder (sensitivity, 0.80; specificity, 0.86), and dependence (sensitivity, 0.92; specificity, 0.80; positive predictive value, 0.25; negative predictive value, 0.99). Validity was not significantly affected by age, sex, or race. The CRAFFT questions are as follows:

C: Have you ever ridden in a car driven by someone (including yourself) who was "high" or had been using alcohol or drugs?

R: Do you ever use alcohol or drugs to relax, feel better about yourself, or to fit in?

A: Do you ever use alcohol/drugs while you are by yourself, alone?

F: Do your family or friends ever tell you that you should cut down on your drinking or drug use?

F: Do you ever forget things you did while using alcohol or drugs?

T: Have you gotten into trouble while you were using alcohol or drugs?

More comprehensive screens include: Drug Usage Screening Inventory – revised (DUSI), the Problem Oriented Screening Instrument for Teenagers (POSIT), and the Teen Addiction Severity Index. All of these comprehensive screens can be obtained in manual by Rahdert and Czechowicz (1995). Instead of screening for substance use alone as the CRAFFT does, each of these more comprehensive assessments screen for more risk domains that may be placing the adolescent at greater risk for substance abuse and relapse. For instance, the POSIT screens for the following ten domains: use/abuse, physical health, mental health, family relations, peer relations, educational status, vocational status, social skills, leisure/recreation, and aggressive behavior. It has 139 questions and takes about 20–30 minutes to complete. It should be pointed out that these screens must be followed by a much more comprehensive biopsychosocial evaluation and by other assessments that may be appropriate, such as educational testing.

The Massachusetts Youth Screening Instrument – second version (MAYSI-2) created by Grisso et al. (2001) is a screening instrument designed for the juvenile justice system and is designed to screen for substance abuse and mental disorders. It has seven domains that include: alcohol/drugs; anger; depression and anxiety; somatic complaints; suicidal ideation; thought disturbances; and traumatic experiences.

Levels of care

Once the evaluation is complete, treatment recommendation can be made at different levels of care. These levels of care include outpatient counseling, intensive outpatient care, partial or day treatment, intensive acute care, and residential treatment. Respite and wrap around services may be incorporated in these levels. An instrument that can be used to determine the level of care needed has been developed by Fallon (2000) and has inter-rater reliability and face validity. It is called the Child and Adolescent Levels of Care Utilization Services (CALOCUS). The instrument has six dimensions, which include: risk of harm; functional status; co-morbidity including medical, substance abuse, developmental disability and psychiatric diagnosis; recovery environment, including stress and support; resiliency and treatment history; and acceptance and engagement of the child and parents.

The levels of care that may be utilized are:

Level 0 – basic services (prevention and health maintenance)

Level 1 – recovery maintenance and health management (for those stepping down from higher levels)

Level 2 – outpatient services (once/week visits)

Level 3 – intensive outpatient services (two or more sessions/week)

Level 4 – intensive integrated services without 24-hour medical monitoring (day treatment, partial hospitalization, or "wrap around services")

Level 5 – non-secure, 24-hour, medically monitored services (group homes, foster care or residential facility, or very intensive "wrap around services")

Level 6 – secure, 24-hour medically managed services (inpatient psychiatric or highly programmed residential facilities, or "wrap around" with security measures)

The instrument, the CALOCUS, compared to the American Society of Addiction Medicine Adolescent Patient Placement Criteria, is much more user friendly, has reliability, and the levels of care indicated are applicable to services available in both the private and public sectors.

Treatment

Youth who come in contact with police may be better served in a healthcare system than a juvenile justice system. In a study by Feeney *et al.* (2005), the General Health Questionnaire (GHQ-28) was administered to young cannabis users who had a criminal record after being diverted to a treatment hospital and drug service. Sixty percent of these participants were substance dependent. As compared to normative data, these participants had significantly higher levels of anxiety, somatic concerns, social dysfunction, and depression. These high levels of psychopathology suggest that these youth may be better served in a healthcare system, where they would be more accurately assessed for treatment. In fact, youth placed in a modified therapeutic environment, with the juvenile justice system separated from treatment, demonstrated better outcomes.

In data collected over a five-year period (Jainchill *et al.*, 2005), youth in a Recovery House program, designed as above, were polysubstance users whose primary substance was marijuana, and whose secondary substance was alcohol. The sample yielded multiple psychiatric disorders, with conduct disorder being the most prevalent. Post-treatment drug use was infrequent, and there were reductions in the percentage reporting criminal involvement. Although females were less likely to complete treatment, their post-treatment outcomes were better.

Motivation enhancement therapy

Motivation is a major factor in determining success with incarcerated substance-abusing youth. Slavet *et al.* (2006) have shown that increased motivation had a positive correlation with treatment engagement and a negative correlation with substance use.

As noted under assessment, motivational enhancement therapy (MET) can be used during the initial evaluation. This technique helps to create an alliance between the clinician and the patient. The five parts of motivational enhancement therapy are referred to as FRAMES and include:

Feedback on personal risk

Emphasis on personal **R**esponsibility to change

Clear **A**dvice to change

A **M**enu of change options or treatment options

Empathy as an intervention approach

Self-efficacy (Miller & Sanchez, 1994; Miller & Rollnick, 1991)

During the evaluation and intervention, feedback may include comparisons between prior high functioning behavior and behaviors that have resulted in impairments in school work or personal relationships, injury, and trouble with the law, and the impact of these behaviors on future goals. Issues concerning responsibility include recognizing that only the individual can decide whether to get help. If the patient decides to enter treatment, it should be noted that everyone would be there to support him/her. Menu options can include the suggestions discussed under assessments, which included a method of intervention for each stage of use. It should also include a list of treatment options. These options can be determined by using the CALOCUS as discussed above. Empathy requires the clinician to avoid anger and confrontation, to include statements of hope, and to emphasize that the patient has the strength to recover.

Brief motivational treatment has been studied in regard to adolescent smoking (Monti *et al.*, 1998). In this study, over two-thirds of the teens reported significant reductions in smoking rate and dependence. The stage of change predicted subsequent smoking outcomes. A higher stage of change predicted higher serious quit attempts and longer duration of abstinence from cigarette smoking.

Motivational enhancement therapy has been incorporated into Jaffe's workbook on the first five steps based on a twelve-step program. This is discussed under 12 step treatment approaches.

Family therapy

There are three types of family therapy that have been found to be helpful in the treatment of adolescent substance abusers and their families (Riggs & Whitmore, 1999). The three types are: behavioral therapy; family systems therapy; and multiple systems therapy.

An approach used in family systems therapy is called structural-strategic therapy (Stanton *et al.*, 1982). This therapy is problem focused. Insight is not needed to do this therapy, wherein it is felt that problems arise from unclear boundaries. Substance abuse is seen as a maladaptive behavior in response to a dysfunctional family.

Functional family therapy employs structural-strategic techniques, as well as behavioral and cognitive interventions directed at the substance-abusing adolescent (Alexander & Parsons, 1982). Functional family therapy is one of three types of multiple systems therapy approaches using the above combined techniques. The other two include multisystemic therapy (Henggeler *et al.*, 2002) and multidimensional family therapy (Liddle & Hogue, 2000). Multidimensional therapy, when compared to adolescent group therapy and a family educational group showed more consistent improvements (Liddle *et al.*, 2001). In a four-year outcome study using multisystemic therapy (MST), treatment completion (98 percent), school attendance, and cost savings were all positive. However, criminal behavior, substance abuse, and mental health functioning did not demonstrate the significant effects MST had shown in previous randomized trials where the juvenile offenders did not have substance abuse (Henggeler *et al.*, 2002). Henggeler and Randall feel that increased emphasis on treatment integrity and focusing on drug use may improve these findings.

In a more recent review of MST with community services (MST/CS), CS alone, drug court (DC), family court (FC), DC/MST/CS, and DC/MST the following was observed. Drug court was more effective in decreasing alcohol and drug use in juvenile justice offenders than FC. Drug court/multisystemic therapy was slightly more effective than DC, and DC/MST/ CS was slightly more effective than DC/ MST. Self report of status offenses and crimes were decreased more in DC/MST/ CS and DC/MST than FC. However, arrest data showed no between-group differences. Drug court/multisystemic therapy/community services and DC/MST experienced a more rapid decrease than did FC and DC alone (Henggeler *et al.*, 2006). Combining therapies does seem to be a more effective way of reducing substance abuse, but more needs to be done to target behaviors that lead to further arrests.

Behavioral therapy employs the use of parent management techniques. Here, only the parents are seen in therapy and are taught such things as contingency contracting and reinforcement.

Cognitive behavioral therapy

Cognitive behavioral therapy (CBT) focused either at the individual level (Waldron, 1998) or at the group level (Kaminer, 1994) has been used with adolescent substance abusers. Waldron and Kaminer have incorporated motivational enhancement techniques into these approaches.

Waldron (1998) uses functional analysis, to target substance use or non-use, and relapse. For each of these domains, the adolescent is focused on the antecedents (internal and external triggers) as well as the positive and negative consequences (short term and long term) of use, non-use, or relapse. Waldron also incorporates such CBT interventions as: anger management, techniques for coping with urges and cravings to use, communication, drug-refusal, and problem-solving skills, into the individual sessions.

Kaminer has developed 12 CBT group sessions targeting relapse prevention. A three-month follow-up comparing the use of interactional therapy (which focuses on interpersonal relationships, self-care, affect, and self-esteem) demonstrated a significant reduction in severity of substance use compared to interactional therapy (Kaminer et al., (1998). Kaminer has also developed CBT for the treatment of cannabis abuse. In this model, the first two sessions involve MET and the next ten involve group CBT. The CBT sessions include such things as: alcohol and drug refusal skills; coping with cravings; managing thoughts about use; coping with negative moods; problem solving; emergency preparation; awareness and management of negative thinking; enhancement of support systems; anger management; and development of skills for handling criticism (Kaminer, 1998).

Comparisons were also made between cognitive behavior treatment (CBT) and psychoeducational treatment (PET). On three-month follow-up, adolescents who were in the CBT group improved on severity of peer problems, as compared to adolescents in the PET group. A trend toward improvement on the drug and alcohol severity measures was observed for adolescents in the PET group (Kaminer, 1999).

The use of contingency management MET and CBT has been positive. Carroll et al. (2006) randomized marijuana dependent youth to one of four treatment modalities: MET/CBT, MET/CBT with incentives contingent on session attendance and submission of marijuana-free urine specimens (CM), individual drug counseling (DC) and CM, and DC without CM. There was a significant main effect of CM on treatment retention and marijuana-free urine specimens. The combination of MET/CBT plus CM was significantly more effective than MET/CBT without CM, or DC with CM, as measured by treatment attendance and percentage of marijuana-free urine specimens. Participants assigned to MET/CBT continued to reduce the frequency of their marijuana use through six-month follow-up.

Individual behavior therapy

Behavioral therapy involves stimulus control, which helps adolescents to avoid triggers of substance use and to replace these activities with activities that don't involve substance use; urge-control, which helps adolescents to recognize and change thoughts, feelings, and plans that lead to substance use; and social-control, which involves family members and/or influential people who can help the adolescent avoid drugs. Azrin *et al.* (1996) demonstrated that when supportive therapy was compared to behavioral therapy, more favorable results occurred with behavioral therapy. Results were especially favorable if family members were involved, and if drug abstinence was rewarded after each negative urine analysis. At six months, 73 percent of the adolescents participating in the behavioral program were abstinent compared to 7 percent in the supportive therapy.

12 steps

There has been little research to demonstrate the effectiveness of 12 step programs. Two studies have looked at 12 step programs in connection with adolescents. Alford *et al.* (1991) followed adolescents for two years while in 12 step-based inpatient treatment or halfway houses. Follow-up occurred at 6, 12, and 24 months.

At six months, 71 percent of boys and 79 percent of girls who completed the program were abstinent, while 37 percent of girl and 30 percent of boy non-completers were abstinent. Forty-five percent of completers and abstinent youth had successful functioning in school, while this was true for only 25 percent of non-completers.

At 12 months, the abstinence rates for boys who completed the program fell to 48 percent and increased for non-completers to 44 percent. For girl completers, there was a small decrease in abstinence to 70 percent, and for girl non-completers it fell to 28 percent. Twenty-nine percent of completers and abstinent youth were functioning well, while 18 percent of non-completers were functioning well.

At 24 months, non-completer and completer boys showed no difference in abstinence – 30 percent vs. 40 percent. Girl completers fell slightly to 61 percent and non-completers to 27 percent. Regardless of program completion status, 72 percent of those who did not use at 24 months were functioning well. Only 33 percent of those who used intermittently, and 37 percent of those who used frequently were socially adaptive.

By two years, 84 percent of high frequency Alcoholics Anonymous/Narcotics Anonymous (AA/NA) attendees were abstinent or essentially abstinent.

Therefore, in this study, girls who completed the program, and high frequency attendees, had the best chance of recovery. The percentage of abstinent/essentially abstinent male and female completers at six months was greater than the number of abstinent/essentially abstinent at one or two years. Abstinence rates decreased more for boys than girls. This emphasizes the need for targeting relapse prevention, especially in males.

In another study, the acceptance of 12 step ideology (including frequent and lifelong attendance, and a need to "surrender" to a higher power) was a significant predictor of weekly or more frequent attendance at 12 step meetings (Fiorentine & Milhouse, 2000). This acceptance of ideology may predict frequent attendance and, thus, a better chance for recovery.

In another study, 142 adolescents (ages 12–18) were followed at 6, 12, and 24 months in a 12 step program. Teens with less drug and alcohol use post-treatment improved in their functioning emotionally, interpersonally with families, and in school, work, and recreational activities. Abstainers displayed the best psychosocial functioning. Those who returned to substance abuse and those who became more severe with use accounted for the majority of dropouts (Brown, 1993). This concurs with the above Alford et al. study that demonstrated that abstinent teens had the best psychosocial functioning. Therefore complete abstinence would be a better goal for adolescents in treatment programs.

Jaffe (1990) has developed a workbook for adolescents using the first five steps. In a revision of the workbook in 2001, he incorporated MET into these steps. Simkin has written about the psychodynamics of 12 steps from a developmental prospective for adolescents, and Jaffe has summarized his approach for the first five steps (Jaffe & Simkin, 2002).

Treatment accountability and safer communities program

Research shows that relapse to drug use and recidivism to crime are significantly lower if the drug offender remains in treatment. Combining criminal justice sanctions with treatment can be effective in decreasing drug use and related crime. The Treatment Accountability and Safer Communities (TASC) program provides an alternative to detention. The key features of TASC involve: (1) coordination of criminal justice and drug treatment; (2) early identification, assessment and referral of drug-involved offenders; (3) monitoring offenders through drug testing; and (4) use of legal sanctions as inducement to remain in treatment. A judge can order these services for first time offenders in drug court (Inciardi et al., 1997).

Psychopharmacology

The most commonly asked question is whether to treat adolescents with stimulants if they have a co-occurring substance abuse problem. Both wellbutrin and cylert have been found to be effective in treating ADHD (Riggs et al., 1996; 1998). However, liver complications may make the use of cylert less attractive.

Venlafaxine is helpful in the treatment of co-morbid alcohol/cocaine abuse and ADHD in adults, but has not been studied in adolescents (Upadhyaya *et al.*, 2001). Attention-deficit/hyperactivity disorder with tics can be treated with nortriptyline or guanfacine. In a comparison of methylphenidate and atomoxetine (a norepinephrine re-uptake inhibitor) in the treatment of ADHD, both drugs were associated with marked improvement and no statistical difference was found (Kratochvil *et al.*, 2002).

When considering whether to treat a known substance-abusing adolescent with a stimulant, the clinician should clarify with the adolescent that use of a stimulant cannot occur until she or he is ready to enter a treatment agreement. Even then, it may be wise to treat the adolescent with a drug that has no real abuse potential. Treating someone with ADHD early on in development is very different from treating someone with a history of substance abuse and ADHD as an adolescent. Treating an adolescent with a recent history of substance abuse with stimulants for ADHD may not allow the system to revert to normal. In humans, methamphetamine damage caused to dopamine transporters, with consequent reduction of motor and cognitive skills, did not recover until nine months after abstinence occurred (Volkow, 2001a; 2001b). The time it takes for the mesolimbic system to recover for each substance of abuse is unclear. Until such recovery it may be better to treat ADHD substance abusers with such substances as atomoxetine, buproprion, tenex, and effexor. Stimulants may be reserved for sub-clinical treatment, after at least 6–12 months of sobriety.

Although, modafinil has been shown to be effective in children in the treatment of ADHD in an open-label trial (Rugino & Copley, 2001), it has been shown to possess weak reinforcing effects in drug experienced individuals (Jasinski, 2000). However, it is not easily abused because its low water solubility is not compatible with intravenous injection, it is broken down by increased temperature and therefore can't be smoked, and it does not break down to a drug of abuse.

Atomoxetine has been compared to methylphenidate in light drug users. At higher doses (90 mg) atomoxetine seemed to cause aversive effects, whereas, at higher doses of methylphenidate, subjects produced higher scores on tests that measured the desirable effect of the drug. Therefore, atomoxetine would not seem to have the abuse liability of methylphenidate (Heil *et al.*, 2002).

Most early onset bipolar patients are more likely to have rapid cycling. Valproate is usually the treatment of choice for rapid cycling. However, for adolescents with bipolar disorder and secondary SUD, a double blind and placebo-controlled study of lithium not only alleviated the symptoms of the bipolar disorder, but also decreased the use of alcohol (Geller *et al.*, 1998). Lithium increases serotonin levels and seems to be associated with a decreased risk for suicide (Baldessarini *et al.*, 2001). Important research is needed to determine if lithium treats bipolar effectively, decreases the intake of alcohol, and decreases the risk of suicide, solely due to increasing levels of serotonin during lithium treatment.

For early onset alcoholics, (less than 25 years of age) odansetron in combination with cognitive behavior therapy reduced alcohol cravings. In this study, a reduction of plasma carbohydrate-deficient transferrin, a biochemical marker, was associated with decreased drinking. Platelet analysis was used to identify different serotonin transporter functions in alcoholic subgroups. Odansetron (an antinausea medication) was thought to work by correcting a serotonin imbalance. A dose of 4 µg/kg resulted in the best response. Johnson (2002) reported that the response in this subgroup indicated that these individuals were genetically predisposed, with a strong family history of alcoholism. They started using earlier and had a more severe course than late onset alcoholics who did not respond to the drug odansetron. Dr. Johnson feels that early-onset alcoholics may differ from late-onset in that their disease may be due to complex interactions between serotonin, glutamate, and opioids rather than just a serotonin deficiency. Alcohol interacts with all three of these receptors at the nucleus accumbens.

Fluoxentine has been shown to effectively treat drug dependent delinquents with depression (Riggs et al., 1997). However, other selective serotonin re-uptake inhibitors may be equally effective since a serotonin imbalance is suspected to play a role in SUD and depression.

Research on drugs that have been used to ward off withdrawal effects, or used to prevent further use, have been limited in adolescents. In regards to aversion therapy, one case study of naltrexone has been reported as helpful in a 17-year-old alcoholic male (Wold & Kaminer, 1997). There is no research on the use of mecamlamine for smoking cessation, nor on the use of acupuncture for cocaine withdrawal in adolescents.

The use of bupropion in a case report for an adult with amphetamine withdrawal, relieved symptoms of withdrawal in two to three days after starting bupropion SR 150 mg per day (Chan-Ob et al., 2001). The sensitization to cocaine has been reversed in rats using a D-class agonist, and an NMDA antagonist and a D2 agonist. The latter combination consisted of pergolide and memantine, which is approved for human use, and the effect continued for two weeks after cessation of the drugs (Li et al., 2000). It is hoped that research may be able to discern means of reversing the effects of repeated cocaine abuse.

Proper psychopharmacological interventions should be made for psychiatric disorders. If one drug has not been found to be effective, another untreated psychiatric disorder may be present and it is always important to tease out which remaining symptoms are present after a therapeutic trial has been tried.

It should be noted that before a child is labeled with oppositional-defiant disorder (ODD) or conduct disorder, every effort should have been made to detect any underlying psychiatric disorder that has not been treated and therefore may look like a conduct disorder (e.g., bipolar disorder).

Prenatal exposure to alcohol

Prenatal exposure to alcohol/fetal alcohol syndrome is the most common non-hereditary cause of mental retardation. The prevalence varies from 0.5–3.0 per 1000 live births (Streissguth, 1999). Fetal alcohol syndrome has shown a sixfold increase between 1979 and 1993 (Ebrahim *et al.*, 1998). This is primarily due to the fact that drinking has become more socially acceptable among women.

Children without the facial features commonly associated with fetal alcohol syndrome are referred to as having fetal alcohol effects. Unfortunately, without the facial features, it becomes more difficult to identify these children, and 60–90 percent escape identification in the normal population (Mattson *et al.*, 1998). The percentage of adolescents with fetal alcohol syndrome in juvenile justice forensic units is three–ten times greater than the accepted worldwide incidence. The percentage of these youths with any alcohol-related diagnosis is 10–40 times greater than the accepted worldwide incidence (Fast *et al.*, 1999).

Children with fetal alcohol syndrome or fetal alcohol effects suffer not only because diagnosis is often missed, but also because the disease is accompanied by many mental health and social problems. In a study of 415 children with fetal alcohol syndrome or fetal alcohol effects, Ann Streissguth *et al.* (1997) reported that 94 percent had mental health problems, 45 percent demonstrated inappropriate sexual behavior, 43 percent had disrupted school experiences, and 42 percent had been in trouble with the law.

There are four cognitive areas affected by fetal alcohol syndrome and fetal alcohol effects: learning and memory, visual-spatial processes, executive function, and attention (Coles *et al.*, 1997; Uecker & Nadel, 1996; Mattson *et al.*, 1996; Mattson & Riley, 1999; Mattson *et al.*, 1999). Mattson *et al.* (1996) noted that the cognitive effects found in children with fetal alcohol syndrome or fetal alcohol effects lead to breaking rules more often secondary to their impulsivity during testing. These behaviors are consistent with impulsive behaviors that lead to arrest and incarceration.

Streissguth *et al.* (1998) have emphasized that any evaluation of children and adolescents should include questions helpful in determining if fetal alcohol syndrome or fetal alcohol effects are a possibility. A careful review of the mother's pregnancy history and the child's developmental history, as well as a clinical examination of the child (if fetal alcohol syndrome or fetal alcohol effects are suspected), should take place. The underlying mechanisms of alcohol (or acetaldehyde) induced damage to the fetus in the central nervous system seem to be related to the timing of exposure, blood alcohol concentrations and pattern of drinking, duration of exposure, levels of susceptibility related to the genetic makeup of mother and fetus, other drugs used, and the poor nutrition of the mother. Binge drinking seems to be the most damaging. However, having one ounce of drink per day, seven or more drinks per week, or five or more drinks per occasion, is highly associated with fetal alcohol syndrome and fetal alcohol effects. In fact, the Frequency Binge Aggregate Score (F-BAS) can be used to help identify fetal alcohol syndrome and fetal alcohol effects. It requires either a once per month frequency of five or more drinks daily or almost-daily. The combination of these two had 100 percent sensitivity and 90 percent specificity. Any physical alcohol-related birth defects, such as kidney or cardiac defects, should be examined. Cognitive and language assessment and a miniature neurological examination are recommended.

Pre-natal alcohol use, which may not result in FAS/FAE, may nonetheless cause a significant risk of alcoholism in offspring related to effects on brain growth. This risk may be due to genetic and/or environmental factors. Gilman *et al.* (2007) studied intracranial volume (ICV) in early onset and late onset alcoholics with a positive and negative family history (FH) of heavy alcohol use. The FH positive patients had smaller ICV than the FH negative patients, suggesting less pre-morbid brain growth. Late onset FH positive patients had significantly lower IQ scores than late onset FH negative patients; IQ scores correlated with ICV. Late onset alcoholics showed a greater difference in ICV between FH positive and FH negative parents than early onset alcoholics.

Conclusions

The key to the prevention of juvenile offenders lies in early detection and treatment for risk factors that increase the risk for becoming involved in the juvenile justice system. Many adolescents who had a long history of missed opportunities for intervention and a history for severe crimes may be more difficult to treat because of the complexity of the psychological, social, and biological problems associated with these adolescents. Clearly, all agencies involved with the juvenile justice system must continue to educate themselves about the mental health issues of these youth, and work to coordinate services and follow-up in order to, hopefully, turn negative risk factors into protective factors. In this way, these adolescents may not continue to move in a direction that leads to a lifelong history of crime and recidivism.

References

Abram, K. M. (2004). Posttraumatic stress disorder and trauma in youth in juvenile justice. *Archives of General Psychiatry*, **61**(4), 403–410.

Alexander, J. F. & Parsons, B. V. (1982). *Functional Family Therapy*. Monterey, CA: Brooks/Cole.

Alford, G. S., Koehler, R. A. & Leonard, J. (1991). Alcoholics anonymous-narcotics anonymous model for inpatient treatment of chemically dependent adolescents: a two year study. *Journal of Studies on Alcohol*, **52**(2), 118–261.

Azrin, N. H., Acierno, R., Kogan, E., *et al.* (1996). Follow-up results of supportive versus behavioral therapy for illicit drug abuse. *Behavioral Research and Therapy*, **34**(1), 41–46.

Babor, T. F., Hoffman, M., Del Boca, F. K. *et al.* (1992). Types of alcoholics I. Evidence for an empirically derived topology based on indicators of vulnerability and solvent. *Archives of General Psychiatry*, **47**, 599–608.

Baldessarini, R. T., Tondo, L. & Hennen, J. (2001). Treating suicidal patients with bipolar disorder. Reducing suicide risk with lithium. *Annals of the New York Academy of Science* **932**, 24–28.

Baumrind, D. (1983). Familial antecedents of adolescent drug use. A developmental perspective. In C. L. Jones and R. J. Battjes, eds., *Etiology of Drug Abuse: Implications-Prevention*. NIDA Research Monographs, **56**, 13–44.

Bennett, E. M. & Kempfer, K. J. (1994). Is abuse during childhood a risk factor for developing substance abuse problems as an adult? *Journal of Development and Behavioural Pediatrics*, **15**(6), 426–429.

Brent, D. A., Perper, J. A. & Allman, C. J. (1987). Alcohol, firearms, and suicide among youth. *Journal of the American Medical Association*, **257**, 3369–3372.

Bukstein, O. G., Brent, D. A., Perper, J. A. *et al.* (1993). Risk factors for completed suicide among adolescents with a lifetime history of substance abuse: a case control study. *Acta Psychiatrica Scandinavica*, **88**(6), 403–408.

Carroll *et al.* (2006). The use of contingency and motivational/skills-building therapy to treat young adults with marijuana dependence. *Journal of Consulting and Clinical Psychology*, **74**(5), 955–956.

Castellanos, F. (2002). Developmental trajectories of brain volume abnormalities in children and adolescents with ADHD. *Journal of the American Medical Association*, **28**(14), 1740–1748.

Chambers, R. A., Taylor, J. R. & Potenza, M. N. (2003). Developmental neurocircuitry of motivation in adolescence: a critical period of addiction vulnerability. *American Journal of Psychiatry*, **160**, 1041–1052.

Chan-Ob, T., Kuntawongse, N. & Boonyanaruthee, V. (2001). Bupropion for amphetamine withdrawal syndrome. *Journal of the Medical Association of Thailand*, **84**(12), 1763–1765.

Clark, D. B., Kirisci, L. & Tarter, R. E. (1998). Adolescent versus adult onset and the development of substance use disorders in males. *Drug and Alcohol Dependence*, **49**(2), 115–121.

Cloniger, C. R., Bohman, M. C., Sigvardisson, S. *et al.* (1985). Psychopathology in adopted out children of alcoholics. The Stockholm Adoption Study. In M. Galanter, ed., *Recent Developments in Alcoholism*. New York: Plenum Press, 37–50.

Cocozza, J. & Skowyra, K. (2000). Youth with mental health disorders: issues and emerging responses. Office of Juvenile Justice and Delinquency Prevention. *Juvenile Justice Journal*, (**7**)1, 1–5.

Coffey, C., Wolfe, R., Lovett, A. W. *et al.* (2004). Predicting death in young offenders: a retrospective cohort study. *The Medical Journal of Australia*, **181**(9), 473–477.

Coles, C. D., Platzman, K. A., Raskind-Hood, C. L. *et al.* (1997). A comparison of children affected by prenatal alcohol exposure and attention deficit hyperactivity disorder. *Alcoholism: Clinical and Experimental Research*, **21**(1), 150–161.

Costello, E. J., Erkanli, A. & Federman, E. (1999). Development of psychiatric co-morbidity with substance abuse in adolescents: effects of timing and sex. *Journal of Clinical Child Psychology*, **28** (3), 298–311.

Couwenbergh, C. *et al.* (2006). Comorbid psychopathology in adolescents and young adults treated for substance use disorders: a review. *European Child & Adolescent Psychiatry*, **15**(6), 319–328.

DeWitt, D. J., Adlaf, E. M., Offord, D. R. *et al.* (2000). Age of first alcohol use: a risk factor for the development of alcohol disorders. *American Journal of Psychiatry*, **157**, 745–750.

Dishion, T. J., Spracklin, K. M., Andrews, D. W. *et al.* (1996). Deviancy training in male adolescent friendships. *Behavior Therapy*, **27**, 373–390.

Disney, E. R., Elkins, I. J., Mc Gue, M. *et al.* (1997). Effects of ADHD, conduct disorder and gender on substance use abuse in adolescents. *American Journal of Psychobiology*, **156**(10), 1515–1521.

Duncan, T. E., Biglan, A. & Ary, D. V. (1998). Contributions of the social context to the development of adolescent substance use: a multivariate latent growth modeling approach. *Drug and Alcohol Dependence*, **50**, 57–71.

Ebrahim, S. H., Luman, E., Floyd, R. L. *et al.* (1998). Alcohol consumption by pregnant women in the United States 1988–95. *Obstetrics and Gynecology*, **92**(2), 187–192.

Fallon, T. & Pumariega, A. (2000). The child and adolescent levels of care utilization services for psychiatric and addiction services. Presented at the American Academy of Child and Adolescent Psychiatry's Annual Conference.

Fast, D. K., Conry, J. & Loock, C. A. (1999). Identifying Fetal Alcohol Syndrome among youth in the criminal juvenile justice system. *Journal of Developmental and Behavioural Pediatrics*, **20**(5), 370–372.

Feeney, G. F. *et al.* (2005). Cannabis dependence and mental health perception amongst people diverted by police after arrest for cannabis-related offending behavior in Australia. *Criminal Behavior and Mental Health*, **15**(4), 249–260.

Fiorentine, R. & Milhouse, M. P. (2000). Exploring the addictive effects of drug misuse treatment and twelve step involvement: does twelve-step ideology matter? *Substance Use and Misuse*, **35**(3),367–397.

Geller, B., Cooper, T. B., Sein, K. *et al.* (1998). Double blind and placebo controlled study of lithium for adolescent bipolar disorders with secondary substance dependence. *Journal of the American Academy of Child and Adolescent Psychiatry*, **37**(2), 171–178.

Gilman, J. M., Bjork, J. M. & Hommer, D. W. (2007). Parental alcohol use and brain volume in early and late onset alcoholics. *Biological Psychiatry*, in press.

Grella, C., Stein, J. & Greenwell, L. (2005). Association among childhood trauma, adolescent problem behaviors and adverse adult outcomes in substance abusing women offenders. *Psychology of Addictive Behaviors*, **19**(1), 43–53.

Grisso, T., Barnum, R. & Fletcher, J. (2001). Massachusetts's youth screening instrument for mental health needs of juvenile justice youth. *Journal of the American Academy of Child and Adolescent Psychiatry*, **40**(5), 541–548.

Hambrecht, M. & Hafner, H. (2000). Cannabis, vulnerability and onset of schizophrenia: an epidemiological perspective. *Australian and New Zealand Journal of Psychiatry*, **34**, 468–475.

Hansen, W. B. (1996). Prevention programs: What are the critical factors that spell success? National Conference on Drug Prevention Research: Presentations, Papers and Recommendations, Plenary session. National Institute of Drug Abuse.

Harrell A. V. & Wirtz, P. W. (1989). Screening for adolescent problem drinking: validation of a multi-dimensional instrument for case identification. *Psychological Assessment*, **1**, 61–63.

Harrington, R., Kroll, L., Rothwell, J. *et al.* (2005). Psychosocial needs of boys in secure care for serious or persistent offending. *Journal of Child Psychology and Psychiatry*, **46**(8), 859–866.

Hartney, C., Wordes, M. & Krisberg, B. (2002). Health care for our troubled youth: provision of services in the foster care and juvenile justice systems of California. National Council on Crime and Delinquency, available at www.Calendow.org/reference/publications/pdf/mental/TCE0315-2002_Health_Care_Fo.pdf.

Heil, S. H., Holmes, W. K., Bickel, S. T. *et al.* (2002). Comparison of the subjective, physiological and psychomotor effects of atomoxetine and methylphenidate in light drug users. *Drug and Alcohol Dependency*, **67**, 149–156.

Henggeler, S. W., Clingempeel, W. G., Brondino, M. J. *et al.* (2002). Four-year follow-up of multisystemic therapy with substance-abusing and substance-dependent juvenile offenders. *Journal of the American Academy of Child and Adolescent Psychiatry*, **41**(7), 868–874.

Henggeler, S. W., Halliday-Boykins, C. A., Cunningham, P. B. *et al.* (2006). Juvenile drug court: enhancing outcomes by integrating evidence-based treatment. *Journal of Consulting and Clinical Psychology*, **74**(1), 42–54.

Hops, H. A., Davis, B. & Lewin, L. M. (1999). The development of alcohol and other substance use: a gender study of family and peer context. *Journal of Studies on Alcohol Supplement*, **13**, 22–31.

Inciardi, J. A., Martin, S. S., Butzin, C. A. *et al.* (1997). An effective model of prison-based treatment for drug-involved offenders. *Journal of Drug Issues*, **27**(2), 261–278.

Jaffe, S. L. (1990). *Step Workbook for Adolescent Chemical Dependency Recovery: A Guide to the First Five Steps*. Washington, DC: American Psychiatric Press, Inc.

Jaffe, S. & Simkin, D. (2002). Alcohol and drug abuse in children and adolescents. In Lewis, ed., *Child and Adolescent Psychiatry Textbook*.

Jainchill, N., Hawke, J. & Messina, M. Post-treatment outcomes among adjudicated adolescent males and females in modified therapeutic community treatment. *Substance Use & Misuse*, **40**(7), 975–976.

Jasinski, D. R. (2000). An evaluation of the abuse potential of modafinil using methylphenidate as a reference. *Psychopharmacology*, **14**(1), 53–60.

Johnson, B. (2002). Odansetron curbs drinking in some alcoholics. *Clinical Psychiatry News*. September, 12.

Johnston, L. (2005). *Monitoring the Future*. University of Michigan, News and Information Services.

Johnston, L. (2006). *Monitoring the Future*. University of Michigan, News and Information Services.

Kaminer, Y. (1999). Addictive disorders in adolescents. *Psychiatric Clinics of North America*, **22**(2), 275–288.

Kaminer, Y. (1994). *Adolescent Substance Abuse: A Comprehensive Guide to Theory and Practice.* Plenum Medical Press.

Kaminer, Y., Burleson, J. A., Blitz, C. *et al.* (1998). Psychotherapies for substance abusers: a pilot study. *Journal of Nervous and Mental Disease*, **186**, 684–690.

Kandel, D. B., Kessler, R. & Marguiles, J. (1978). Antecedents of adolescent initiation into stages of drug abuse. *Journal of Youth and Adolescence*, **7**, 13–40.

Kandel, D. B., Yamaguchi, K. & Chen, K. (1992). Stages of progression in drug involvement from adolescence to adulthood: further evidence for the gateway theory. *Journal of Studies on Alcohol*, **53**(5), 447–457.

Kendler, K. S. & Presscott, C. A. (1998a). Genetic and environmental risk factors for cannabis use, abuse, dependence: a study of female twins. *American Journal of Psychiatry*, **155**(8) 1016–1022.

Kendler, K. S. & Presscott, C. A. (1998b). Genetic and environmental risk factors for cocaine use, dependence: a study of female twins. *British Journal of Psychiatry*, **173**, 345–350.

Kirk, J. & Reid, G. (2001). An examination of the relationship between dyslexia and offending in young people and its implications. *Dyslexia*, **7**(2), 77–84.

Knight, J. R. (1997). Adolescent substance use: screening, assessment, and intervention in medical office practice. *Contemporary Pediatrics*, **14**(4), 45–72.

Knight, J. R., Shrier, L. A., Bravender, T. D. *et al.* (1999). CRAFFT: A new brief screen for adolescent substance abuse. *Archives of Pediatric and Adolescent Medicine*, **153**(6), 591–596.

Knight, J. R., Sherritt, L., Shier, L. A. *et al.* (2002). Validity of the CRAFFT substance abuse screening test among adolescent clinic patients. *Archives of Pediatrics and Adolescent Medicine*, **156**(6), 607–614.

Koppelman, J. (2005). Mental health and juvenile justice: moving toward more effective systems of care. *Natonal Health Policy Forum*, Issue Brief, No. 805, July 22.

Kratochvil, C. J., Heiligenstein, J. H., Dittman, R. *et al.* (2002). Atomoxetine and methylpheni-date treatment in children with ADHD: a prospective, randomized, open-label trial. *Journal of the American Academy of Child and Adolescent Psychiatry*, **41**(7), 776–784.

Lee, G. P. & DeClemente, C. C. (1985). Age of onset versus duration of problem drinking on the alcohol use inventory. *Journal of Studies on Alcohol*, **46**, 298–402.

Lennings, C. J., Kenny, D. T. & Nelson, P. (2006). Substance use and treatment in young offenders on community orders. *Journal of Substance Abuse Treatment*, **31**(4), 425–432.

Li, Y., White, F. J. & Wolf, M. E. (2000). Pharmacological reversal of behavioral and cellular indices of cocaine sensitization in the rat. *Psychopharmacology*, **151**(2–3), 175–183.

Liddle, H. A. & Hogue, A. A. (2000). A family-based, developmental-ecological preventive intervention for high-risk adolescents. *Journal of Marital and Family Therapy*, **26**(3), 265–279.

Liddle, H. A., Dakof, G. A., Parker, K. *et al.* (2001). Multidimensional family therapy for adolescent drug abuse: results of a randomized trial. *American Journal of Drug and Alcohol Abuse*, **27**(4), 651–658.

Luna, B. & Sweeney, J. A. (2004). The emergence of collaborative brain function: FMRI studies of the development of response inhibition. *Annals of the New York Academy of Sciences*, **21**, 296–309.

Mattson, S. N. & Riley, E. P. (1999). Implicit and explicit memory functioning in children with heavy prenatal alcohol exposure. *Journal of the International Neuropsychological Society*, **5**(5), 462–471.

Mattson, S. N., Riley, E. P., Delis, D. C. *et al.* (1996). Verbal learning and memory in children with fetal alcohol syndrome. *Alcoholism: Clinical and Experimental Research*, **20**(5) 810–816.

Mattson, S. N., Riley, E. P., Gramling, L. *et al.* (1998). Neuropsychological comparison of alcohol-exposed children with or without physical features of fetal alcohol syndrome. *Neuropsychology*, **12**(1), 146–153.

Mattson, S. N., Goodman, A. M., Caine, C. *et al.* (1999). Executive functioning in children with prenatal alcohol exposure. *Alcoholism: Clinical and Experimental Research*, **23**(11), 1808–1815.

Miller, W. R. & Rollnick, S. (1991). *Motivational Interviewing.* New York, NY: Guilford Press.

Miller, W. R. & Sanchez, V. C. (1994). Motivating young adults for treatment and lifestyle change. In G. Howard ed., *Issues in Alcohol Use and Misuse by Young Adults.* Notre Dame IN: University of Notre Dame Press, pp. 51–81.

Monti, P., Colby, S., Barnett, N. & Rohsenow, D. (1998). Brief motivational interviewing in a hospital setting for adolescent smoking: a preliminary study. *Journal of Consulting and Clinical Psychology*, **66**(3), 574–578.

National Institute for Drug Abuse (2003). *Preventing Substance Abuse Among Children and Adolescents – A Researched-Based guide*, 2nd edn. NIH pub. no. 04-4212(A).

Newcomb, M. D. (1997). Psychosocial predictors and consequences of drug use: a developmental perspective within a prospective study. *Journal of Addictive Disorders*, **16**(1), 51–89.

Nowinski, J. (1990). *Substance Abuse in Adolescents and Young Adults, A Guide to Treatment.* New York, NY: N. N. Norton and Company, 59–61.

Prinz, R. J. & Kerns, S. E. (2003). Early substance use by juvenile offenders. *Child Psychiatry and Human Development*, **33**(4), 263–277.

Prochaska, J. O. & DiClemente, C. (1982). Transtheoretical theory: toward a more integrated model of change. *Psychotherapy: Theory, Research, and Practice*, **19**, 276–288.

Rahdert, E. & Czechowicz, D. (1995). *Adolescent Drug Abuse: Clinical Assessment and Therapeutic Interventions.* Rockville, MD: National Institute on Drug Abuse.

Rao, U., Ryan, N., Dahl, D. E. *et al.* (1999). Factors associated with the development of substance use disorders in depressed adolescents. *Journal of the American Academy of Child and Adolescent Psychiatry*, **38**(9), 1109–1117.

Riggs, P. & Whitmore, E. (1999). Substance use disorders and disruptive behavior disorders. In R. Henderson, ed., *Disruptive Behavior Disorders in Children and Adolescents.* Review of Psychiatry Series Vol. 18.

Riggs, P., Thompson, L., Mikulich, S. *et al.* (1996). An open trial of pemoline in drug-dependent delinquents with attention deficit hyperactivity disorder. *Journal of the American Academy of Child and Adolescent Psychiatry*, **35** (8), 1018–1024.

Riggs, P., Mikulich, S., Coffman, L. M. *et al.* (1997). Fluoxentine in drug-dependent delinquents with major depression: an open trial. *Journal of Child and Adolescent Psychopharmacology*, **7**(2), 87–95.

Riggs, P., Leon, S. L., Mikulich, S. *et al.* (1998). An open trial of buproprion for ADHD in adolescents with substance abuse disorders and conduct disorders. *Journal of the American Academy of Child and Adolescent Psychiatry*, **37**(12), 1271–1278.

Rugino, T. A. & Copley, T. C. (2001). Effects of modafinil in children with attention deficit hyperactivity disorder: an open label trial. *Journal of the American Academy of Child and Adolescent Psychiatry*, **40**(2), 230–235.

Scheier, L. M., Botvin, C. J., Drag, T. *et al.* (1999). Social skills, competence and drug refusal efficacy as predictors of adolescent alcohol use. *Journal of Drug Education*, **29**(3), 251–278.

Schuckit, M. A. (1999). New findings in the generics of alcoholism. *Journal of the American Medical Association*, **281**(20), 1875–1876.

Shelton, D. (2001). Young offenders with emotional disorders. *Journal of Nursing Scholarship*, (**33**)3, 259–263.

Simkin, D. R. & Graves, L. (2001). The association between ADHD and processing problems and learning disorders. Presented at the American Academy of Child and Adolescent Psychiatry's annual conference, Honolulu, Hawaii.

Slavet, J. D. *et al.* (2006). The Marijuana Ladder: measuring motivation to change marijuana use in incarcerated adolescents. *Drug and Alcohol Dependence*, **83**(1), 42–48.

Stacy, A. W., Newcomb, M. D. & Bentler, P. M. (1993). Cognitive motivations and sensation seeking as long term predictors of drinking problems. *Journal of Clinical Psychology*, **12**, 1–24.

Stanton, M. D., Todd, T. C. *et al.* (1982). *The Family Therapy of Drug Abuse and Addiction*. New York, NY: Guilford.

Streissguth, A. (1999). Fetal alcohol syndrome and alcohol and pregnancy: new findings. *The Union Signal: A Journal of Social Welfare*, **CXXV**(2), 9–15.

Streissguth, A. P. & O'Malley, K. D. (1997). Fetal alcohol syndrome/fetal alcohol effects, secondary disabilities and mental health approaches. *Treatment Today*, Spring, 16–17.

Streissguth, A. P., Boolstein, F. L., Barr, H. M. *et al.* (1998). A fetal alcohol behavior scale, *Alcoholism: Clinical and Experimental Research*, **22**(2), 325–333.

Swan, N. (1995). Early childhood behavior and temperament predict later substance abuse. *National Institute on Drug Abuse Notes*, **10**(1).

Tapert, S. F., Baratta, B. S., Abrantes, B. A. *et al.* (2002). Attention dysfunction predicts substance involvement in community youth. *Journal of the American Academy of Child and Adolescent Psychiatry*, **41**(6), 690–696.

Teplin, L. A. (2002) Psychiatric disorders in youth in juvenile detention. *Archives of General Psychiatry*, **59**(12), 1133–1139.

Turner, A. P. *et al.* (2005). Identifying a negative mood subtype in incarcerated adolescents: relationship to substance use. *Addictive Behaviors*, **30**(7), 1442–1448.

Uecker, A. & Nadel, L. (1996). Spatial locations gone awry: object and spatial memory deficits in children with fetal syndrome. *Neuropsychologia*, **34**(3), 209–223.

Upadhyaya, H. P., Brady, K. T., Sethuraman, G. *et al.* (2001). Venlafaxine treatment of patients with co-morbid alcohol/cocaine abuse and attention-deficit/hyperactivity disorder: a pilot study. *Journal of Clinical Psychopharmacology*, **21**, 116–118.

Volkow, N. D. (2001a). Association of dopamine transporter reduction with psychomotor impairment in methamphetamine abusers. *American Journal of Psychiatry*, **158**(3), 377–382.

Volkow, N. D. (2001b). Loss of dopamine transporters in methamphetamine abusers recovers with protracted abstinence. *Journal of Neuroscience*, **21**(23), 9414–9418.

Volkow, N. D., Goldstein, R. Z. *et al.* (2002a). Drug addiction and its underlying neurobiological basis: neuroimaging evidence for the involvement of the frontal cortex. *American Journal of Psychiatry*, **159**(10), 1642–1652.

Volkow, N. D., Thanos, P. K., Freimuth, P. *et al.* (2002b). Overexpression of dopamine D2 receptors reduces alcohol self-administration. *Journal of Neurochemistry*, **78**(5), 1094–1103.

Volkow, N. D., Fowler, J. S. & Wang, G. J. (2002c). Role of dopamine in drug reinforcement and addiction in humans: results from imaging studies. *Behavioral Pharmacology*, **13**(5–6), 355–366.

Waldron, H. B. (1998). Adolescent substance abuse disorders. In A. Bellack and M. Hersen, eds., *Comprehensive Clinical Psychology* (Vol. 5: *Children and Adolescents: Clinical Formulation and Treatment*).

Wasserman, G. A. & McReynolds, L. S. (2006). Suicide risk at juvenile justice intake. *Suicide & Life-Threatening Behavior*, **36**(2), 239–249.

Whitmore, E. A., Milulick, S. K., Thompson, L. L. *et al.* (1997). Influences on adolescent substance dependence, conduct disorders, depression, attention deficit hyperactivity disorder, and gender. *Drug and Alcohol Dependence*, **47**(2), 87–97.

Wilens, T. E., Biederman, J., Millstein, R. B. *et al.* (1999). Risk for substance use disorders in youth with child and adolescent onset bipolar disorder. *Journal of the American Academy of Child and Adolescent Psychiatry*, **38**(6), 680–685.

Wold, M. & Kaminer, Y. (1997). Naltrexone for alcohol abuse. *Journal of Child and Adolescent Psychiatry*, **30**(11), 6–7.

Wright, B. (2004). Learning problems, delayed development and puberty. *Proceeding of the National Academy of Sciences*, **10**(6), 9942–9946.

8

Suicide and delinquent adolescents

Amer Smajkic and David C. Clark

Introduction

According to the Surgeon General of the United States, youth suicide is a national tragedy and a major public health problem (US Department of Health and Human Services, 1999). From 1950–2001, the suicide rate for young people (ages 15–24) tripled from 2.7 per 100 000 to 9.9 per 100 000 (Arias *et al.*, 2003). In 2002 the rates were unchanged at 9.9 per 100 000 (Kochanek *et al.*, 2002). The 2001 rate translated to 13 435 deaths of adolescents ages 15–19 years.

From 1952–1994, the incidence of suicide among adolescents approximately tripled, although there has been a general decline in youth suicides since 1994. In 1950 the death rate for adolescent suicide was 2.7 per 100 000, in 1990 it was 11.1 per 100 000, with a decline to 7.4 per 100 000 in 2002. From 1950–1990 the suicide rate among adolescents increased by 411 percent. From 1990–2002 the suicide rate for 15- to 19-year-olds decreased by 33%. See Fig. 8.1.

Over the same period (1950 to present), unintentional injury has remained the leading cause of death for adolescents. In 2001 unintentional injury accounted for approximately 48 percent of all deaths among adolescents ages 15–19 years. Homicide and suicide have consistently ranked as the second and third leading causes of death, accounting for 14 and 12 percent, respectively, of all deaths among 15 to 19-year-olds (National Center for Health Prevention and Injury Control, 2001). A recent US survey found that three million adolescents are at risk for suicide each year in the community, with 37 percent of surveyed subjects reporting a suicide attempt during the past 12 months (Substance Abuse and Mental Health Services Administration, 2001).

Studies of suicide among delinquent children and adolescents have unfortunately been limited to studies in juvenile correction facilities. To review suicide and suicide attempt trends in jails and prisons, it is important to begin with an explanation of the distinction between "jails" and "prisons." These words have different meanings.

The word *jail* traces back through the Middle English words *jaiolem, gaiol*, and *gaol*; to the Old North French *gaiole*; to the Vulgar Latin *gaviola*; and finally to the

The Mental Health Needs of Young Offenders: Forging Paths toward Reintegration and Rehabilitation, eds. Carol L. Kessler and Louis J. Kraus. Published by Cambridge University Press. © Cambridge University Press 2007.

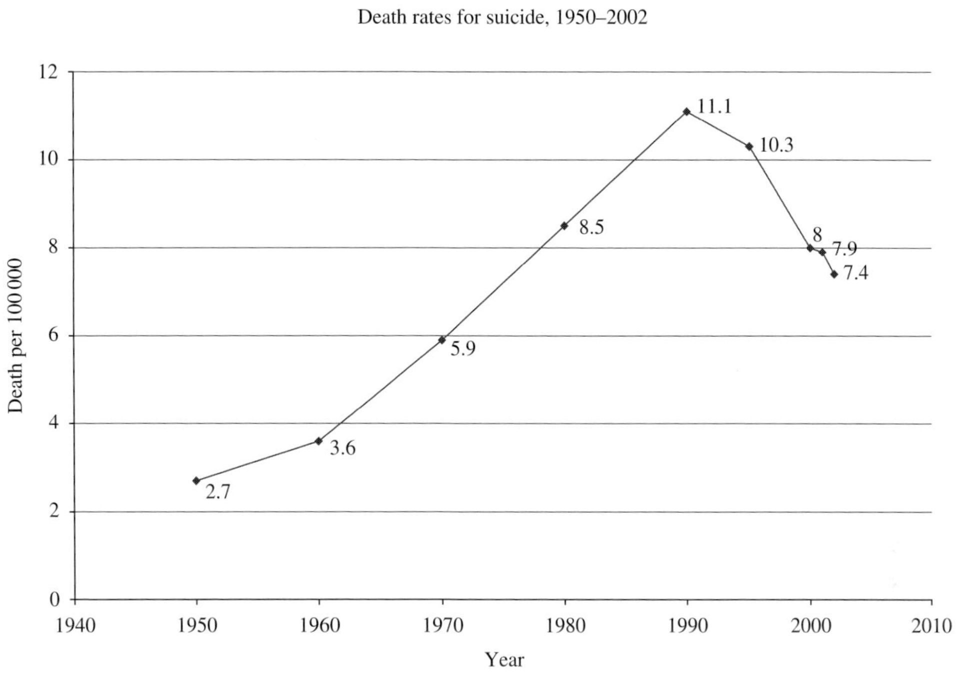

Death rates for suicide, 1950–2002

Figure 8.1   Suicide among adolescents, 1952–1994.

Latin *caveola*, diminutive of *cavea*, which referred to a cage or hollow. In modern usage, jail is a place of confinement for persons awaiting trial and for persons sentenced to shorter terms of confinement for misdemeanors.

The word *prison* originates with the Latin word *prēnsiō*, which labeled the action or power of making an arrest. *Prēnsiō* then surfaces in the Old French of the twelfth century with the form *prison* and the senses of "capture" and "place of imprisonment." From Old French as well as the Medieval Latin word *priso*, meaning "prison," came our Middle English word *prisoun*, first recorded before 1121 with the sense of "imprisonment." In modern usage, prison is a place of confinement for the punishment and rehabilitation of criminals. By the end of the eighteenth century, imprisonment was the chief mode of punishment for all but capital crimes. While jail and prison are both places of confinement, jail refers to institutions of shorter stays, while prison refers to long-term stay institutions.

Suicide in US jails and prisons

Suicide is a leading cause of death within the jails in USA. More than 400 inmates take their lives each year, and the jail suicide rate is estimated to be five times greater than that of the general population (Bureau of Justice Statistics, 2001).

Suicide is the third leading cause of death in prisons, just behind natural causes and HIV/AIDS (Bureau of Justice Statistics, 2000). Close to 200 inmates commit suicide in state and federal prisons each year (Criminal Justice Institute, 2000). While the rate of suicide within prisons is far below that for jail suicides, prison rates are still greater than general population rates (Hayes, 1995).

Among all children and adolescents, those incarcerated in the juvenile or criminal justice systems are at the highest risk for serious suicide attempts (Gray et al., 2002; Sanislow et al., 2003).

In Canada too, adolescents involved in the child welfare and juvenile justice systems are associated with higher suicide rates. They committed at least one-third of all completed suicides in their age group in 1995 and 1996. Their risk of suicide, standardized for age and sex, was five times that of the general adolescent Canadian population, and female juvenile delinquents showed the highest relative risk of suicide (36.1) (Farand et al., 2004).

Psychiatric risk factors for fatal suicide in the delinquent youth population

A number of studies of suicide by delinquent adolescents focus on individual psychological and psychiatric risk factors, past suicide attempts and thoughts, sexual victimization, and gang affiliation, as well as demographic factors (Battle et al., 1993; Evans et al., 1996; Messier & Ward, 1998; Morris et al., 1995; Rohde et al., 1997).

Several clinically oriented studies indicate that depression is an important risk factor when assessing suicide risk in juvenile detainees (Rohde et al., 1997). Cole (1989) and colleagues reported that for both adolescent juvenile detainees and public high school students, depression is a more important risk factor for suicidal behaviors than hopelessness. Overall clinical studies of suicide in juvenile detainees point to depression as a consistent risk factor, but other potential risk factors are less well established.

Other risk factors for fatal suicide in the delinquent youth population

Most jail suicide victims are young white males arrested for non-violent offenses who were found to be intoxicated at the time of arrest. Many are isolated in jail and are typically found dead within 24 hours of incarceration. The overwhelming majority of victims are found hanging by either bedding or clothing (Hayes, 1989). Studies of prison suicide found that the majority of victims had been convicted of personal crimes, housed in cells alone, and had prior histories of suicide attempts and/or mental illness (Bonner, 1992; White & Schimmel, 1995).

Hayes' survey on juvenile suicide in confinement

Lindsay Hayes' report on "Juvenile suicide in confinement: a national survey" (2004), commissioned by the Office of Juvenile Justice and Delinquency Prevention, was the first comprehensive study of the scope and distribution of suicides by youth confined in American public and private juvenile facilities. The study identified 110 juvenile suicides occurring between 1995 and 1999, and analyzed data for 79 of these cases. Of these suicides, 42 percent occurred in secure facilities, 37 percent in short-term detention centers, 15 percent in residential treatment centers, and 6 percent in reception diagnostic centers.

Almost half (48 percent) of the 79 suicides occurred in facilities administered by state agencies, 39 percent took place in county facilities, and 13 percent in private programs. Sixty-eight percent of the victims were Caucasian and 80 percent of victims were male. The mean age of the suicide victims was 16 years, with over 70 percent between the ages of 15–17. Thirty-eight percent of the victims were living with one parent at the time of confinement.

Seventy percent of the 79 suicide victims were confined for non-violent offenses. Two-thirds (67 percent) of victims were being held in confinement at the time of death, and the other 33 percent were on detained (in jail) status. The vast majority (88 percent) of victims held in detention centers were on detained status.

Seventy-eight percent of the suicide victims had a prior history of offenses, and most of these (73 percent) were of a non-violent nature. All of the detention center suicides occurred within the first four months of confinement, and over 40 percent of these occurred within the first 72 hours. Excluding suicides in (short-stay) detention centers, only 4 percent of suicides occurred within the first 24 hours of confinement. The remainder of the non-detention suicides were evenly distributed from the first three days of confinement to more than 12 months of confinement.

It will come as no surprise to those familiar with detention suicides, that 99 percent of the juvenile detention suicides in Hayes' series were effected by hanging. Seventy-two percent of the hanging victims utilized sheets or blankets. The victims used a variety of anchoring devices to hang themselves: door hinge/knob (20 percent), air vent (19 percent), bed frame (19 percent), and window frame (14 percent). Most interestingly, none of the victims were under the influence of alcohol and/or drugs at the time of the suicide.

Seventy-five percent of the 79 suicide victims were assigned to single-occupancy rooms. Forty-one percent of the victims were found dead within 15 minutes of last observation. Slightly more than 15 percent of the suicide victims were found after more than one hour since last observation.

Sixteen percent of the victims were on suicide precaution status at the time of suicide. Most of them were required to be observed at 15-minute intervals. Despite these requirements, almost half of the suicide victims had not been observed for more than 15 minutes prior to the suicide. Seventy percent of victims were assessed by a qualified mental health professional (QMHP) prior to their death, though only 34 percent of the detention center victims received such assessments. Slightly less than half (44 percent) of all victims had never been assessed by a QMHP or had not been assessed by a clinician within 30 days of their deaths (Hayes, 2004).

Gallagher studied the association between suicide screening practices and attempts requiring emergency care in the juvenile justice facilities. His findings show that the most attempts occurred in facilities screening just some of their population over a seven-day window, and the fewest attempts occurred in facilities screening older children and adolescents in the first 24 hours following admission (Gallagher & Dobrin, 2005).

Psychological distress in incarcerated youth

Mental disorder and substance abuse are the most important pair of risk factors for adolescent suicide in the general population (Brent, 1995). Other risk factors include impulsive aggression, depression in family members, substance abuse, family discord and abuse, and the absence of family support. Life stressors, specifically interpersonal conflict and loss, as well as legal and disciplinary problems, are also associated with adolescent suicidal behavior. Many of the afore-mentioned risk factors are prevalent in youth confined in juvenile facilities (Alessi, et al., 1984; Rohde, Seeley & Mace, 1997).

Sanislow et al. (2003) found that confined youth show levels of depression, hopelessness, and situational stress similar to those shown by severely disturbed adolescents hospitalized on an acute psychiatric inpatient unit. Juveniles in con-finement had life histories predisposing them to suicide (including mental dis-orders; substance abuse; physical, sexual, and emotional abuse; and current and prior history of self-harming behavior). The same author concluded that correlates of suicide in juvenile detainees might be different from those in other high risk groups, and (in particular) impulsivity and history of drug abuse might have a stronger relationship with suicide in detained adolescents (Sanislow et al., 2003).

Psychiatric disorders and fatal suicide in delinquency

Multiple research studies are looking into prevalence of mental disorders among incarcerated youth. A study published by Steiner et al. (1997) reports that 32 percent of confined male delinquents met the criteria for posttraumatic stress disorder (PTSD), and that these PTSD youth had increased levels of distress, anxiety, and depression, while exhibiting lower levels of restraint, impulse control, and suppression of aggression. Another study reported that at least 66 percent of confined youth met the DSM-IV diagnostic criteria for a mental disorder, with over half of the youth suffering from multiple disorders including conduct and substance abuse (Robertson & Husain, 2001).

Teplin and colleagues conducted a longitudinal study of mental disorders among 1830 youth confined in an Illinois county juvenile detention center. The study reports that two-thirds of the youth had one or more alcohol, drug, or mental disorders (Teplin *et al.*, 2002).

It has been estimated that the following rates of mental disorders are experienced by youth in confinement: 50–90 percent for conduct disorders, up to 46 percent for attention deficit disorders, 6–41 percent for anxiety disorders, 25–50 percent for substance abuse or dependence, 32–78 percent for affective disorders, 1–6 percent for psychotic disorder, and more than 50 percent for co-morbid mental health and substance abuse disorder (Otto *et al.*, 1992; Edens & Otto, 1997).

The National Survey on Juvenile Suicide in Confinement reports that history of mental illness was found in 66 percent of suicide victims, with the majority (65 percent) suffering from depression at the time of their deaths (Hayes, 2004). Other types of mental illnesses reported include attention-deficit/hyperactivity disorder, conduct disorder, posttraumatic stress disorder, and psychotic disorder (Hayes, 2004). In addition 54 percent of the victims were taking psychotropic medication at the time of their deaths. The same study reports that 73 percent of the victims had a history of substance abuse.

Approximately one third (33 percent) of the victims with a substance abuse history used alcohol, marijuana, and cocaine prior to their confinement. These rates are consistent with or higher than other recent data, suggesting that two-thirds of confined youth have one or more alcohol, drug, or mental disorders (Teplin *et al.*, 2002).

Physical, sexual, emotional abuse, and fatal suicide

Delinquent youth have higher rates of physical, sexual, and emotional abuse compared to the adolescents in the community. High rates of both physical (35 percent) and sexual (18 percent) abuse were reported among confined youth in Maryland (Shelton, 2000). In a study done by Esposito and Clum (2002), the authors found even higher rates of physical (58 percent) and sexual (24 percent) abuse for confined youth.

Confined youth who reported a history of sexual abuse had a 42 percent incidence of suicidal ideation and a 35 percent incidence of one or more suicide attempts, as compared to adolescents who reported no history of sexual abuse – with an

18 percent rate of suicidal ideation and a 12 percent rate of suicide attempts (Morris *et al.*, 1995).

In another study by Hayes, 44 percent of confined youth reported a history of emotional abuse. The most frequent examples of this abuse were excessive punishment, neglect, abandonment, verbal abuse, or similar types of family dysfunction. Morris and colleagues reported a history of physical abuse in 34 percent of confined youth, the perpetrator being an immediate family member (father or stepfather) in the vast majority (20 of 27) of cases. History of sexual abuse was found in 28 percent of the confined youth, the perpetrator being an immediate family member (e.g., father or stepfather) in many of the cases (Hayes, 2004).

Non-fatal suicidal attempts and self-harm behavior

According to the one national study, more than 11 000 adolescents engage in more than 17 000 incidents of suicide behavior in juvenile facilities each year (Parent *et al.*, 1994). A large percentage of detained youth had previous histories of suicide attempts (Dembo *et al.*, 1990) and current suicidal behavior (Robertson & Husain, 2001; Shelton, 2000; Davis *et al.*, 1991; Woolf & Funk, 1985).

Morris and colleagues reported the results from a 1991 national survey. They administered a modified version of the Center for Disease Control's Youth Risk Behavior Surveillance System (YRBSS) survey to over 1800 confined youth in 39 juvenile institutions throughout the country. They found that almost 22 percent of confined youth seriously considered suicide, 20 percent had made a plan, 16 percent made at least one attempt, and 8 percent were injured during an attempt in the previous 12 months (Morris *et al.*, 1995).

Another study found that 31 percent of confined youth self-reported a prior suicide attempt, and that 9 percent were currently suicidal with either ideation and/or a plan to act on suicidal thoughts (Robertson & Husain, 2001).

There is evidence of racial differences with regard to suicide attempts in confinement. White youth attempt suicide in confinement at a higher rate than African American youth (Kempton & Forehand, 1992; Alessi *et al.*, 1984). Morris *et al.* (1995) found that Native American (29 percent) and white (25 percent) youth reported higher rates of suicidal ideation than Hispanic (15 percent), Asian (12 percent), or African American (8 percent) youth. Other researchers have reported similar findings of higher rates of suicidal behavior (Duclos, LeBeau & Elias, 1994) and psychiatric disorders (Duclos *et al.*, 1998) among Native American youth confined in juvenile facilities.

One study reported that among juvenile delinquents, conduct disorder is associated with higher rates of suicidal ideation and attempts. The authors suggest that a combination of intrinsic and extrinsic factors associated with conduct disorder create vulnerability to stressors, which interact with situational factors to produce suicidal thoughts and acts (Ruchkin *et al.*, 2003).

Some researchers have reported that imprisoned youth with either major affective disorders or borderline personality disorders have a higher degree of suicidal ideation and more suicide attempts than adolescents in the general population (Alessi *et al.*, 1984). A more recent report indicated that over half (52 percent) of detained youth self-reported current suicidal ideation, with 33 percent showing a history of suicidal behavior (Esposito & Clum, 2002). These researchers concluded that a history of sexual abuse directly affects the development of suicidal ideation and behavior in incarcerated adolescents.

Suicidal behavior in males has been significantly associated with depression, major life events, and poor social connections. Suicidal behavior in females has been associated with impulsivity, current depression, instability, and younger age (Mace, Rohde & Gnau, 1997; Rohde, Seeley & Mace, 1997). For both males and females, suicidal behavior was associated with not living with a biological parent before detention (Rohde, Seeley & Mace, 1997). One of the more recent reports of confined youth found that 30 percent reported suicidal ideation or behavior and 30 percent reported self mutilative behavior while incarcerated (Penn *et al.*, 2003).

An interesting study done in Russia by Ruchkin examined suicidal ideation and attempts in Russian male juvenile delinquents with conduct disorder (CD). The study reports that 34 percent of those diagnosed with CD (92 subjects) reported a lifetime history of either suicidal thoughts or attempts. Suicidal ideators and attempters did not differ significantly on any variable of interest, but both reported significantly higher rates of psychopathology and exposure to violence than the non-suicidal group. Juvenile delinquents with CD had high rates of suicidal ideations and attempts, related to a wide spectrum of psychopathology and specific personality traits. These findings reinforce the idea that a combination of intrinsic and extrinsic factors create vulnerability to stressors, which under the influence of situational factors may lead to suicidal thoughts and acts (Ruchkin *et al.*, 2003).

The most recent data about suicidal behavior in delinquent adolescents found that a history of suicidal behavior was found in 70 percent of completed suicides. The most frequent type of suicidal behavior was a suicide attempt (46 percent), followed by suicidal ideation and/or threat (31 percent) and suicidal gesture and/ or self mutilation (24 percent) (Hayes, 2004). The same study suggests that the vast majority of confined youth who commit suicide, evidence a higher percentage of prior suicidal behavior than those confined youth who engage in suicidal behavior, but do not die.

Mental health services in juvenile facilities

Mental health services available to adolescent delinquents, and their living conditions within the juvenile system has recently become a focus of research. The study *Conditions of Confinement: Juvenile Detention and Corrections Facilities* included a survey of 984 public and private detention centers, reception and diagnostic centers, training schools, and ranches throughout the United States (Parent *et al.*, 1994). This study was sponsored by the US Justice Department's Office of Juvenile Justice and Delinquency Prevention.

On a daily basis, these facilities held almost 65 000 juveniles or 69 percent of all youth confined in the United States. Serious and widespread problems in living space, healthcare, security, and the control of suicidal behavior were found in the facilities surveyed. In regard to the provision of mental health services in juvenile facilities, the survey found that the availability and use of phones for staff improved their communication about inmate risk for suicide. The survey also showed that 64 percent of facilities provided initial mental health screening, 74 percent had the capability to provide clinical valuations by mental health staff, 82 percent had provisions for psychotropic medication, and 69 percent provided onsite access to psychiatrists, psychologists, and/or master's level social workers (Goldstrom *et al.*, 2001).

In this survey, Hayes defines "qualified mental health professional" as an individual, who by virtue of his/her education, credentials, and experience is permitted by law to evaluate and care for the mental health needs of patients. This list of professionals includes, but is not limited to, psychiatrists, psychologists, clinical social workers, and psychiatric nurses. The same report shows that the majority (70 percent) of suicide victims were assessed by a qualified mental health professional prior to death. A much smaller percentage (34 percent) of suicide victims housed in detention centers receive mental health assessments prior to their deaths, compared to those in other types of facilities.

Slightly over half (52 percent) of all detention center suicide victims committed suicide during the first six days of confinement, suggesting the possibly that intake or early assessment might have important prevention value (Hayes, 2004). Only 20 percent of victims assessed were not assessed by a QMHP within 30 days prior to their death. Overall, a little less than half (44 percent) of the suicide victims in the study had never been assessed by a QMHP, or had not been assessed by a clinician within 30 days of their death (Hayes, 2004).

National juvenile correctional standards and standard correctional practices recommend that all confined youth should be assessed as early as possible during their confinement by a QMHP (National Commission on Correctional Health Care, 1995, 1999; Underwood & Berenson, 2001), and performance standards require an assessment within seven days of entry into the facility (Council of Juvenile Correctional Administrators, 2003).

Does suicide rate vary by the type of juvenile institution?

The national survey of juvenile suicide in confinement found that 42 percent of juvenile suicides took place in training school/secure facilities, while 37 percent occurred in detention centers, 15 percent in residential treatment centers, and 6 percent in reception/diagnostic centers. Almost half (48 percent) of the suicides occurred in facilities administered by state agencies, while 39 percent took place in county facilities, and 13 percent in private programs. Interestingly, the study did not find any evidence to suggest that overcrowding was a contributing factor to juvenile suicide (Hayes, 2004).

National juvenile correctional standards recommend that all juvenile facilities should have a written suicide prevention policy that details methods for the identification and management of suicidal youth (American Correctional Association, 1991; Council of Juvenile Correctional Administrators, 2003; Hayes, 1999). Hayes reported that the majority (79 percent) of correctional facilities responding to his survey indicated that their facility maintained a written suicide prevention policy at the time of the suicide, although detention centers maintained suicide prevention policies to a lesser degree (62 percent). Regarding intake screening for suicide risk, the majority (71 percent) of facilities reported that they maintained an intake screening process to identify suicide risk of youth entering their facility, although less than half (48 percent) of the detention centers maintained an intake screening process to identify suicide risk.

More than half (57 percent) of facilities reported that they provided some type of suicide prevention training to all of their direct care staff. The overwhelming majority (90 percent) of facilities reported that they maintained a suicide precaution protocol for the observation of youth known to be at risk. However, less than half (48 percent) of facilities responded that constant observation was the highest level of suicide precaution in the facility, with 37 percent reporting 15-minute interval observation as their highest suicide precaution level. Only 28 percent of detention center respondents indicated that constant observation was the highest level of suicide precaution in their facilities (Hayes, 2004).

Gallagher and Dobrin (2005) examined the association between suicide screening practices and the outcome of attempts requiring emergency care in juvenile justice facilities. This study reports that controlling for facility characteristics, screening the entire facility population within the first 24 hours after arrival is significantly associated with a lower rate of serious suicide attempts. This author concludes that the level of risk for serious suicide attempts may be reduced by screening every child and adolescent within the 24-hour window directly follow-ing arrival, regardless of facility size, and by treating transfer between institutions as new admissions (Gallagher & Dobrin, 2005).

Special issues and future directions

We do have to question why suicide rates are so high in institutions that are supposed to be secure and safe. Further research should perhaps focus on factors that may contribute to the rates of suicide in juvenile confinement.

While there are some published studies on the prevention of youth delinquency, there are few evaluations of treatment programs for incarcerated youth. Available studies on the prevention of delinquency support the conclusion that primary prevention efforts have real impact and decrease the risk of relapse up to three years after intervention (Woolfenden et al., 2001). Family interventions can even significantly reduce delinquency in siblings (Klein et al., 1977).

We found reports on family interventions for delinquent youth associated with good outcomes. Such interventions include functional family therapy (FFT), multisystemic therapy (MST) and multidimensional treatment foster care (MTFC) (Alexander & Parsons, 1982; Bronfenbrener, 1979; Borduin et al., 1995; Henggeler et al., 1993; Chamberlain & Reid, 1998; Chamberlain, 1990; Chamberlain & Reid, 1994). One task force on community preventive services recommended this intervention for prevention of violence in adolescents with a history of chronic delinquency (Hahn et al., 2005).

In one Australian study, parent education groups were offered to volunteers from 14 high schools that were closely matched to 14 comparison schools, to evaluate the impact of an empowerment-based parent education program on suicide risk factors in eighth grade students (aged 14 years). The professionally led groups aimed to empower parents to assist one another by improving com-munication skills and relationships with adolescents. The students responded to classroom surveys repeated at baseline and after three months. Students in the intervention schools demonstrated increased maternal care, reductions in conflict with parents, reduced substance use, and less delinquency. The study concluded that a whole-school parent education intervention demonstrated promising impact on a range of risk behaviors and protective factors relevant to youth self-harm and suicide (Toumbourou & Gregg, 2002).

Because impulsivity and anxiety are hypothesized to be crucial clinical features of at-risk behavior among adolescents, another French study examined the poten-tial value of sorting high-risk groups based on these qualities. The study reported that subtyping adolescents with at-risk behavior into four groups according to their level of anxiety and impulsivity showed that mood disorders, delinquency with conduct disorder, and anorexia were associated with high scores on both variables. Substance abuse was associated with high impulsivity but not high anxiety levels. It is likely that this approach to subtyping at-risk youth may be useful for prevention and therapeutics (Askenazy *et al.*, 2003).

Problem-solving ability was the focus of a controlled clinical trial done by Biggam and colleagues in Scotland. Three groups of vulnerable incarcerated young offenders displayed impoverished problem-solving abilities: those at risk for suicidal behavior, those under protection due to their inability to assimilate into the mainstream, and those who bullied but remained in normal circulation. Deficits in problem-solving skills were significantly correlated with the levels of anxiety, depression, and hopelessness. This study evaluated the effectiveness of a time-limited group-based problem-solving training intervention compared with a non-treatment control for vulnerable incarcerated young offenders. A total of 46 young offenders were assigned to either intervention or control groups. Intervention participants experienced significant reductions in their levels of anxiety, depression, and hopelessness, and improvement in their self-assessed social problem-solving abilities. Gains in problem-solving ability and mental health associated with the intervention group continued to be evident at three month follow-up (Biggam & Power, 2002).

The effectiveness of suicide prevention programs in jails

Studies have documented reductions in the number of suicide attempts and deaths in confinement systems that have implemented suicide prevention programs. These prevention programs typically include training for correctional officers and health professionals, intake screening, psychiatric evaluation for at risk inmates, communication among staff, special safe housing units, observation of inmates by officers, medical intervention procedures, and systematic retrospective review of completed suicide as they occur (Hayes, 1989; Winkler, 2002). As a result, national juvenile correctional standards and standard correctional practice require that all juvenile facilities have a written suicide prevention strategy that includes several key components (American Correctional Association, 1991; Council of Juvenile Correctional Administrators, 2003; Hayes, 1999; National Commission on Correctional Health Care, 1999).

One national survey on juvenile suicide in confinement reported that only 20 percent of facilities had written policies encompassing seven key suicide prevention elements at the time of the suicide. The degree to which facilities had documented all seven suicide prevention elements varied considerably by facility type – detention centers (10 percent), training schools/secure facilities (24 percent), reception/diagnostic centers (40 percent), and residential treatment centers (25 percent). These findings are consistent with the trends noted in the Office of Juvenile Justice and Delinquency Prevention's conditions of confinement study. While all types of facilities documented individual suicide prevention strategies more than any other type, few facilities had applied all seven components of a comprehensive suicide prevention program (Hayes, 2004).

The same study suggests a strong relationship between juvenile suicide and room confinement. Sixty-two percent of suicide victims had a history of room confinement prior to their deaths and 50 percent of victims were on room confinement status at the time of their deaths. What may be more interesting from a prevention perspective is that 85 percent of victims who committed suicide while on room confinement status died during daytime hours. The relationship between suicide and isolation has been described in the adult prisoner suicide literature (Bonner, 1992; Hayes, 1989).

Suicidal youth in confinement appear to feel more isolated, receive fewer visits, write fewer letters, and miss loved ones more than non-suicidal youth in custody (Liebling, 1993). Another study reported that 77 percent of all confined youth are in facilities that permit the use of isolation, and that the rates of suicidal behavior are higher for those isolated from their peers or assigned to single-room housing (Parent et al., 1994). With regard to non-fatal suicidal attempts, the studies and prevention programs surveyed suggest that it is optimal to screen every child and adolescent admitted to a juvenile justice facility within 24 hours of arrival, regardless of the type of facility, and regardless of whether the new admission is a transfer or not. Screening children and adolescents *as deemed necessary* (rather than systematically) was associated with higher rates of suicide attempts requiring emergency care. It may not be clinically reasonable or efficient to expect a troubled child or adolescent to communicate his/her dysphoria, suicidal thoughts, or need for screening during the highly stressful period of transition into a new facility (Gallagher & Dobrin, 2005).

National correctional standards and practices identify critical components that all juvenile facilities, regardless of size and type, should document in detailed suicide prevention policies and procedures (Council of Juvenile Correctional Administrators, 2003; Hayes, 1999, 2004; National Commission on Correctional Health Care, 1999). These critical components include: training, identification/screening, communication, housing, levels of supervision, intervention, reporting, and follow-up/mortality review.

The American Academy of Child and Adolescent Psychiatry (AACAP) has recently started an official action with the aim of building the practice parameters for the assessment and treatment of youth in juvenile detention and correctional facilities. The practice parameters do pay special attention to the problem of suicide in juvenile confinement and detention. In this article AACAP recommends that all youths entering a juvenile justice detention or correctional facility should be screened for mental or substance use disorders, suicide risk factors and behaviors, and other emotional or behavioral problems. All youths held in a juvenile justice detention or correctional facility should receive continued monitoring for mental or substance abuse disorders, emotional or behavioral problems, and especially for suicide risk. Any youth with recent/current suicidal ideation, attempts, or symptoms of a mental or substance-related disorder during the period of incarceration should be referred for additional evaluation by a mental health clinician (AACAP, 2005).

Conclusions

To address the multidimensional nature of suicide by delinquent adolescents, it is important to establish a systematic approach to the problem. There is very little research reported in the area of the primary prevention of suicide in delinquent adolescents. Most of the literature consists of retrospective reviews or intervention studies.

The literature on delinquent suicide is primarily focused on youth who are confined in jail or prison. There are no studies about suicide in delinquents who are not in confinement. It is likely that there is a sizable at-risk young delinquent population outside of jails and prisons.

The existence of juvenile institutions and their underlying missions are based in part on the belief that delinquents are amenable to behavior change. The juvenile justice system has evolved around the idea of individual rehabilitation. The institutions that facilitate this rehabilitation are supposed to be safe. This assumption may not be warranted. There are still open questions about environmental safety in the juvenile facilities. Other concerns include the absence or underutilization of suicide prevention policies, the unavailability or underutilization of mental health treatment, and insufficient interest in the value of primary prevention programs.

In some ways it appears that the American juvenile system has some of the same problems as the broader American healthcare system. Both offer excellent secondary and tertiary care, but come up short in the areas of prevention research studies and primary prevention programs. One could imagine that preventing mental illness, family dysfunction, and substance abuse by interventions in families, schools, and communities would be much more helpful in reducing the rate of adolescent suicide. Further research is needed.

References

AACAP (2005). Practice parameter for the assessment and treatment of youth in juvenile detention and correctional facilities. *Journal of the American Academy of Child and Adolescent Psychiatry*, **44**(10), 1085–1098.

Alessi, N., McManus, M., Brickman, A. & Grapentine, L. (1984). Suicidal behavior among serious juvenile offenders. *American Journal of Psychiatry*, **141** (2), 286–287.

Alexander, J. F. & Parsons, B. V. (1982). *Functional Family Therapy*. Monterey, CA: Brooks/Cole.

American Correctional Association (1991). *Standards for Juvenile Detention Facilities and Standards for Juvenile Correctional Facilities*. Laurel, MD: Author.

Arias, E., Anderson, R., Kung, H., Murphy, S. & Kochanek, K. (2003). Deaths: final data for 2001. *National Vital Statistics Report*, **52**(3). Hyattsville, MD: National Center for Health Statistics.

Askenazy, F. L., Sorci, K., Benoit, M. *et al.* (2003). Anxiety and impulsivity levels identify relevant subtypes in adolescents with at-risk behavior. *Journal of Affective Disorders*, **74** (3), 219–227.

Battle, A. O., Battle, M. V. & Tolley, E. A. (1993). Potential for suicide and aggression in delinquents at Juvenile Court in a southern city. *Suicide and Life-Threatening Behavior*, **23**(3), 230–244.

Biggam, F. H. & Power, K. G. (2002). A controlled, problem-solving, group-based intervention with vulnerable incarcerated young offenders. *International Journal of Offender Therapy and Comparative Criminology*, **6**(6), 678–698.

Bonner, R. (1992). Isolation, seclusion, and psychological vulnerability as risk factors for suicide behind bars. In R. Maris *et al.*, eds., *Assessment and Prediction of Suicide*. New York, NY: Guilford Press, pp. 398–419.

Borduin, C. M., Mann, B. J., Cone, L. *et al.* (1995). Multisystemic treatment of serious juvenile offenders: long-term prevention of criminality and violence. *Journal of Consulting and Clinical Psychology*, **63**, 569–578.

Brent, D. (1995). Risk factors for adolescent suicide and suicidal behavior: mental and substance abuse disorders, family environmental factors, and life stress. *Suicide and Life Threatening Behavior*, **25** (Supplement), 52–63.

Bronfenbrener, U. (1979). *The Ecology of Human Development: Experiments by Nature and Design*. Cambridge, MA: Harvard University Press.

Bureau of Justice Statistics (2000). *Correctional Populations in the United States, 1997*. Washington, DC: US Department of Justice.

Bureau of Justice Statistics (2001). *Census of Jails, 1999*. Washington, DC: US Department of Justice.

Chamberlain, P. (1990). Comparative evaluation of specialized foster care for seriously delinquent youth: a first step. community alternatives. *International Journal of Family Care*, **2**, 21–36.

Chamberlain, P. & Reid, J. B. (1994). Differences in risk factors and adjustment for male and female delinquents in treatment foster care. *Journal of Child and Family Studies*, **3**, 23–39.

Chamberlain, P. & Reid, J. B. (1998). Comparison of two community alternatives to incarceration for chronic juvenile offenders. *Journal of Consulting and Clinical Psychology*, **66**(4), 624–633.

Cole, D. A. (1989). Psychopathology of adolescent suicide: hopelessness, coping beliefs, and depression. *Journal of Abnormal Psychology*, **98**, 248–255

Council of Juvenile Correctional Administrators (2003). *Performance-based Standards (PbS) for Youth Correction and Detention Facilities: PbS Goals, Standards, Outcome Measures, Expected Practices and Processes*. Braintree, MA: Author.

Criminal Justice Institute (2000). *The 2000 Corrections Yearbook: Adult Corrections*. Middletown, CT: Author.

Davis, D., Bean, G., Schumacher, J. & Stringer, T. (1991). Prevalence of emotional disorders in a juvenile justice institutional population. *American Journal of Forensic Psychology*, **9**, 1–13.

Dembo, R., Williams, L., Wish, E. *et al.* (1990). Examination of the relationships among drug use, emotional/psychological problems, and crime among youths entering a juvenile detention center. *The International Journal of the Addictions*, **25**, 1301–1340.

Duclos, C., LeBeau, W. & Elias, G. (1994). American Indian suicidal behavior in detention environments: cause for continued basic and applied research. *Jail Suicide Update*, **5**(4), 4–9.

Duclos, C. W., Beals, J., Novins, D. K. *et al.* (1998). Prevalence of common psychiatric disorders among American Indian adolescent detainees. *Journal of the American Academy of Child and Adolescent Psychiatry*, **37**(8), 866–873.

Edens, J. & Otto, R. (1997). Prevalence of mental disorders among youth in the juvenile justice system. *Focal Point*, Spring, 1–8.

Esposito, C. & Clum, G. (2002). Social support and problem-solving as moderators of the relationship between childhood abuse and suicidality: applications to a delinquent population. *Journal of Traumatic Stress*, **15**(2), 137–146.

Evans, W., Albers, E., Macari, D. & Mason, A. (1996). Suicide ideation, attempts space and abuse among incarcerated gang and non gang delinquents. *Child and Adolescent Social Work Journal*, **13**, 115–126.

Farand, L., Chagnon, F., Renaud, J. & Rivard, M. (2004). Completed suicides among Quebec adolescents involved with juvenile justice and child welfare services. *Suicide and Life-Threatening Behavior*, **34**(1), 24–35.

Gallagher, C. A. & Dobrin, A. (2005). The association between suicide screening practices and attempts requiring emergency care in juvenile justice facilities. *Journal of the American Academy of Child and Adolescent Psychiatry*, **44**(5), 485–493.

Goldstrom, I., Jaiquan, F., Henderson, M., Male, A. & Manderscheid, R. (2001). The availability of mental health services to young people in juvenile justice facilities: a national survey. In *Mental Health, United States, 2000*. Washington, DC: Substance.

Gray, D., Achilles, J., Keller, T. *et al.* (2002). Utah Youth Suicide Study, Phase I: Government agency contact before death. *Journal of the American Academy of Child and Adolescent Psychiatry*, **41**, 427–434.

Hahn, R. A., Bilukha, O., Lowy, J. *et al.* (2005). Task force on community preventive services. The effectiveness of therapeutic foster care for the prevention of violence: a systematic review. *American Journal of Preventative Medicine*, **28**(1), 72–90.

Hayes, L. (1989). National Study of Jail Suicides: seven years later. *Psychiatric Quarterly*, **60**(1), 7–29.

Hayes, L. (1995). Prison suicide: an overview and a guide to prevention. *The Prison Journal*, **75**(4), 431–455.

Hayes, L. (1999). *Suicide Prevention in Juvenile Correction and Detention Facilities: A Resource Guide*. South Easton, MA: Council of Juvenile Correctional Administrators.

Hayes, L. (2004). Juvenile suicide in confinement: a national survey. NCIA.

Henggeler, S. W., Melton, G. B., Smith, L. A., Schoenwald, S. K. & Hanley, J. (1993). Family preservation using multisystemic therapy: long-term follow-up to a clinical trial with serious juvenile offenders. *Journal of Child and Family Studies*, **2**, 283–293.

Kempton, T. & Forehand, R. (1992). Suicide attempts among juvenile delinquents: the contribution of mental health factors. *Behavior Research and Therapy*, **30**(5), 537–541.

Klein, N. C., Alexander, J. F. & Parsons, B. V. (1977). Impact of family systems intervention on recidivism and sibling delinquency: a model of primary prevention and program evaluation. *Journal of Consulting and Clinical Psychology*, **45**(3), 469–474.

Kochanek, K. D., Murphy, S. L., Anderson, R. N. & Scott, C. (2002). Deaths: final data for 2002. *National Vital Statistics Report*, **53**(5), 1–115.

Liebling, A. (1993). Suicides in young prisoners: a summary. *Death Studies*, **17**, 381–409.

Mace, D., Rohde, P. & Gnau, V. (1997). Psychological patterns of depression and suicidal behavior of adolescents in a juvenile detention facility. *Journal for Juvenile Justice and Detention Services*, **12**(1), 18–23.

Messier, L. P. & Ward, T. J. (1998). The coincidence of depression and high ability in delinquent youth. *Journal of Child and Family Studies*, **7**, 97–105.

Morris, R., Harrison, E., Knox, G. *et al.* (1995). Health risk behavioral survey from 39 juvenile correctional facilities in the United States. *Journal of Adolescent Health*, **17**(6), 334–344.

National Center for Health Prevention and Injury Control (2001). Suicide fact sheet, 2001. (www.cdc.gov/ncipc/factsheets/suifacts.htm)

National Commission on Correctional Health Care (1995). *Standards for Health Services in Juvenile Detention and Confinement Facilities*. Chicago, IL: Author.

National Commission on Correctional Health Care (1999). *Standards for Health Services in Juvenile Detention and Confinement Facilities*. Chicago, IL: Author.

Otto, R., Greenstein, J., Johnson, M. & Friedman, R. (1992). Prevalence of mental disorders among youth in the juvenile justice system. In *Responding to the Mental Health Needs of Youth in the Juvenile Justice System*. Seattle, WA: National Coalition for the Mentally Ill in the Criminal Justice System, pp. 7–48.

Parent, D., Leiter, V., Kennedy, S. *et al.* (1994). *Conditions of Confinement: Juvenile Detention and Corrections Facilities*. Washington, DC: Office of Juvenile Justice and Delinquency Prevention, US Department of Justice.

Penn, J. V., Esposito, C. L., Schaeffer, L. E., Fritz, G. K. & Spirito, A. (2003). Suicide attempts and self-mutilative behavior in a juvenile correctional facility. *Journal of the American Academy for Child and Adolescent Psychiatry*, **42**(7), 762–769.

Robertson, A. & Husain, J. (2001). *Prevalence of Mental illness and Substance Abuse Disorders Among Incarcerated Juvenile Offenders*. Jackson, MS: Mississippi Department of Public Safety and Mississippi Department of Mental Health.

Rohde, P., Seeley, J. & Mace, D. (1997). Correlates of suicidal behavior in a juvenile detention population. *Suicide and Life-Threatening Behavior*, **27**(2), 164–175.

Ruchkin, V. V., Schwab-Stone, M., Koposov, R. A., Vermeiren, R. & King, R. A. (2003). Suicidal ideations and attempts in juvenile delinquents. *Journal of Child Psychology and Psychiatry, and Allied Disciplines*, **44**(7), 1058–1066.

Sanislow, C., Grilo, C., Fehon, D., Axelrod, S. & McGlashan, T. (2003). Correlates of suicide risk in juvenile detainees and adolescent in-patients. *Journal of the American Academy of Child and Adolescent Psychiatry*, **42**(2), 234–240.

Shelton, D. (2000). Health status of young offenders and their families. *Journal of Nursing Scholarship*, **32**(2), 173–178.

Steiner, H., Garcia, I. & Matthews, Z. (1997). Posttraumatic stress disorder in incarcerated juvenile delinquents. *Journal of the American Academy of Child and Adolescent Psychiatry*, **36**(3), 357–365.

Substance Abuse and Mental Health Services Administration (2001). *Summary of Findings from the 2000 National Household Survey on Drug Abuse*. NHSDA Series: H-13, DHHS Publication No. SMA 01-3549. Rockville, MD: Author.

Teplin, L., Abram, K., McClelland, G., Dulcan, M. & Mericle, A. (2002). Psychiatric disorders in youth in juvenile detention. *Archives in General Psychiatry*, **59**, 1133–1143.

Toumbourou, J. W. & Gregg, M. E. (2002). Impact of an empowerment-based parent education program on the reduction of youth suicide risk factors. *Journal of Adolescent Health*, **31**(3), 277–285.

Underwood, L. & Berenson, D. (2001). *Mental Health Programming in Youth Correction and Detention Facilities: A Resource Guide*. South Easton, MA: Council of Juvenile Correctional Administrators.

US Department of Health and Human Services (1999). *The Surgeon General's Call To Action To Prevent Suicide*. Washington, DC: Author.

White, T. & Schimmel, D. (1995). Suicide prevention in federal prisons: a successful five-step program. In L. Hayes, ed., *Prison Suicide: An Overview and Guide to Prevention*. Washington, DC: National Institute of Corrections, US Department of Justice, pp. 46–57.

Woolf, A. & Funk, S. (1985). Epidemiology of trauma in a population of incarcerated youth. *Pediatrics*, **75**(3), 463–468.

Woolfenden, S. R., Williams, K. & Peat, J. (2002). Family and parenting interventions for conduct disorder and delinquency in children and adolescents aged 10–17. *Archives of Disease in Childhood*, **86**(4), 251–256.

9

Juvenile sex offenders

Corinne Belsky, Wade C. Myers, and Daniel Bober

Definition

A juvenile sex offender can be defined as a youth who commits a sexual act upon a victim without consent, against the person's will, or in an exploitative, threatening, or aggressive manner. Due to variations in county, state, and federal statutes, what legally constitutes a sex offense or offender in one jurisdiction may not hold for another. Likewise, the sexual actions of minors in different countries will be acceptable or not depending on prevailing laws, culture, and local customs. Thus, it is important to consider the historical and cultural setting in which sexual offenses occur. For example, in some cultures masturbation is considered deviant.

Historical comment

Given the magnitude of juvenile sexual offenses and the toll they take on society, it is surprising they were not consistently taken seriously until at least the 1970s. Prior to that time the offenses were often regarded as exploratory, temporary behaviors that would resolve with age (Ryan & Lane, 1997). Other changes took place in the 1970s: civil and criminal statutes addressing sexual offenses were broadened, the accumulation of research on adult sex offenders began to accelerate, and adolescent sex offender programs were developed (Ryan & Lane, 1991). However, by the early 1980s there were still few studies of adequate sample size addressing the success rates for managing youths' sexually deviant behavior (Mayer, 1988).

Demographic data

As will be evident from the material presented in this chapter, perhaps the most overarching principle pertaining to juvenile sex offenders is that they are a

The Mental Health Needs of Young Offenders: Forging Paths toward Reintegration and Rehabilitation, eds. Carol L. Kessler and Louis J. Kraus. Published by Cambridge University Press. © Cambridge University Press 2007.

heterogeneous population. Having said this, they do share some commonalties. Most of them, about 90 percent, are male (Badgley, 1984). They generally have a history of non-sexual as well as sexual offenses (Greenfield, 1997). Their racial, socioeconomic, and religious distribution is similar to that of the general population in the United States (Ryan *et al.*, 1996). About one-half of adult sex offenders report they committed their first sexual transgression prior to age 18 (Groth, Longo & McFadin, 1982). Similarly, Fehrenbach, Smith, Monastersky, and Deisher found that half of convicted rapists and child molesters committed their first offense before age 18 (Fehrenbach *et al.*, 1986).

Juveniles commit a significant proportion of sexual crimes. It is estimated adolescents account for 20 percent of arrests for all sexual offenses excluding prostitution (Snyder, 1997), 20–25 percent of rapes (Hunter, 2000; Weinrott, Riggin & Frothingham, 1997), 14 percent of aggravated sexual assaults (Greenfield, 1996), and up to 50 percent of child molestation (Hunter, 2000).

Etiology

A number of theories have been proposed to explain the cause of sexual offending in juveniles. Key theories include those centering on such areas as family systems, cognitive patterns, learning, developmental influences, physiological mechanisms, psychosis, and deviant sexual fantasies (Ryan & Lane, 1991). For example, family systems theory postulates that disturbed family dynamics can contribute to sexual offending in children through pathological role modeling or exposure to deviant parental behaviors.

Cognitive explanations typically rest on the premise that juvenile offenders hold distorted beliefs they use to rationalize their behavior. There are perhaps developmental influences on minors' cognitive beliefs. It has been observed they are less likely than adults to use power, control, and violence during their offenses (Saunders & Awad, 1991). Moreover, they are more likely to endorse sex-role stereotypes, male dominance, rape-supportive myths, and to hold negative stereotypes regarding women (Epps, Haworth & Swather, 1993; Segal & Stermac, 1984). In a study of 1600 juvenile sex offenders, Ryan *et al.* (1996) found that only one-third perceived sex as a way to show love, one-quarter believed it was a way to feel power, one in ten thought of it as a way to dissipate anger, and just under one in ten identified it as a way to degrade or punish others (Ryan *et al.*, 1996).

Learning mechanisms suggest a child's early experiences of sexual arousal may have occurred in exploitative relationships and thus led to the formation of a pathological substrate for future sexual behavior. Developmental influences explain sexual offending through factors like child abuse, undefined family boundaries, and exposure to unhealthy sexual material.

From a physiological standpoint, testosterone, the sex hormone with the greatest effect on male sexual behavior, clearly plays a significant role in the etiology of most sex offenses. There also is substantial neurobiological literature indicating traumatic experiences like sexual abuse are associated with changes in the brain's chemical and structural integrity (Grant, 2000; Weber & Reynolds, 2004). Whether these alterations contribute to the potential for later sexual offending is unclear. Regarding psychosis, only a very small percentage of offenders have a psychotic illness impacting their behavior. In general, this latter group will be best served through traditional mental health treatment.

Obsessive deviant sexual fantasy has been implicated as a driving force for these types of offenses. Sex offenders typically become aware of their deviant predilections around the time of puberty; in some cases much earlier. Fantasies of abnormal sexual behavior often pre-date their acting upon them by several years. In a sample of 87 male adolescent sexual offenders it was discovered their deviant fantasies throughout treatment exceeded their normal sexual fantasies, and were more frequently paired with masturbation (Aylwin, Reddon & Burke, 2005). However, as treatment progressed, the proportion of deviant fantasies that were interrupted versus those coupled with masturbation grew from about 20 percent to 70 percent. They also experienced an overall decrease in deviant fantasies.

Categorization of abusers

A number of sex offender categorization schemes have been described. Several of them will be briefly outlined here. Becker (1988) suggested four types of sexual abusers: the antisocial; the paraphiliac; the adolescent with a psychiatric, biological, or neurological disorder; and the youth with impaired social skills. The antisocial youth has a broad range of exploitative behaviors. The paraphiliac has an established deviant pattern of arousal. The juvenile with a medical or psychiatric disorder may have poor impulse control. The youth lacking social skills may turn to younger children because sexual outlets are not available to him within his peer group.

Graves *et al.* (1996) reported three categories of juvenile sex offenders: pedophilic; sexual assault offender; and mixed offender. Pedophilic offenders were described as lacking confidence in their social ability and isolated from peers. Sexual assault offenders were those whose first offenses were commonly reported between the ages of 13–15, who victimized more females than males, and who offended against victims of various ages. The mixed offenders had committed a variety of offenses involving younger children. Their offenses included exhibitionism, voyeurism, frotteurism, and other behaviors. This last group was identified as having the most severe social and psychological problems.

O'Brien and Bera (1986) classified juvenile male sex offenders into seven sub-groups: naïve experimenter; undersocialized child exploiter; pseudosocialized child exploiter; sexual aggressive; sexual compulsive; disturbed impulsive; and group influenced (O'Brien & Bera, 1986). These categories are largely self-explanatory.

Female offenders

A study by Fehrenbach and Monastersky (1988) looked at 28 girls with an average age of 13. Seventy percent offended while baby-sitting and 50 percent had a history of having been victimized. The average age of their victims was five.

Hirshberg and Riskin (1994) studied 20 female adolescent sex offenders at a residential program. As this was a residential population it can be assumed that the girls had more serious or more frequent offending behaviors than would be seen in an outpatient population. In this sample, 80 percent initiated their offending prior to age 13, 90 percent had been sexually abused, 55 percent had been physically abused, and 100 percent had been either physically or sexually abused. None of the girls came from an intact family. Their victims were evenly split between boys and girls. Of the 48 victims, 28 were family members, 3 were relatives outside of the house, 5 were children for whom they baby-sat, and 12 were neighborhood children. There was an average age difference of five years between the victim and perpetrator. Regarding sexual acts performed by the girls upon their victims, 75 percent carried out genital contact without penetration, 45 percent committed oral sex, 30 percent penetrated the victim's vagina with a finger or object and 10 percent had intercourse with their victims.

Very young offenders

In the juvenile population, it is not only teenagers who commit sex offenses. In a study of 616 juveniles who were referred for treatment after the age of 12, 26 percent had been abusing others prior to age 12 (Ryan *et al.*, 1996). In the very young age group, the percentage of female offenders is higher than in the adolescent group (Araji, 1997).

Studies by English and Ray comparing pre-adolescent and adolescent offenders indicate the adolescents were more aggressive and coercive, less empathic, and more likely to minimize.

In Johannesburg, South Africa, The Teddy Bear Clinic has established a special treatment track for rapists in the age range of six–nine years old (Johnston, 2004).

The curriculum for these child offenders includes creating victim empathy, anger management, appropriate sexual behavior, and impulse control. One of their tasks is to re-enact their crimes while putting themselves in the victim role. This clinic was conceived when the courts became overwhelmed with pre-pubescent rapists too young to be prosecuted.

Risk factors

There are many risk factors for the development of juvenile sex offending. Perpetrators often have a history of victimization, including physical or sexual abuse, and have often witnessed domestic violence (Becker & Kaplan, 1988). Twenty to 50 percent have been physically abused and 40–80 percent have been sexually abused. These rates are even higher for female abusers (Hunter & Becker, 1998). Other risk factors include deviant sexual interests, an impaired capacity for empathy, poor impulse and anger control, social skills deficits, disturbed inter-personal relationships, low self-esteem, psychiatric illness, having divorced parents, developmental delay, poor academic performance, neuropsychiatric deficits, non-sexual conduct disordered behavior, and inadequate sex education (Becker & Kaplan, 1988; Becker & Hunter, 1993). Sexually offending youths also have a higher rate of exposure to hard-core pornography (Ford & Linney, 1995). In terms of peer relationships, Fehrenbach *et al.* (1986) noted two-thirds of juvenile sex offenders experienced significant social isolation, one-third had no close friends, and one-third were friendless.

A Canadian study examined 852 subjects, 6 percent of whom had been convicted of a sexual offense. The average age was 17. The sex offenders were significantly more likely than the non-sexual offenders to have been sexually abused, have higher depression scores, and to have failed a school grade (Correctional Service of Canada, 1995). Additionally, the juveniles who had also been physically abused were 7.6 times more likely to rape or sodomize other children than those who were sexually abused or neglected (Widom, 1995).

Factors that contribute to sexual abuse victims becoming perpetrators include sexual arousal at the time of the abuse, confusion about sexual identity, compensatory hypermasculinity, and a readiness to re-enact the abuse in the role of the victimizer (Friedrich, 1995; Watkins & Bentovim, 1992). Yates (1982) found that children victimized between the ages of two and six exhibited excessive erotization and had trouble differentiating erotic touching from affectionate touching. The younger the child when his first sex offense occurred, the more likely he was sexually victimized himself. Seventy-two percent of offenders younger than 6, 42 percent of those 7–10, and 35 percent of those 11–12 were sexually victimized (Johnson, 1988). Physical abuse by fathers and sexual abuse by males increased the likelihood of later sexual aggression. Having a bond with the mother was found to be a protective factor for sexual aggression (Kobayashi *et al.*, 1995).

A literary example of developmental influences in a sex offender

William Faulkner (1931) portrayed keen insight into the development of sexual offending behavior in his 1931 novel *Sanctuary*. In this novel, the impotent character Popeye rapes a young woman with a corncob. Popeye's father abandoned his mother while she was pregnant, suggesting the presence of paternal antisocial traits and contributing to an unstable, single-parent household. Popeye's development showed signs of disturbance early on. His mother's pregnancy was complicated by illness. She mistakenly thought he was blind when he was an infant, based on his lack of visual interest in his surroundings and lack of eye contact. He did not learn to walk or talk until he was four years old; further evidence of developmental delay. When Popeye was three years old he was described as looking like a one-year-old. His maternal grandmother left him in a stranger's car while she purchased matches and then returned home and intentionally burned the house down. A further description in the words of Faulkner:

Popeye might well have been dead. He had no hair at all until he was five years old, by which time he was already a kind of day pupil at an institution: an undersized, weak child with a stomach so delicate that the slightest deviation from a strict regimen fixed for him by the doctor would throw him into convulsions . . . . "Alcohol would kill him like strychnine," the doctor said. "And he will never be a man, properly speaking." (William Faulkner, 1931)

One day, when a woman threw a birthday party for Popeye, he locked himself in the bathroom and engaged in animal cruelty:

On the floor lay a wicker cage in which two lovebirds lived; beside it lay the birds themselves, and the bloody scissors with which he had cut them up alive. Three months later . . . Popeye was arrested and sent to a home for incorrigible children. He had cut up a half-grown kitten the same way. (William Faulkner, 1931)

As he got older he was described as uncommunicative. He moved from town to town. Faulkner described that Popeye "had no friends and never known a woman and knew he could never . . . ." He later killed two people.

In summary, Popeye had numerous risk factors for sexual offending and violence in general. He likely had an antisocial father, came from a single-parent family, was a high-risk pregnancy, had developmental delays, suffered from an apparent neurological disorder (convulsions), exhibited childhood aggression, had a grandmother who was an arsonist (she possibly suffered from a paranoid disorder), engaged in delinquent behaviors, lacked friends, and suffered from low self-esteem due to his impotence and small stature.

Psychiatric co-morbidity

Mental disorders are commonly present in juvenile sex offenders. About 80 percent have a diagnosable psychiatric disorder (Kavoussi, Kaplan & Becker, 1988). Roughly 25–35 percent have some degree of intellectual disability (Stermac & Mathews, 1989). Males are more likely to be diagnosed with paraphilias or conduct disorder, whereas females are most commonly diagnosed with mood disorders and engage in self-mutilation (Matthews, Hunter & Vuz, 1997). In one study, 92 percent of male adolescent sex offenders had conduct disorder, 67 percent had a narcissistic personality disorder, and 72 percent had a borderline personality disorder (Shaw, Applegate & Rothe, 1996). Those adolescents who abused children had higher rates of schizoid, dependent, and avoidant personality disorders (Carpenter, Peed & Eastman, 1995).

The law: registration, sexually violent predator, and civil commitment issues

Legal issues

Statutes generally define penetrating offenses (oral, vaginal, or anal) as felonies, and crimes not involving physical contact (voyeurism, exhibitionism, obscene phone calls) as misdemeanors (Myers, Burgess & Nelson, 1998; Kole, 1994; Office of Juvenile Justice, 1999). All states have mandated reporting laws for suspected child abuse. Physicians must report knowledge of juvenile as well as adult child sexual abusers (SIECUS, 1998).

There are a number of reasons why the juvenile justice system exists separately from the adult system. One issue is the concern that children would be preyed upon by adults in adult correctional settings. Second, the adults, who have had more time to perfect criminal behavior, might be a negative influence on children. Also, children are regarded as having diminished responsibility, and a special court atmosphere is necessary to ensure this matter is considered. Furthermore, it is believed juveniles are more amenable to rehabilitation than adults. The minimum age at which a juvenile can be tried for criminal activity varies from 6–12 years old by state (Kole, 1994; Office of Juvenile Justice, 1999; SIECUS, 1998).

There have been many legal changes to the juvenile justice system with regard to sexual offending. More juveniles are being waived to adult courts (Szymanski, 1998). The age at which a juvenile can be tried has been lowered in the majority of states (Szymanski, 1998). Many states do not have a minimum age at which they can be tried as adults (National Center for Juvenile Justice, 1998).

Unfortunately, the adult system does not provide the same supervision, treatment, or protections that are available in the juvenile system (Becker & Hicks, 2003). Many states permit public hearings without regard to the crime. More than half of states permit public access to juvenile court records with few restrictions (Szymanski, 1998). Yet analyses have shown that treatment programs are six times less expensive than incarceration (Donato & Shanahan, 1999). Furthermore, if an adolescent is imprisoned, then suddenly released, he is more likely to reoffend than one who is gradually exposed to the community while in a treatment program (National Institute of Correction, 1988).

Sexually violent predator laws

The Jacob Wetterling Act of 1994 allows for registration and tracking of those convicted of violent sex crimes and sex crimes against minors. The Act was amended in 1996 with Megan's Law, which requires law enforcement agencies to release information needed to protect the public. This was a change from the prior laws that authorized, but did not require, the release of this information. In 1996, the Pam Lynchner Sexual Offender Tracking and Identification Act laid out criteria for lifetime registration of dangerous offenders, penalties for failure to register, and a requirement that a national offender registry be created by the FBI (US Department of Justice, 1999).

Registration

States may require juvenile offender registration if they so choose. However, juveniles convicted as adults must register (US Department of Justice, 1999). Some states have the same registration requirements for juveniles and adults. In other states, juveniles only have to register until age 18 or 21 (Center for Sex Offender Management, 1999).

Arkansas' juvenile assessment and registration laws will be reviewed as an example. Arkansas *requires* sex offender screening and risk assessment for those juveniles charged with rape, sexual assault in the first or second degree, incest, or for those who "engaged children in sexually explicit conduct for use in visual or print medium." A juvenile *may* be screened and assessed for any offense that is sexually motivated. Registration may be required on the recommendation of the Sex Offenders Assessment Committee and following a hearing. Reassessment may be ordered at any time while the court has jurisdiction over the juvenile. The court must conduct a hearing within 90 days of the registration motion. The juvenile is represented by counsel and the court considers the following in making a decision to require registration: the seriousness of the offense, the protection of society, the level of planning and participation in the offense, the juvenile's previous sex offender history, whether there are programs available for rehabilitation, and the sex offender assessment or other information deemed relevant. The court may not use the juvenile's right against self-incrimination, right to a hearing or appeal, or refusal to admit to offenses in their consideration of whether or not to require registration. If the juvenile is required to register, the Division of Youth Services of the Department of Human Services or a juvenile probation officer must then complete the registration form, provide a copy to the juvenile and his or her parents, mail a copy to the Sex Offender Registry Manager, provide a copy to the local law enforcement agency, and forward copies to the court for placement in the court file.

The juvenile may petition the court to have his or her name removed from the registry at any time while the court has jurisdiction over him or her, or when the juvenile turns 21 years of age, whichever is later. The judge shall have the name removed upon proof, by a preponderance of the evidence, that the juvenile no longer poses a threat to the safety of others. If the court does not order for the name to be removed, it will remain on the registry for ten years from the last date on which the juvenile was adjudicated as an adult for a sex offense or until the juvenile turns 21, whichever is longer (National Center on Sexual Behavior of Youth).

Civil commitment

As of 2004, 16 states and Canada had laws pertaining to the involuntary civil commitment of sexually violent adult predators. A sexually violent predator is defined as a person who is a repeat sexually violent offender, and suffers from a behavioral abnormality that makes him or her likely to engage in a predatory act of sexual violence. A predatory act is defined as one whose purpose is victimization (Texas Council on Sex Offender Treatment and the National Center for Prosecution of Child Abuse, 2004). The US Supreme Court's 1997 ruling in *Kansas v. Hendricks* upheld the constitutionality of violent sexual predator commitment for inmates who completed their sentences. The ruling has allowed commitment for an undetermined period of treatment, rather than parole into the community, for those deemed a danger to society. The American Academy of Child and Adolescent Psychiatry has recommended several factors to be taken into account before juveniles are civilly committed in this manner: the juvenile's developmental level; the influences of family and peers as contributory to the behavior; and the fact that placing them in an environment with adult offenders may exacerbate their behavior or put them at risk in other ways (American Academy of Child and Adolescent Psychiatry Task Force on Juvenile Justice Reform, 2001).

Types of sex offenders and case examples

In this section some different types of juvenile sex offenders will be briefly reviewed along with selected case vignettes. It is recognized at the outset that presenting youthful perpetrators in a categorical way has limitations, given that many offenders will engage in more than one form of sexual offending. On the other hand, lumping sex offenders into one group does not allow for the elucidation of certain intraclass characteristics that may be germane to a particular group.

Sibling incest

It is generally believed that limited sexual exploration by close aged siblings is not necessarily pathological. One definition of incest is sexual interaction that goes beyond age-appropriate exploration such that "older siblings, who differ significantly in age or by virtue of their power and resources, may be considered abusive" (Tower, 1996). For siblings close to the same age, incest may merely be sexual exploration that is a part of normal development but socially unacceptable or undesired. When there is coercion or a significant age difference it is considered abuse. Generally, a difference of five or more years between the siblings would constitute abuse by the older child, even if the younger child was willing. Incestuous families are often dysfunctional and disorganized, with their members lacking role definition (Ascherman & Safier, 1990).

Emotional detachment or physical absence on the part of parents may set the stage for sibling abuse. Often, when abuse is occurring, the parents do not want to believe the child's report (Peterson, 1992). Those children who commit incest are more likely to come from families with higher rates of marital discord, parental rejection, and physical discipline, and are likely to have been sexually victimized (Worling, 1995).

O'Brien (1991) compared 170 juveniles who offended against siblings with those who offended against children outside of the family, those who victimized peers, and those who had a mix of sibling and non-sibling victims. The sibling offenders engaged in the most episodes of abuse (18 vs. 4.2 for non-sibling offenders, 7.4 for peer offenders, and 8.5 for mixed offenders). The sibling offenders also committed abuse over the longest duration of time. They were more likely to penetrate their victims (46 percent vs. 28 percent for the non-sibling offenders, and 13 percent for the peer offenders). Furthermore, they were more likely to have multiple victims. Despite these statistics, only about one-third were court-ordered to receive treatment, versus three-quarters of the non-sibling offenders. The sibling offenders had an increased rate of physical abuse (61 percent vs. 45 percent in non-sibling offenders, and 37 percent for peer offenders). They also had higher rates of sexual abuse by their fathers.

Rape

Those juveniles who commit rape more commonly select strangers as their victims (Snyder & Sickmund, 1995). As noted earlier, juveniles are responsible for roughly

20–25 percent of rapes. According to the National Center for Juvenile Justice, of the 95 136 forcible rapes committed in 2002, 23 percent of the offenders who committed them were under the age of 18. This amounts to about 22 000 juvenile perpetrated rapes for that year.

Cowan and Campbell (1995) examined the attitudes of adolescents towards rape in 453 Black, Asian, Hispanic, and White high school students. Subjects rated five factors that they believed were the most likely causes of rape (male dominance, female precipitation, society, male sexuality, and male pathology). There was a gender difference in responses. The female students ranked male pathology as the most likely cause, whereas males ranked female precipitation as most likely.

Rape case example

Jack, a 15-year-old male, was arrested for sexual battery on a 9-year-old neighbor. Jack sodomized this youth during a sleepover. The parents of the two youths were friends and there was no suspicion beforehand that Jack was capable of such behavior. During the act Jack wore a condom and used lotion for lubrication. A physical examination of the victim revealed a small anal tear. In an interview with police, Jack placed the blame for the sexual contact squarely on the victim. He said this boy disrobed in the bedroom where they were to sleep that night and pestered him for sex. At last, Jack relented and, in his words, obtained no enjoyment from it. In sharp contrast was the victim's description: he described Jack entering the bedroom naked, pulling his pajama bottoms down, and physically coercing him into complying with the act. The victim appeared frightened and tense as he recalled the event. On evaluation it was discovered Jack was mildly mentally retarded and also had attention-deficit/hyperactivity disorder (ADHD) and a language disorder. He had been suspended from school on several occasions for fighting. There was no known history of sexual abuse in Jack's past and he denied previous sexual contact with anyone.

Sexual homicide

Juveniles commit approximately one percent of sexual homicides annually (Myers, 2002). In a study by Myers and Blashfield (1997) of 14 juvenile sexual murderers, it was found that two-thirds reported violent sexual fantasies prior to their crimes, obtained erections, and experienced orgasms at the crime scene, used cutting weapons in the commission of their crimes (predominantly knives), and generally knew their victims, acted alone, and chose low-risk victims. All had academic problems despite an average intelligence quotient (IQ) of 101. Ninety-three percent had a previous history of violent behavior, 86 percent had conduct disorder, 43 percent had a substance abuse disorder, 21 percent had ADHD, and 21 percent had an anxiety disorder. Two-thirds had at least one personality disorder, more commonly from Cluster A or B. Myers (2002) identified ten risk factors in this population: impaired capacity to feel guilt; neuropsychiatric vulnerabilities; serious school problems; child abuse; family dysfunction; history of interpersonal violence; prior arrests; sadistic fantasies; psychopathic personality traits; and the presence of a personality disorder. The first three factors were present in 100 percent of the youths studied. Surprisingly, only 13 percent of the boys reported having been sexually abused.

These crimes fell into one of four categories: explosive, predatory, revenge, and displaced matricide. The explosive type was the most common, characterized by a sudden release of sexual and aggressive feelings with little planning involved. The predatory sexual homicide was planned; the juvenile fantasized about the sexual excitement and domination that he was going to experience. The revenge perpetrator was angry at his victim for a perceived wrong and sought to punish him or her. The predatory and revenge offenders generally had markedly elevated psychopathy scores. Sadistic fantasy was unusual in the revenge offender. The displaced matricide type was hypothesized to have acted on unconscious erotic and destructive urges toward the mother that were displaced onto the victim. These youths were found to be less psychopathic and aggressive than the other types. They also were unsuccessful in raping their victims (Myers, 2002).

Sexual homicide by youths is not just a phenomenon seen in the United States. In December 2003, a 14-year-old boy was sentenced by an Israeli court to 15 years incarceration for the rape and murder of a five-year-old girl. When he was 13 he chased the girl as she was leaving a store, caught her, picked her up, and forced her into his room. There he sodomized her. He reported he was unable to silence her crying so he grabbed a kitchen knife and stabbed her 31 times (www. haaretz.com, 2003).

Paraphilias

Paraphilias are recurrent, intense, sexually arousing fantasies, urges, or behaviors involving sexual activity with either non-human objects, children, or other non-consenting people, or involving suffering or humiliation of oneself, or a victim. The symptoms must be present for at least six months and cause distress or impairment in functioning (DSM-IV-TR, 2000). It is a minority of sexually offending youth who manifest paraphilic sexual arousal. The highest levels of deviant sexual arousal are found in those juveniles who exclusively target young male children, particularly when penetration occurs (Hunter & Becker, 1994).

Pedophilia

This disorder consists of fantasies, urges, or behaviors involving sexual activity with a prepubescent child. The offender must be at least 16 years old and five years older than the victim (DSM-IV-TR, 2000). The very definition precludes many juveniles due to the age requirement. Nevertheless, Huizinga (1977) found four out of 21 adult pedophiles claimed awareness of their pedophilic propensity prior to age six and another six offenders were aware of it by age 12 (Huizinga, 1977). Other research suggests more than a third of pedophiles begin their sexual offending *before* the age of 12, and 60–80 percent of them began offending as adolescents.

Although most adolescent molesters are male and their victims female, those adolescents who abuse very young children are more likely to choose male victims (Ryan *et al.*, 1996; Matthews, Hunter & Vuz, 1997). Of those who offend against much younger children, almost half assault at least one male victim. About 40 percent of victims are relatives. These offenders rely on opportunity, guile, and bribes to obtain victims (Hunter, Hazelwood & Slesinger, 2000). They often have low self-esteem and lack social competence (Awad & Saunders, 1989). This is in contrast to youths who offend against peers or adults; usually their victims are female strangers or acquaintances, and their sex crimes are more likely to be committed in conjunction with other criminal activity (Hunter, Hazelwood & Slesinger, 2000). A study by Awad and Saunders (1991) discovered 40 percent of juvenile child molesters had a history of previous child molestation.

Zolondek *et al.* (2001) examined the self-reported characteristics of juvenile sexual offenders. Four hundred and eighty-five male adolescents aged 11–17 years completed the Abel Questionnaire for Boys, a standardized instrument that measures sexual interests. More than 60 percent reported involvement in child molestation. Of the boys who reported never being accused of child molestation, 42 percent reported they had indeed molested a child.

Voyeurism

Voyeurism involves the act of observing unsuspecting individuals, usually strangers, who may be naked, disrobing, or engaging in sexual activity. Masturbation usually occurs during or shortly after voyeuristic activities. One study of 78 university men, who professed interest only in adult women, indicated the age of extinction for their interest in child nudity was on average 11.7 years (Freund & Kuban, 1993). The onset of voyeurism is typically before the age of 15, and the individual may become so invested in the voyeuristic activity that it becomes the sole sexual behavior. It is often a chronic condition.

From a developmental perspective, about one-third of parents reported voyeurism in their two- to five-year-olds and one-fifth reported it in their 10- to 12-year-old children (Schoentjes, Deboutte & Friedrich, 1999). Moll (1908), presented a case of a voyeur who began looking under servants' petticoats at age five or six. His voyeuristic tendency was considered firmly established by age 13.

Exhibitionism

Exhibitionism consists of fantasies, urges, or behaviors involving the exposure of one's genitals to an unsuspecting stranger (DSM-IV-TR, 2000). A certain degree of exhibitionism is normal in children. One study found that parents reported they had observed their children showing sex parts to other children in 13 percent of children age 2–5 and in 7 percent of children age 6–9 (Schoentjes, Deboutte & Friedrich, 1999).

Jones and Frei (1979) described 24 exhibitionists who recalled an early adolescent onset. Most could give an account of the mode of onset, and six were rated by the authors as "single incidents which could plausibly have triggered off a predisposition in a person at a critical stage of sexual development."

Saunders and Awad (1991) found in their clinical assessment of 19 male adolescent sexual offenders who had committed exhibitionism or telephone scatalogia that the majority were maladjusted, had committed numerous sexual offenses, and came from multiproblem families. Antisocial traits, sexual deviance in the family, homosexual conflicts, repressed sexuality, and sexual deviance were considered to be contributory factors.

Sadism

Sadism entails fantasies, urges, or behaviors involving acts in which the psychological or physical suffering, including humiliation, of the victim is sexually exciting to the person (DSM-IV-TR, 2000). Dekkers (2000) related this case: "A 42-year-old engineer remembers that in his boyhood he had enjoyed watching the slaughtering of domestic animals and particularly of pigs. It often gave him a very strong sexual feeling and an ejaculation. Later, he sought out slaughterhouses to enjoy watching the spurting blood and the death throes of the animals, which always gave him a counting feeling of sexual pleasure." There is a lack of systematic research in this area involving juveniles, although clinical case reports over the years are not uncommon (e.g., see De River, 1950; Myers, 2002; Myers, 2004).

Fetishism

This paraphilia is defined as fantasies, urges, or behaviors involving the use of non-living objects for sexual pleasure (DSM-IV-TR, 2000). While in and of itself fetishism is not harmful to others, it may be associated with other sexual deviancies. Extreme examples exist. For instance, serial killer and necrophile Jerry Brudos' abnormal sexual behaviors began at the age of five when he was reprimanded by his mother for playing with her shoes. As an adolescent he became entranced by black stiletto heels. In his later teens he would sneak outside at night to steal women's underwear from clotheslines (Blundell & Blackhall, 2004). In one of the authors' clinical caseloads was an adopted boy who was treated for his need to pilfer

underwear and hosiery from females' bedrooms in the surrounding neighborhood. He would take the underwear back to his bedroom and masturbate into
them. There was a vague history of him having been sexually abused as a very
young boy, but he had no memory of it and records were not available.

Transvestic fetishism

This is a disorder in which a heterosexual male has fantasies, urges, or behaviors
involving cross-dressing (DSM-IV-TR, 2000). Benjamin, as cited in Janssen
(2003), found that in 200 cross-dressers, most of them recalled the onset of their
condition as strikingly early in their childhood. In a non-clinical sample of
504 self-identified transvestites, Prince and Bentler found that 14 percent began
cross-dressing before age five, and 40 percent began between five–ten years old
(Janssen, 2003).

Paraphilias not otherwise specified

These consist of paraphilias that do not meet criteria for any of the specific
categories. Included are telephone scatalogia (obscene phone calls), necrophilia
(corpses), partialism (exclusive focus on a part of the body), zoophilia (animals),
coprophilia (feces), klismaphilia (enemas), and urophilia (urine) (DSM-IV-TR,
2000). It is too broad of a task to cover each of these in detail here, but some
background and case examples will be presented.

Zoophilia

Also referred to as bestiality or buggery, this perversion is the occurrence of
recurrent, intensely sexually arousing fantasies, urges, or behaviors involving
sex with animals. Fleming, Jory and Burton (2002) studied the family characteristics, victimization histories, and number of offenses of juvenile bestiality
offenders to juvenile human sex offenders. Of 381 institutionalized male youth
offenders, 6 percent admitted to having performed a sexual act with an animal.
The average age at the time of the animal contact was 11.3 years old. Twenty-three
of the 24 juveniles (96 percent) who admitted to bestiality also admitted to sexually
offending with a human victim. Fourteen of the 24 had rubbed their
genitals against an animal, ten had intercourse with an animal, four had oral sex
with an animal, and eight inserted a finger or object. The animal offenders were
also found to have a higher rate of victimization histories compared to the human
offenders.

When family characteristics were compared between animal and human sex
offenders, a statistically significant difference was found in the areas of affirming
communication and positive environment: the animal offenders' families were less
affirming and less positive. The animal offenders were also found to have

experienced more neglect and emotional abuse than the human sex offenders. Furthermore, the animal offenders reported more sexual victimization in their histories, as well as more offending events against humans than the purely human offenders (Fleming, Jory & Burton, 2002).

The first juvenile death penalty case in America was for a conviction of bestiality. The year was 1642 in Plymouth Colony, Massachusetts and 16-year-old Thomas Granger had been convicted of buggery. William Bradford, the governor of the colony, described the trial in the *History of Plymouth Plantation*:

He (Thomas Granger) was this year detected of buggery, and indicted for the same, with a mare, a cow, two goats, five sheep, two calves, and a turkey. Horrible it is to mention, but the truth of the history requires it. He was first discovered by one that accidentally saw his lewd practice towards the mare. (I forbear particulars.) Being upon it examined and committed, in the end he not only confessed the fact with that beast at that time, but sundry times before and at several times with all the rest of the forenamed in his indictment. And this his free confession was not only in private to the magistrates (though at first he strived to deny it) but to sundry, both ministers and others; and afterwards, upon his indictment, to the whole Court and jury; and confirmed it at his execution. And whereas some of the sheep could not so well be known by his description of them, others with them were brought before him and he declared which were they and which were not. And accordingly he was cast by the jury and condemned, and after executed about the 8th of September 1642. A very sad spectacle it was. For first the mare and then the cow and the rest of the lesser cattle were killed before his face, according to the law, Leviticus XX.15; and then he himself was executed. The cattle were all cast into a great and large pit that was digged of purpose for them, and no use made of any part of them. (Bradford, 1650)

Leviticus 20:15–16 states, "If a man has carnal relations with a beast, he shall be put to death; and you shall kill the beast. If a woman approaches any beast to mate with it, you shall kill the woman and the beast; they shall be put to death – their bloodguilt is upon them (*The Torah*)." (The Jewish Publication Society of America, 1962)

The German serial killer of the 1920s, Peter Kurten, was introduced to bestiality at the age of nine by a dogcatcher (Blundell & Blackhall, 2002). Below are two case reports involving adolescent bestiality from *The Sexual Criminal: A Psychoanalytic Study* (De River, 1950).

Zoophilia case example one

Betsy was a teenage student who lived with her parents and brothers. She was raised on a cattle and dairy farm and was skilled in the ways of ranch life. Betsy enjoyed the outdoor activities of riding horses, hunting, and fishing. Her health had been good, and her psychiatric history was negative except for a recent onset of depressive symptoms, e.g., decreased sleep and appetite, restlessness, loss of interest, anxiety, and occasional crying spells. At school she never cared much for her studies, and she found the girls at a city school she briefly attended to be "stuck up." She reported smoking cigarettes, but did not use alcohol or drugs. She denied a history of sexual activity with humans, explaining, "They don't interest me." There was no family history of mental illness. Mental status revealed an average or above level of intelligence and no evidence of psychosis.

Betsy first learned of sexual matters as a young girl when she watched – with "great interest" – a stallion aggressively fornicate with and hurt a mare. Both animals suffered minor injuries with bleeding during the union. Following this experience she enjoyed watching other animals engage in sex about the farm. She admitted to fondling the penises of colts on the farm, which caused them to have erections. Her masturbatory fantasies involved such topics as the stallion and mare mating episode, and dogs she had seen copulating. On one occasion the family dog, a Shepherd mix, humped her leg, and she recalled becoming sexually excited during this event. That night she let the dog into her room and allowed him to lick her genitals until she reached orgasm. This activity progressed to her having intercourse with the dog. Betsy recalled a sense of thrill when the dog would growl and snarl during the sex act. If he became overly aggressive she had learned to squeeze his testicles; this caused him to leave the room. She estimated her sexual relationship with the dog lasted two–three years.

Zoophilia case example two

Chico was raised primarily by his father. His mother died when he was seven. There was no family history of mental illness. Mental status revealed a below average level of intelligence and no evidence of psychosis.

Chico reported beginning regular masturbation at the age of six or seven. His first sexual contact with another living creature was with chickens, hens in particular, on his father's farm. He would insert his penis into their cloaca and stifle their sounds by wringing their necks. He estimated he engaged in sex with chickens three times a week, and this practice persisted for years. At the age of 18 he began having sex with a mare by standing on a box behind it. This happened "many times." When Chico was a young adult the neighbors complained he was having sex with his pet Collie. He had some relationships with women, and married once, but he preferred sexual intercourse with animals to human beings. Even the sight of animals sexually excited him. While he did not dislike people, he never got along well with them.

Necrophilia

Necrophilia consists of behaviors, fantasies, or urges to have sexual relations with a corpse. In 2003, CBS News ran the story of 16-year-old Daniel Robbins. He was accused of running down a jogger in hopes of having sex with her corpse. A year earlier he had written a list of New Year resolutions for a typing class assignment that included tasting human flesh, and shooting someone on a camping trip, as well as, "Get a driver's license so I can do those horrible things people like to read about in the paper." Robbins picked the jogger at random and hit her deliberately. He told a friend who was with him that he planned to have sex with the body (CBSNews.com, 2003).

Necrophilia case example

From the work of De River (1950) is a case example of necrophilia with a child-hood onset. This youth began working as a grave digger at a very young age. At the age of 11 he discovered his enjoyment of masturbating while touching the dead bodies of young, attractive women. Over time this behavior escalated to where he was having oral and vaginal sex with the corpses. He later went on to work in a mortuary as a body washer. As an adult he began posing as a mourner at funeral parlors. He would inquire as to how long the body was to be kept there. If the body was to be kept there overnight, he would return later in the evening and have sex with it. He was eventually arrested during the course of one of these outings and placed in an institution. He estimated he had sexual relations with hundreds of dead bodies beginning at age 11.

Evaluation of the juvenile sex offender
Interview and collateral information

Psychiatrists and other mental health professionals may be asked to evaluate the offender immediately following the offense, at the sentencing phase, or for treatment or disposition planning. They are generally asked to assess risk of recidivism, identification of treatment goals, and required level of care (Hunter, 1999). Due to difficulties in obtaining full disclosure, collateral information is imperative. Victim and witness statements, police reports, interviews with family, prior arrest records, and mental health records should be reviewed. Some key behaviors to assess during the interview include a history of sexually acting out, sexually provocative behavior, and being overly attentive to younger children. The clinician should always assess the child's motivation to change and willingness to receive professional help (Hunter, 1999).

At times, it can be a challenge to determine whether sexual activity was normal or exploitative. Areas to be considered in elucidating the motivation include: the age difference between the participants, whether it was consistent with developmental level, whether the participants had the same motivation (young children are more often curious, while adolescents' motives may be sexual pleasure), and whether or not the activity was coercive (De Jong, 1989). It is important to keep in mind that infrequently the younger child will be the abuser.

Some of the questions that may be covered in the evaluation are listed as follows. What was your family's attitude toward sex? How did you learn about sex? Do you or have you had a boyfriend or girlfriend? What was your age at first intercourse? Has any older person tried to do anything with you sexually? Have you ever been forced to have sex by someone threatening to harm you? Have you had sexual contact with someone of the same sex? Have you ever been in trouble for sexual behavior? Has anyone in your family been in trouble with the police for sexual behavior? What were your earliest sexual experiences? How frequently do you masturbate and to what fantasies? Do you view pornography? Do you have any troubles functioning sexually?

Some typical questions that examine criminal history and modus operandi might include any of the following. Have you committed any crimes in the past similar to this one? How long did you consider performing the crime? What was your relationship to the victim? How did you choose your victim? Did you fantasize about the crime beforehand? Did you ever see a movie or read a book with a similar crime? Were you alone or with others? How did you plan to get away with it? Did you have a weapon? How did you feel before, during, and after the crime? Was there a precipitating stressor? What sexual act(s) was committed? What type of force was used? Did you make threats? What was the location? How old was the victim?

If the juvenile is deemed appropriate for a community-based program, his or her living situation should be assessed. It is critical to take note of the location of the home, the level of parental supervision, whether other children reside there, and whether other children or adults in the neighborhood might be at risk if the youth remains in the community (Hunter, 1999).

Psychological and actuarial testing

Various assessment instruments can supplement the clinical interview process by providing information on a juvenile's psychological, behavioral, and sexual functioning. Some examples of tests that might be used in a sex offender evaluation are the MMPI-A (Archer, 1997), the Multiphasic Sex Inventory (Nichols & Molinder, 1984), the Child Sexual Behavior Inventory (Friedrich *et al.*, 1985), and the Adolescent Sexual Interest Card (Hunter *et al.*, 1991). The Juvenile Sex Offender Assessment Protocol-II (J-SOAP-II) and ERASOR-2 (Worling & Curwen, 2001) were developed to assess risk for future sex offenses by adolescents. The J-SOAP-II, designed by Prentky and Righthand (2003), is a checklist of risk factors associated with sexual and criminal offending designed to be used with boys between 12 and 18 years old who have been adjudicated for sexual offenses, or who have a history of sexually coercive behavior. Its purpose is to facilitate risk assessment and management, and to help guide treatment decisions. The checklist is divided into four sections. The first is a sexual drive/preoccupation scale that assesses such items as prior legally charged sex offenses, number of victims, and degree of planning. Scale two is the impulsive/antisocial behavior scale that takes into account pervasive anger, history of conduct disorder, and multiple types of offenses. Scale three is the intervention scale that includes acceptance of responsibility, internal motivation to change, and empathy. The last scale measures community stability/adjustment and includes the stability of the offender's living situation and evidence of a positive support system. The first two scales are combined to form a score of static factors. The second two scales combine to score dynamic factors. If an offender scores high on scale one, but not on scale two, he may benefit from more sex-offense specific treatment and less delinquency interventions. An adolescent who scores high on scale two, but low on one may have more antisocial and less sexually deviant behavior, and might benefit from more delinquency-focused treatment. Those who score high on both scales may require more intensive supervision, such as a residential program addressing both sex-offense treatment and more generalized delinquent intervention. Those who score low on scales one and two may have offended in a very specific situation, and might require limited intervention and have a lower chance of reoffending (Prentky & Righthand, 2003).

The ERASOR also is designed to assess the risk of sexual reoffending in adolescents, and employs both dynamic and static factors related to sexual transgressions. Specific areas it covers are a history of sexual assaults, sexual interests, attitudes and behaviors, psychosocial functioning, family and environmental functioning, and treatment (Worling & Curwen, 2001). It is important to keep in mind that psychological/actuarial testing is only supplementary to the clinical evaluation. None of these instruments should be relied on independently and outside of a clinical context. They each have weaknesses. For instance, the Multiphasic Sex Inventory lacks data on validity in adolescents (Becker & Hunter, 1997). The Adolescent Sexual Interest Card Sort correlates poorly with phallometric assessments (Hunter, Becker & Kaplan, 1995). The Child Sexual Behavior Inventory is limited by its reliance on parent reporting (Shaw, 1999).

Physiological assessment

The two primary physiological assessments used in sex offenders are phallometry and polygraphy. Phallometric assessment measures blood flow to the penis, and thus erectile changes, during presentation of potentially erotic visual and auditory stimuli. It is used to detect deviant sexual arousal that the individual may not have disclosed. While it has fair sensitivity in detecting pedophilia, it is less effective in evaluating other offenders. It can have a high rate of false positives, or for that matter, false negatives in those who are able to suppress arousal during the test. It is generally not used in youth under 14 years of age because of less reliable response patterns. Phallometry results are more accurate in older adolescent males with deviant sexual interest, or with extensive histories of offending (Hunter, 1999).

During polygraphy, an individual is asked questions regarding his sexual interests while a machine measures his physiological response. It is a tool to verify the individual's stated history. There is little research regarding its validity in juvenile sex offenders. Most polygraphers do not use it in youth under 14 years of age. Plethysmography and polygraphy should only be performed with informed consent of the youth, his parents, or by order of the court (Hunter, 1999). Physiological assessments can be helpful additions to the interview, but should never be used in lieu of it.

Treatment

Much of the treatment used for juvenile sex offenders has not been tested on this population, and is adapted from that tested on adults (Pratt *et al.*, 2001).

Biological treatments

Selective serotonin re-uptake inhibitors (SSRIs) and anti-androgens are the mainstays of pharmaceutical treatment. The SSRIs work by helping to curb obsessive thinking and compulsive behaviors of the sex offender (McConaghy, 1990). Antihormone therapies include the antiandrogens (e.g., leuprolide, cyproterone, and medroxyprogesterone) and may help certain sex offenders by decreasing libido. However, the use of these agents and chemical castration with leuteinizing hormone-releasing hormone (LHRH) raise ethical issues in the adolescent population due to potential developmental consequences and other side effects. Surgical castration is not done in the juvenile population (and it is exceedingly rare even among adult offenders).

Cyproterone acetate (CPA) has antiandrogenic, antigonadotropic, and progestational effects. It has a half-life of 72 hours in the injectable form, and 38 hours orally. It rapidly reduces sexual drive and deviant fantasies. Side effects include liver dysfunction, adrenal suppression, and feminization with gynecomastia (Bradford & Kaye, 1999).

Medroxyprogesterone acetate (MPA) is the hormone used most frequently for sexual offenders in the United States. It works by inducing the enzyme that accelerates intracellular testosterone metabolism and reduces plasma testosterone (Sedlak & Broadhurst, 1996). Side effects include weight gain, decreased sperm production, hyperinsulinemic response to glucose, and gallbladder and gastrointestinal dysfunction. It decreases sex drive, deviant fantasies, sexual activity, and possibly aggressiveness (Bradford & Kaye, 1999).

Leuteinizing hormone-releasing hormone (LHRH) analogs produce pharmacological castration by exhausting the hypothalamic pituitary axis (Bradford & Kaye, 1999).

SSRIs were first tried based on the idea that paraphilias were part of the obsessive-compulsive disorder spectrum. The SSRIs allow females to be treated and are a more commonly used option for male offenders in light of the serious side effects of the aforementioned medications.

Psychosocial therapies

Treatment programs generally employ a combination of individual, group, family, social skills, behavioral, and educational therapies in a multisystemic approach. Acceptance of at least some responsibility for the offenses is an important prognostic factor for therapy. Those who maintain their innocence and show no remorse are less likely to benefit from therapy. Motivation is also crucial. While internal motivation is ideal, the external motivation of the legal system is more common and can be helpful in some cases. Using program completion as a contingency of suspension of the sentence is a powerful motivator (Hunter, 1999). The clinician administering treatment should maintain open lines of communication with probation officers, family, social workers, and any other personnel involved in the offender's care and management. Residential treatment ensures community safety and permits intensive treatment for those juveniles at high risk to sexually reoffend. These programs work best when there is a gradual reduction in supervision, and treatment is based on compliance and appropriate application of learned material (Virginia Commission on Youth, 2003). Aggressive juveniles, those with psychiatric illnesses that cannot be managed by the program, and those who are uninterested in receiving help should not be admitted to community programs (Hunter, 1999).

Cognitive-behavioral therapy is considered the most useful therapeutic modality (American Academy of Child and Adolescent Psychiatry Task Force on Juvenile Justice Reform, 2001). Cognitive behavioral programs focus on taking responsibility for behavior, developing victim empathy, and developing skills to prevent reoffending (Virginia Commission on Youth, 2003). The overall purpose is to reduce deviant sexual arousal and increase appropriate arousal. Research suggests most sex offenders have ideas and beliefs about sexuality that condone taking sexual gratification from others (Connolly & Wolf, 1995).

Aversion therapy, a form of behavior therapy, is a technique pairing sexual behavior or events that led to offending with negative stimuli such as images of being arrested, foul odors, or electric shocks.

As in most work with adolescents, family therapy is a useful and important modality. This is especially true for juvenile sex offenders given their families have high rates of instability, tend to deny sexual problems, and lack knowledge regarding sexual information (Blaske *et al.*, 1989). One-quarter of offenders parents have sexual pathology of their own (Kaufman, Hilliker & Daleiden, 1996).

The general goals of psychosocial treatment can be broad and may aim to help the offender gain control of the deviant behavior; learn impulse control and coping skills in order to manage sexual impulses; improve conflict resolution skills, anger management techniques, and social skills; enhance empathy in order to appreciate the negative effects of sexual abuse on victims and their families; improve understanding of the cycle of thoughts, feelings, and events that lead to inappropriate sexual behavior in order to identify the circumstances and thoughts that should be avoided; promote respect in male–female relationships; and provide sex education that teaches healthy sexual behavior (Virginia Commission on Youth, 2003).

Fernandez and Marshall (2003) studied empathy in adult rapists and came up with some interesting results that could be relevant for the treatment of youths as well. They found that rapists and non-sexual offenders did not differ in empathy on a sexual assault victim scale. The rapists obtained higher empathy scores than the non-sexual offenders on an accident victim scale. Nevertheless, the rapists showed the least sympathy to their own victims. The results indicated that victim-specific empathy deficits, rather than a generalized lack of empathy, were the issues that needed to be addressed. Not surprisingly, denial, minimization, and rationalization were significant problems in this offender population.

A description of psychoeducational/therapeutic modalities

Shaw (1999) summarized the major interventional techniques:

Victim awareness/empathy.   The focus is on understanding the effects of sexual assault on the victim, identifying cognitive distortions and myths that support the sexual assault, and promoting participation in therapeutic endeavors.

Values clarification.   The therapist clarifies sexual values as they relate to the cessation of exploitative sexual relationships.

Cognitive restructuring.   An effort is made to correct the cognitive distortions and the irrational beliefs that support the sexual offending behavior and to replace them with reality-focused and culturally acceptable beliefs.

Anger management.   Instruction is provided to facilitate the recognition and the development of appropriate coping strategies for managing anger.

Assertiveness training.   Training is provided to promote more appropriate self-assertive behavior to have one's needs satisfied in a reality-oriented and culturally acceptable manner.

Social skills training. The therapist facilitates the acquisition of more effective prosocial behaviors, communication skills, and interpersonal awareness.

Sexual education. The therapist provides information regarding human sexuality, myths, sex roles, and variations of sexual behaviors.

Stress reduction/relaxation management. Techniques for coping and reducing stress, anxiety, and frustration are made available.

Autobiographical awareness. Emphasis is on the individual developing an understanding of his or her own life trajectory and how the pattern of sexual offending behavior evolved over time.

An example of a juvenile sex offender program from Colorado is summarized (Hunter, 1999). Arrested juvenile sex offenders are assessed and are screened for risk, which determines whether the youth will be detained or will remain in the community. Treatment can start before sentencing. The offender is sentenced to probation for no more than two years. A process is used to determine appropriate treatment. Probation officers may attend treatment sessions to determine progress. Polygraphs and plethysmography are performed when deemed appropriate. A case management team consisting of the probation officer, treatment providers, a child advocacy center representative, staff from the prosecutor's office and the schools meet monthly to review each case.

Recidivism issues

There are limited recidivism studies addressing child and adolescent offender populations. This is also a difficult area to study given the true rate of recidivism can never be confidently determined as most offenses go undiscovered and self-report measures may be inaccurate. The latter are dependent on responder honesty that can be adversely affected by antisocial characteristics in this population, as well as by a lack of trust for the assurance of confidentiality (American Academy of Child and Adolescent Psychiatry Task Force on Juvenile Justice Reform, 2001). Also, different types of offenders have different risk levels for further offenses, and the methodology in a number of studies does not take this into account.

Different sexual offender pathways are an interesting concept to consider when looking at risk of recidivism. Becker and Kaplan (1988) described three paths the juvenile sex offender can take: dead-end, delinquency, and sexual interest paths. The dead-end path implies no further crimes. In the delinquency path, the juvenile continues to commit sexual offenses, but also commits non-sexual crimes. The juvenile following a sexual interest path continues to commit sex offenses. Another potential pathway is that of youth who drop out of treatment programs. Hunter and Figueredo (1999) found that up to 50 percent of juveniles in a community-based treatment program were expelled. These youths also had higher levels of sexual maladjustment and were at greater risk to recidivate.

Some research indicates there may be an offense-specific pattern for recidivism. Fehrenbach *et al.* (1986) evaluated 297 adolescent male offenders and found that the offenses, in order of frequency, were indecent liberties (touching), rape, exposure, and non-contact offenses including exhibitionism, peeping, and making obscene phone calls. Fifty-eight percent had committed a prior sexual offense, and of that group about three-quarters of them had engaged in the same type of offense. Along these lines, in a study of 112 adolescent sex offender males, over a 29-month follow-up period, 14 percent recidivated (Smith & Monastersky, 1986). The rates of reoffending were higher for those convicted of indecent liberties and hands-off offenses, as well as for those males who offended against strangers and those who offended against a male.

Studies vary on recidivism rates. Sipe, Jensen & Everett (1998) found that non-violent juvenile sex offenders had only a 9.7 percent rate of recidivism. The authors' results supported the concept that violent adolescent sexual offenders are at greater risk of recidivism. A study hampered by a very small number, but nonetheless occasionally quoted, found that juveniles receiving multisystemic therapy had recidivism rates of 12.5 percent compared to rates of 75 percent in those treated with individual therapy alone (Borduin *et al.*, 1990).

Long-term residential treatment or custodial placement is necessary for those at higher risk of recidivism. Risk factors for recidivism include multiple sexual offenses, multiple non-sexual offenses, clear interest in children, failure to comply with probation requirements, obvious signs such as statements of intent to reoffend or uncontrolled behaviors, and family resistance to supervision. For those juveniles who offend against children, several caveats for their management are important: no baby-sitting, no access to children without direct supervision by an adult who is aware of the problem, no supervisory role over young children, and no possession of pornographic material (Chaffin, Bonner & Pierce, 2003).

Conclusion

Juvenile sex offenses comprise a wide range of behaviors. Certain factors may help to identify youths at risk to offend or reoffend. Co-morbid psychiatric illness is common. Various treatment modalities exist: from the less restrictive community treatment models, to more restrictive residential programs, to the most restrictive involving the correctional system. In general, offenders may benefit from a multi-modal approach that combines cognitive-behavioral treatment, other psychosocial therapies, possible biological approaches, and community supervision. For most sex offenders a "cure" is not realistic, and instead, an ongoing management strategy is required.

References

American Academy of Child and Adolescent Psychiatry Task Force on Juvenile Justice Reform (2001). Recommendations for Juvenile Justice Reform. American Academy of Child and Adolescent Psychiatry.

Araji, S. (1997). *Sexually Aggressive Children: Coming To Understand Them*. Thousand Oaks, CA: Sage Publications.

Archer, R. P. (1997). *MMPI-A: Assessing Adolescent Psychopathology*, 2nd edn. Mahwah, NJ: Lawrence Erlbaum Associates.

Ascherman, L. & Safier, E. (1990). Sibling incest: a consequence of individual and family dysfunction. *Bulletin of the Menninger Clinic*, **54**(3), 311–323.

Awad, G. A. & Saunders, E. B. (1989). Adolescent child molesters: clinical observations. *Child Psychiatry and Human Development*, **19**, 195–206.

Awad, G. & Saunders, E. B. (1991). Male adolescent sexual assaulters, clinical observations. *Journal of Interpersonal Violence*, **6**, 446–460.

Aylwin, A., Reddon, J. & Burke, A. (2005). Sexual fantasies of adolescent male sex offenders in residential treatment: a descriptive study. *Archives of Sexual Behavior*, **34** (2), 231–239.

Badgley, R. (1984). *Report of the Committee on the Study of Sexual Offenses Against Children and Youths*. Ottawa: Ministry of Supply and Services.

Becker, J. V. (1988). Adolescent sex offenders. *Behavioral Therapy*, **11**, 185–187.

Becker, J. V. & Hicks, S. J. (2003). Juvenile sexual offenders: characteristics, interventions, and policy issues. *Annals of the New York Academy of Sciences*, **989**, 397–410.

Becker, J. V. & Hunter, J. A. (1993). Aggressive sexual offenders. *Child and Adolescent Psychiatric Clinics of North America*, **2**, 477–487.

Becker, J. V. & Hunter, J. A. (1997). Understanding and treating child and adolescent sexual offenders. In *Advances in Clinical Child Psychology*. New York: Plenum, pp. 177–197.

Becker, J. V. & Kaplan, M. S. (1988). The assessment of adolescent sexual offenders. *Advances in Behavioral Assessment of Children and Families*, **4**, 97–118.

Blaske, D. M., Borduin, C. M., Henggeler, S. W. & Mann, B. J. (1989). Individual, family, and peer characteristics of adolescent sex offenders and assaultive offenders. *Developmental Psychology*, **25**(5), 846–855.

Blundell, N. & Blackhall, S. (2002). *The Visual Encyclopedia of Serial Killers*. London: PRC Publishing, pp. 66–250.

Borduin, C. M., Henggeler, S. W., Blaske, D. M. & Stein, R. J. (1990). Multisystemic treatment of adolescent sexual offenders. *International Journal of Offender Therapy and Comparative Criminology*, **34**, 105–114.

Bradford, J. M. W. & Kaye, N. S. (1999). Pharmacological treatment of sexual offenders. *American Academy of Psychiatry and the Law Newsletter*, **24**, 16–17.

Bradford, W. (1650). Capital offences: buggery. In *History of Plymouth Plantation*.

Carpenter, D. R., Peed, S. F. & Eastman, B. (1995). Personality characteristics of adolescent sexual offenders: a pilot study. *Sexual Abuse*, **7**, 195–203.

CBSNews.com (2003). Teen's "To Do" List: Necrophilia. August 7, 2003.

Chaffin, M., Bonner, B. L. & Pierce, K. (2003). NCSBY fact sheet: what research shows about adolescent sex offenders. National Center on Sexual Behavior of Youth. Online at www.ncsby.org.

Connolly, M. & Wolf, S. (1995). Services for juvenile sex offenders: issues in establishing programs. *Australian Social Work*, **48**(3), 3–10.

Correctional Service of Canada (1995). Young sex offenders: a comparison with a control group of non-sex offenders. Correctional Service of Canada. 7:1.

Cowan, G. & Campbell, R. R. (1995). Rape: casual attitudes among adolescents. *Journal of Sex Research*, **32**(2), 145–153.

De Jong, A. R. (1989). Sexual interactions among siblings and cousins: experimentation or exploitation? *Child Abuse and Neglect*, **13**(27), 1–279.

Dekkers, M. (2000). *Dearest Pet: On Bestiality*. New York, NY: Verso.

De River, J. P. (1950). *The Sexual Criminal: A Psychoanalytic Study*. Springfield, IL: Charles C. Thomas.

Diagnostic Statistical Manual-IV-TR (2000). Washington, DC: American Psychiatric Association.

Donato, R. & Shanahan, M. (1999). The economics of implementing intensive in-prison sex-offender treatment programs. *Trends and Issues in Crime and Criminal Justice*, No. 134, November, 1999.

Epps, K. J., Haworth, R. & Swaffer, T. (1993). Attitudes toward women and rape among male adolescents convicted of sexual versus non-sexual crimes. *Journal of Psychology*, **127**, 501–506.

Faulkner, W. (1931). *Sanctuary*. New York, NY: Vintage Books.

Fehrenbach, P. & Monastersky, C. (1988). Characteristics of female adolescent sex offenders. *American Journal of Orthopsychiatry*, **58**, 148–151.

Fehrenbach, P. A., Smith, W., Monastersky, C. & Deisher, R. W. (1986). Adolescent sexual offenders: offender and offense characteristics. *American Journal of Orthopsychiatry*, **56**,(2), 225–233.

Fernandez, Y. M. & Marshall, W. L. (2003). Victim empathy, social self-esteem, and psychopathy in rapists. *Sexual Abuse: A Journal of Research and Treatment*, **15**(1), 11–26.

Fleming, W. M., Jory, B. & Burton, D. L. (2002). Characteristics of juvenile offenders admitting to sexual activity with non-human animals. *Society and Animals Journal of Human–Animal Studies*, **10**, 1.

Ford, M. E. & Linney, J. A. (1995). Comparative analysis of juvenile sexual offenders, violent nonsexual offenders, and status offenders. *Journal of Interpersonal Violence*, **10**, 56–70.

Freund, K. & Kuban, M. (1993). Toward a testable developmental model of pedophilia: the development of erotic age preference. *Child Abuse and Neglect*, **17**, 315–324.

Friedrich, W. N. (1995). *Psychotherapy With Sexually Abused Boys: An Integrated Approach*. Thousand Oaks, CA: Sage.

Friedrich, W. N., Grambsch, P., Damon, L. & Hewitt, S. (1985). Child sexual behavior inventory: normative and clinical comparisons. *Psychological Assessment*, **4**, 303–311.

Grant, A. (2000). The historical development of treatment for adolescent sex offenders. *Australian Institute of Criminology, trends and issues in crime and criminal justice*. Canberra, Australia (www.aic.gov.au/publications).

Graves, R. B., Openshaw, D. K., Ascione, F. R. & Ericksen, S. L. (1996). Demographic and parental characteristics of youthful sexual offenders. *International Journal of Offender Therapy and Comparative Criminology*, **40**, 300–317.

Greenfield, L. A. (1996). *Child Victimizers: Violent Offenders and their Victims*. Washington, DC: Bureau of Justice Statistics, US Department of Justice, Office of Justice Programs, and Office of Juvenile Justice and Delinquency Prevention. NCJ-153258.

Greenfield, L. A. (1997). *Sex Offenses and Offenders: An Analysis of Data on Rape and Sexual Assault*. Washington, DC: US Department of Justice: Bureau of Justice Statistics.

Groth, A. N., Longo, R. E. & McFadin, J. B. (1982). Undetected recidivism among rapists and child molesters. *Crime and Delinquency*, **28**, 450–458.

Hirshberg, D. & Riskin, K. (1994). Female adolescent sexual offenders in residential treatment: characteristics and treatment implications. Online at www.germainelawrence.org.

Huizinga, C. J. (1977). Pedofielen over zichzelf. *Tijdschr Orthopedagog*, Netherlands, **17**(11), 386–392.

Hunter, J. (1999). *Understanding Juvenile Sexual Offending Behavior: Emerging Research, Treatment Approaches and Management Practices*. Center For Sex Offender Management (www. csom.org/pubs).

Hunter, J. (2000). Understanding Juvenile Sexual Offending Behavior: Research Findings and Guidelines for Effective Treatment. Juvenile Justice Fact Sheet, Charlottesville; Institute of Law, Psychiatry and Public Policy, University of Virginia.

Hunter, J. A. & Becker, J. V. (1994). The role of deviant sexual arousal in juvenile sexual offending: etiology, evaluation, and treatment. *Criminal Justice and Behavior*, **21**, 132–149.

Hunter, J. A. & Becker, J. V. (1998). Motivators of adolescent sex offenders and treatment perspectives. In *Sexual Aggression*. Washington, DC: American Psychiatric Press.

Hunter, J. A. & Figueredo, A. J. (1990). Factors associated with treatment compliance in a population of juvenile sexual offenders. *Sexual Abuse: A Journal of Research and Treatment*, **11**, 49–68.

Hunter, J. A. & Figueredo, A. J. (1999). Longer-term recidivism of child molesters. *Journal of Consulting and Criminal Psychology*, **25**(5), 846–855.

Hunter, J. A., Becker, J. V., Kaplan, M. & Goodwin, D. W. (1991). The reliability and discriminative utility of the adolescent cognition scale for juvenile sexual offenses. *Annals of Sex Research*, **4**, 281–286.

Hunter, J. A., Becker, J. V. & Kaplan, M. (1995). The adolescent sexual interest card sort: test-retest reliability and concurrent validity in relation to phallometric assessment. *Archives of Sexual Behavior*, **24**, 219–229.

Hunter, J. A., Hazelwood, R. R. & Slesinger, D. (2000). Juvenile perpetrated sexual crimes: patterns of offending and predictors of violence. *Journal of Family Violence*, **15**, 1.

Janssen, D. F. (2003). Protoparaphilia. Online at www.growingupsexually.tk.

Johnson, T. C. (1988). Child perpetrators – children who molest other children: preliminary findings. *Child Abuse and Neglect*, **12**, 219–229.

Johnston, J. (2004). The boy rapists. Online at www.*Mirror.co.uk*.

Jones, I. H. & Frei, D. (1979). Exhibitionism – a biological hypothesis. *British Journal of Medical Psychology*, **52**(1), 63–70.

Kaufman, K. L., Hilliker, D. R. & Daleiden, E. L. (1996). Subgroup differences in the modus operandi of adolescent sexual offenders. *Child Management*, **1**, 17–24.

Kavoussi, R. J., Kaplan, M. & Becker, J. V. (1988). Psychiatric diagnosis in adolescent sex offenders. *Journal of the American Academy of Child and Adolescent Psychiatry*, **27**, 241–243.

Kobayashi, J., Sales, B. D., Becker, J. V., Figueredo, A. J. & Kaplan, M. S. (1995). Perceived parental deviance, parent–child bonding, child abuse, and child sexual aggression. *Sexual Abuse: A Journal of Research and Treatment*, **7**, 25–44.

Kole, S. M. (1994). Statute protecting minors in a specified age range from rape or other sexual activity as applicable to defendant minor within protected age groups. *American Law Reports (ALR5th) Annotations and Cases*, **18**, 856–890.

Matthews, R., Hunter, J. A. & Vuz, J. (1997). Juvenile female sexual offenders: clinical characteristics and treatment issues. *Sex Abuse: A Journal of Research and Treatment*, **9**, 187–199.

Mayer, A. (1988). *Sex Offenders: Approaches to Understanding and Management*. Holmes Beach, FLA: Learning Publications.

McConaghy, N. (1990). Assessment and treatment of sex offenders: the Prince of Wales Programme. *Australia and New Zealand Journal of Psychiatry*, **24**, 175–181.

Moll, A. (1908). *Sexual Life of the Child*. Leipzig, Germany: p. 135.

Myers, W. (2002). *Juvenile Sexual Homicide*. San Diego, CA: Academic Press.

Myers, W. (2004). Serial murder by children and adolescents. *Behavioral Sciences and the Law*, **22**, 357–374.

Myers, W. & Blashfield, R. (1997). Psychopathology and personality in juvenile sexual homicide offenders. *Journal of the American Academy of Psychiatry and the Law*, **25**(4), 497–508.

Myers, W. C., Burgess, A. W. & Nelson, J. A. (1998). Criminal and behavioral aspects of juvenile sexual homicide. *Journal of Forensic Science*, **43**, 340–347.

National Center for Juvenile Justice. Fact sheet. Online at www.ncjj.org.

National Center on Sexual Behavior of Youth. Sex Offender Registration. Online at www.csom.org.

National Institute of Correction (1988). *Questions and Answers on Issues Related to the Incarcerated Male Sex Offender*. US Department of Justice.

Nichols, H. R. & Molinder, M. A. (1984). *Multiphasic Sex Inventory Manual*. Tacoma, WA.

O'Brien, M. (1991). Taking sibling incest seriously. In M. Q. Patton, ed., *Family Sexual Abuse*. Newbury Park, CA: Sage Publications, pp. 75–92.

O'Brien, M. J. & Bera, W. H. (1986). Juvenile sexual offenders: a descriptive typology. *Preventing Sexual Abuse*, 1.

Office of Juvenile Justice (1999). *Juvenile transfer to criminal court*. Juvenile Justice Reform Initiatives in the States 1994–1996.

Peterson, A. L. T. (1992). Sibling sexual abuse: an emerging awareness of an ignored childhood trauma. *Moving Forward Newsjournal*, **1**(4).

Pratt, H. D., Patel, D. R., Greydanus, D. E. *et al.* (2001). Adolescent sexual offenders: issues for pediatricians. *International Pediatrics*, **16**(2).

Prentky, R. & Righthand, S. (2003). Juvenile Sex Offender Assessment Protocol-II (J-SOAP-II). Online at csom.org/pubs/JSOAP.pdf.

Ryan, G. & Lane, S. (1991). *Juvenile Sexual Offending: Causes, Consequences and Correction*, 1st ed. Massachusetts: Lexington Books.

Ryan, G. & Lane, S. (1997). *Juvenile Sexual Offending: Causes, Consequences and Correction*, 2nd ed. California: Jossy-Bass.

Ryan, G., Miyoshi, T. J., Metzner, J. L., Krugman, M. D. & Fryer, G. E. (1996). Trends in a national sample of sexually abusive youths. *Journal of the American Academy of Child and Adolescent Psychiatry*, **35**, 17–25.

Saunders, E. B. & Awad, G. A. (1991). Male adolescent sexual offenders: exhibitionism and obscene phone calls. *Child Psychiatry and Human Development*, **21**, 169–178.

Schoentjes, E., Deboutte, D. & Friedrich, W. (1999). Child sexual behavior inventory: a Dutch-speaking normative sample. *Pediatrics*, **104**(4), 885–893.

Sedlak, A. J. & Broadhurst, D. D. (1996). US Department of Health and Human Services. Executive summary of the third national incidence study of child abuse and neglect.

Segal, Z. V. & Stermac, L. (1984). A measure of rapists' attitudes towards women. *International Journal of Law and Psychiatry*, **7**, 437–440.

Sexuality Information and Education Council of the United States (SIECUS) (1998). Public Policy Department: *SIECUS looks at states' sexuality laws and the sexual rights of their citizens.* SIECUS Report **26**(6), 4–15.

Shaw, J. A. (1999). Practice parameters for the assessment and treatment of children and adolescents who are sexually abusive of others. *Journal of the American Academy of Child and Adolescent Psychiatry*, **38**, 12.

Shaw, J. A., Applegate, B. & Rothe, E. (1996). Psychopathology and personality disorders in adolescent sex offenders. *American Journal of Forensic Psychiatry*, **17**(4), 19–37.

Sipe, R., Jensen, E. L. & Everett, R. S. (1998). Adolescent sexual offenders grown up – recidivism in young adulthood. *Criminal Justice and Behavior*, **25**(1), 109–124.

Smith, W. & Monastersky, C. (1986). Assessing juvenile sex offenders' risk for re-offending. *Criminal Justice and Behavior*, **13**, 115–140.

Snyder, H. N. (1997). Juvenile arrests 1996. *The Juvenile Justice Bulletin NCJ*. 167578, November.

Snyder, H. N. & Sickmund, M. (1995). *Juvenile Offenders and Victims: A National Report.* Washington, DC: Office of Juvenile Justice and Delinquency Programs, National Center for Juvenile Justice.

Stermac, L. & Mathews, F. (1989). *Adolescent Sex Offenders: Towards a Profile.* Toronto: Central Toronto Youth Services.

Szymanski, L. (1998). *Frequent Questions and Answers.* National Center for Juvenile Justice.

Texas Council on Sex Offender Treatment and the National Center for Prosecution of Child Abuse (2004). State by state comparison of the involuntary civil commitment of sexually violent predators. Online at www.dshs.state.tx.us/csot_comar.shtm.

The Jewish Publication Society of America (1962). *The Torah* Leviticus 20: 15–16. Philadelphia.

Tower, C. (1996). *Child Abuse and Neglect*, 3rd edn. Boston, MA: Allyn and Bacon, pp. 137–189.

US Department of Justice (1999). *Megan's Law; Final Guidelines for the Jacob Wetterling Crimes Against Children and Sexually Violent Offender Registration Act, as Amended.* Federal Register, **64**(2), 572–587.

Virginia Commission on Youth (2003). Maladaptive behaviors – sexual offending. Virginia General Assembly.

Watkins, B. & Bentovim, A. (1992). The sexual abuse of male children and adolescents: a review of current research. *Journal of Child Psychology and Psychiatry*, **33**, 197–248.

Weber, D. A. & Reynolds, C. R. (2004). Clinical perspectives on neurobiological effects of psychological trauma. *Neuropsychology Review*, **14**(2), 115–129.

Weinrott, M. R., Riggan, M. & Frothingham, S. (1997). Reducing deviant arousal in juvenile sex offenders using vicarious sensitization. *Journal of Interpersonal Violence*, **2**(5), 704–728.

Widom, C. S. (1995). Victims of childhood sexual abuse – later criminal consequences. *National Institute of Justice Research in Brief*. Washington, DC: US Department of Justice, Office of Justice Programs, National Institute of Justice.

Worling, J. R. (1995). Adolescent sibling-incest offenders: differences in family and individual functioning when compared to adolescent non-sibling sex offenders. *Child Abuse and Neglect*, **19**, 633–643.

Worling, J. R. & Curwen, T. (2001). *Estimate of Risk of Adolescent Sexual Offense Recidivism*. Lyme Regis: Russell House Publishing.

www.haaretz.com. (December 25, 2003). Minor gets 15 years for rape and murder of 5-year-old girl. Article 1059519.

Yates, A. (1982). Children eroticized by incest. *American Journal of Psychiatry*, **139**, 482–485.

Zolondek, S. C., Abel, G. G., Northey, W. F. & Jordan, A. D. (2001). The self-reported behaviors of juvenile sexual offenders. *Journal of Interpersonal Violence*, **16**(1), 73–85.

10

Educational needs of youth in the juvenile justice system

Malika Closson and Kenneth M. Rogers

Introduction and overview

In 1998, more than 70 million people (26 percent of the total resident population) in the United States were classified as *juveniles*, that is, persons less than 18 years of age. The juvenile population fell to its lowest in 1984, but since that time has been growing gradually. It is estimated that, between now and 2015, the number of juveniles in the United States will increase by approximately eight percent. The number of juveniles ages 15–17, the age group responsible for two-thirds of all juvenile arrests, is in fact expected to have increased by approximately 19 percent by the year 2007 (this figure represents the total increase in this particular population between the years 1995–2007). Because public perceptions of juvenile delinquency have been influenced by the increasing media attention focused on high-profile incidents, some speculate that the incidence of juvenile crimes will increase alongside this projected increase in the general juvenile population.

But do the relatively few high-profile cases accurately reflect the majority of crimes actually committed by juveniles? According to the Office of Juvenile Justice and Delinquency Prevention Program (OJJDP), 2.2 million juveniles were arrested in the United States in 2003, which represents a decrease of 11 percent from 1999 (Snyder & Sickmund, 2006). The Juvenile Residential Facility Census, 2002, indicates an even higher rate of decrease in the number of juvenile arrests nation-wide, citing a 29 percent decrease since 1996 (OJJDP, 2006). Of the juveniles arrested in 2003, 29 percent were female and 32 percent were under the age of fifteen. In 1999, on any given day, approximately 109 000 juveniles were in residential placement throughout the juvenile correctional system. According to the 1997 National Longitudinal Survey of Youth (which surveyed a "nationally representative sample of 9000 youth between the ages of 12 and 16"), less than one-tenth of youth between the ages of 12–16 reported ever having been arrested. Forty percent of those arrested once reported two or more arrests. The most serious charge in over 40 percent of all juvenile arrests in 1997 was larceny/theft, simple

The Mental Health Needs of Young Offenders: Forging Paths toward Reintegration and Rehabilitation, eds. Carol L. Kessler and Louis J. Kraus. Published by Cambridge University Press. © Cambridge University Press 2007.

assault, drug abuse violation, or disorderly conduct. It is clear from these statistics that a relatively small proportion of the juvenile population is engaging in delinquent behavior; however, a large number of those who do so once continue to do so repeatedly.

With regard to demographic variables, 80 percent of juveniles in the general population of the US are either Caucasian or Hispanic, 15 percent are African American, and 5 percent belong to other minority groups. This is in striking contrast to the juvenile justice populations, which contains a greater proportion of minorities, primarily African Americans, when compared to the general population. In 1997, 53 percent of the juveniles arrested were Caucasian, while 44 percent were Black. This overrepresentation of minorities is consistent throughout every phase of the juvenile justice system (arrest, detention, shelter, and residential settings). With regard to overrepresentation in the juvenile justice system, data also show that the majority of youth in juvenile correctional settings are from either urban or rural (compared to suburban) communities (Khattri, Riley & Kane, 1997).

Another demographic trend within the juvenile justice system is the growing number of females involved in delinquent acts. Female juveniles accounted for 20.4 percent of all arrests during 2003 (NCJRS website at www.ncjrs.gov). Additionally, between 1988–1997, the number of delinquency cases involving females under the age of 16 increased by 89 percent, while the number of cases involving females 16 or older increased 74 percent (Scahill, 2000). The number of female juveniles arrested for Violent Crime Index offenses increased by 25 percent between 1992–1996, while there was no increase in male juvenile arrests for the same offenses. According to the Bureau of Justice Statistics 2003 (www.ojp.usdoj.gov/bjs), the likelihood of a woman spending time in prison at some point during her lifetime is six times higher for a woman born in 2001 than a woman born in 1974.

Another trend, which has likely impacted the number of youth in the US who come into contact with the juvenile justice system, is the wide implementation of zero-tolerance policies throughout US school districts. Zero-tolerance refers to a disciplinary policy that is "intended primarily as a method of sending a message that certain behaviors will not be tolerated, by punishing all offenses severely, no matter how minor" (Skiba & Peterson, 1999).

Data show that, beginning in 1989, school districts in several US states began to implement zero-tolerance policies, with mandated expulsion for drugs, fighting, and gang-related activity (Skiba & Noam, 2001). By 1993, zero-tolerance policies had been adopted in school districts nationwide, but oftentimes the policies were broadened to include not only drugs and weapons, but also things such as smoking and school disruption. With the passage of the Gun Free Schools Act in 1994, which instituted a mandatory one-year expulsion for possession of a firearm along with referral of law-violating students to the juvenile justice system, zero-tolerance became a national policy. Originally, the Gun Free Schools Act only applied to the possession of a firearm, but recent amendments have broadened its scope to include any instrument that may be used as a weapon.

A 1997 National Center on Education Statistics (NCES) report found that 94 percent of all schools had zero-tolerance policies for weapons or firearms, 87 percent had such policies for alcohol, and 79 percent had such policies for violence or tobacco. Some critics of zero-tolerance policies have argued that targeting both minor and major disciplinary events for punishment will ultimately result in the punishment of a small percentage of serious infractions and a large percentage of minor infractions, based on data that suggest that truly serious, dangerous behavior occurs infrequently in schools while minor disruptive behavior occurs relatively frequently. It has been argued that zero-tolerance policies in schools have contributed to an increased number of both juvenile arrests and of youth engaging in delinquent behaviors. According to critics, zero-tolerance policies may directly lead to an increase in the number of juveniles arrested as fights, thefts, and vandalism, which have in the past been handled by assistant principals at the school level, will instead increasingly lead to arrest. Additionally, since zero-tolerance policies generally lead to a student's suspension or expulsion, critics express concern that severing a student's connection to school increases the likelihood that a student will engage in delinquent behaviors (Skiba & Noam, 2001; Browne, Losen & Wald, 2001).

For some students, particularly students with disabilities, suspension is a strong predictor of academic failure and subsequent school dropout. Research shows that special education students are disproportionately more likely to drop out of school as a result of suspension or expulsion than regular education students. Additionally, national studies of school dropout indicate that students who have been suspended are three times more likely to drop out of school by tenth grade than students who have not been suspended. Other studies have suggested that the strength of the school social bond is an important predictor in explaining delinquency, with those students who experience multiple breaks in the school social bond (e.g., through suspensions or expulsion) being more at-risk for delinquency. Expulsion may act to further alienate already disengaged youth from the learning environment and those in it, and may intensify the very behaviors that led to the expulsion in the first place (Marrison *et al.*, 2001). Research shows that students with behavior problems who are expelled are in fact at greater risk of engaging in delinquent acts because they are not in school and therefore often left at home unsupervised, do not receive needed treatment, and have more opportunity to associate with deviant peers and use illicit substances, tobacco, and alcohol. Thus, many youth who are expelled from school become involved with the juvenile justice system, and the widespread implementation of zero-tolerance policies in US schools likely exacerbates the situation.

Because the proportion of the general juvenile population engaging in delinquent behavior is relatively small, one begins to consider whether or not there are any common characteristics (beyond the aforementioned demographic variables) among youth who ultimately become involved with the juvenile justice system.

Balfanz *et al.* (2003) examined a cohort of high school students who passed through the educational and justice systems of a large mid-Atlantic city (a city not identified by the authors but felt to have many common features with other cities in the North and Midwest, including Chicago, Detroit, Milwaukee, St. Louis, Baltimore, and Philadelphia). In 1999, that city's juvenile delinquency court handled approximately 9000 cases involving 6205 youths between the ages of 10–17. From 1995–2000, in the city studied, approximately two percent of eighth–twelfth graders were dropped from their schools' rolls due to incarceration. Balfanz *et al.* noted key characteristics of the students most likely to become incarcerated in that particular city. Most were in ninth grade when they became incarcerated and, compared to non-incarcerated ninth graders, the incarcerated students were disproportionately male and African American (80 percent of all incarcerated first-time ninth graders were African American, but African Americans accounted for only 63 percent of all first-time ninth graders). Within the 22 neighborhood high schools in this city, students who became incarcerated were further concentrated in 12 of the highest-poverty high schools. Notably, nearly all of the students who became incarcerated had a history of severe academic and social difficulties; the majority of first-time ninth graders who were incarcerated had attended school only 58 percent of the time during their eighth grade year, failed at least a quarter of their classes and, on average, read at a sixth grade level at the end of eighth grade. Additionally, on average, students who were incarcerated while in the tenth–twelfth grades had a 59 percent attendance rate in ninth grade and an average grade point average of 56, compared with a 75 percent attendance rate and 69 grade point average for all ninth graders in the high schools they attended.

Although Balfanz *et al.* (2003) focus on youth in schools in a large urban area, other research has shown that youth in rural areas face similar challenges when it comes to schooling. The 1993–1994 Schools and Staffing Survey showed that approximately 59 percent of rural and small town students were enrolled in mid- to high-poverty schools (Henke *et al.*, 1996). Data from the National Assessment of Education Progress (NAEP) shows that, in 1998, although eighth grade achievement of rural students in high-poverty schools was higher than that of their urban counterparts, by tenth grade the performance of the rural students was the same as that of the urban students (www.nces.ed.gov/nationsreportcard). Additionally, rural youth have been found to have high school dropout rates similar to urban youth; between 1987–1989, 13.4 percent of rural youth between the ages of 16–24 were found to be out of school without a high school or equivalent degree, compared with 15.3 percent of urban youth. In 1993, the dropout rate for rural youth was 11 percent, compared to 17 percent for urban youth, and 9 percent for suburban youth. Although these dropout rates are concerning, other authors have suggested that the dropout rates are significantly higher in many urban school districts. These numbers are significantly higher for African American and Latino males who have dropout rates as high as 50 percent in some school districts.

One important fact for consideration is that nearly all of the youths who come into contact with the juvenile justice system within a particular city continue to be educated by that city's public school system, either while on probation or after their release from relatively short placements in juvenile justice facilities. In the Balfanz *et al.* (2003) study, within one year of being dropped from their schools' rolls due to incarceration, most of the ninth graders returned to the school system, usually to a different neighborhood school from the one attended prior to incarceration. Within one year of re-enrollment, however, nearly two-thirds of the ninth graders dropped out of school, and only 12 percent of the ninth graders who were incarcerated and attempted to complete high school in the city's school district actually succeeded. Balfanz *et al.* hypothesize that one possible explanation for why so few incarcerated students succeeded in their attempt to complete high school is that, prior to incarceration, very few possessed the academic skill levels that would enable them to easily reintegrate into and successfully complete high school. Even without the added burden of time lost from school due to incarceration, students with very weak educational records in eighth grade, similar to incarcerated students, typically do not make it past the tenth grade, and graduate in extremely low numbers.

It is clear that a large number of juvenile offenders have significant academic difficulties even prior to their incarceration, and that without targeted and significant educational interventions during incarceration and after their return to school, students who become incarcerated appear to have very little chance of obtaining a high school diploma. The question then becomes, what educational services do juvenile offenders actually receive while in the juvenile justice system, whether on probation, in residential settings, or in detention centers? As mentioned previously, many of the youth in the juvenile justice system already have had difficulties in school prior to being arrested, including poor reading performance, truancy, and behavioral difficulties beginning as early as elementary school. Anywhere from 20–70 percent of youth in juvenile detention centers have learning disabilities, compared to only five percent of youth in the general population. Research additionally suggests that juveniles with learning disabilities, mild to moderate mental retardation, and emotional or behavioral difficulties, are over-represented in juvenile justice facilities (Leone *et al.*, 2005; Stenhjem, 2005). One study cites the prevalence of juvenile offenders identified as eligible for special education prior to their arrest at approximately three–five times that seen in the general public school population. By law, all school-aged children are entitled to an educational program while they are held in secure facilities, including special education services for youth with disabilities, general education development (GED) classes, and vocational training.

Individuals with Disabilities Education Act, 1975 (IDEA) guarantees a free appropriate public education for all eligible children and youth with disabilities through the age of 21. This provision ensures access to special education, but does not ensure equity for youth with disabilities through opportunities to achieve positive academic, vocational, and behavioral outcomes commensurate with those provided to youth without disabilities. In addition to IDEA, Section 504 of the Vocational Rehabilitation Act of 1973 (Section 504) and Title II of the Americans with Disabilities Act (ADA) prohibit discrimination against persons with disabilities by any program or activity in the US that receives federal funds, including correctional facilities. Not all children with disabilities require or will be eligible for special education services under IDEA, but they may meet the guidelines for services under Section 504. In such a case a "504 Plan" must be developed that specifies accommodations that will be provided to enable a student to participate in the general curriculum. Section 504 defines students with handicaps as (1) having a physical or mental impairment that substantially limits one or more major life activities, (2) having a record of such an impairment, or (3) being regarded as having such an impairment. Learning is identified as a major life activity subject to Section 504 protections for eligible youth.

It would seem that the educational component of the juvenile justice system should therefore be constructed to meet the needs of the specific population it serves. Unfortunately, this often is not the case, and many youth in juvenile justice facilities do not receive the educational services to which they are entitled. While there is a requirement to apply provisions of IDEA for juvenile offenders in juvenile detention and confinement facilities, the implementation of IDEA in juvenile justice facilities has historically been problematic. Numerous difficulties exist in providing the range and intensity of academic (and vocational) supports needed by youth who become incarcerated, including problems with regard to both access and equity to appropriate educational programming. In fact, special education programs for incarcerated youth often fail to meet legal requirements and accepted professional standards. Furthermore, educational services are not always consistent with what these youth would receive in their zoned public school setting. For example, children with learning disabilities typically receive approximately 20 class periods of special education services per week prior to incarceration. By comparison, juvenile offenders receive on average only between 5–10 class hours of special education services per week. One study found that up to 55 percent of juvenile offenders in detention who require special education services are not receiving them.

Juvenile facilities face several unique challenges in meeting the provisions of special education law and regulations, and there are several reasons juvenile offenders too often do not receive the academic services they require. One reason is a lack of collaboration between the juvenile correctional setting and the public school the youth attended prior to incarceration. Oftentimes, the public school does not transfer the youth's academic records to the juvenile correctional setting, or alternatively, school records have not been requested by the correctional setting. Another challenge is that the juvenile correctional setting may not have the necessary staff to enable testing to be done that would determine a youth's academic ability and diagnose the presence of a learning disability. One study reports that greater than a quarter of juvenile offenders are held in correctional facilities that do not routinely assess a youth's academic, vocational, or personal needs. Due to such limitations, a youth's academic placement within an educational program in the juvenile justice system may be based solely on their last known grade level, irrespective of that youth's actual abilities.

Yet other challenges to adequate educational programming within juvenile correctional settings arise because of the difficulties the juvenile justice system has in attracting and retaining qualified teachers, particularly special education teachers, willing to work in the correctional setting. The teachers who are willing and do work in correctional settings may additionally be unaware of cutting-edge curricula and instructional strategies that have been identified by schools research, largely due to the fact that juvenile correctional education programs are generally isolated from the changes that may have influenced educational programs in the local community. Additional challenges to implementing appropriate educational services in the juvenile correctional setting become apparent when one considers the frequent movement of youth in and out of the various juvenile correctional settings. Lengths of stay for juvenile offenders can range from a few hours for some youth to several months for others, even within the same juvenile correctional placement. It therefore becomes exceedingly difficult for the educational staff to accurately judge how much time they would even have to complete any educational/psychological assessments of these youth, which directly impacts their ability to address each youth's individual educational needs. Also, due to court appearances, meetings with family members or with probation officers or lawyers, and medical appointments, a youth's school day is frequently interrupted, allowing little time for the educational staff to actually work effectively with the youth.

Overcrowding, additionally, has a negative impact on the delivery of appropriate educational programs to youth in juvenile correctional settings, and allocation of resources for educational programs has not kept pace with the number of youth confined in these settings. In a survey of US juvenile justice facilities in 2002, 34 percent of all juvenile offenders being held were in facilities that indicated they were operating either at or above their standard bed capacity (Sickmund, 2006). With regard to funding for juvenile correctional education programs, the largest federal programs responsible for funding are the Carl D. Perkins Vocational and Applied Technology Act and IDEA. States contribute only a small portion of the funding for juvenile correctional education programs; one 1993 study reported that only a third of all states surveyed spent $2001 or more per student annually (Miles, 1993; Meisel et al., 1998). According to another study, it is this combination of overcrowding and lack of funding for educational programs that contributes to a "one size fits all" approach to service delivery, with resultant decreases in scheduled instructional time due to youth attending school in shifts, as well as lack of sufficient space for school-related activities.

This reduction in appropriate educational services typically means that juvenile offenders are not prepared for the transition back to their community schools following their release from the correctional setting. Youth who come into contact with the juvenile justice system will often miss a significant number of school days, as many are placed in preadjudication detention and most experience several hearing postponements prior to actually appearing before a judge for adjudication. For these youth, many of whom already have a history of school difficulties, missing school days further decreases the likelihood that they will graduate high school or obtain a GED. One study found that 43 percent of youth participating in a correctional remedial program chose not to return to school after their release. In addition, 16 percent of youth who re-enrolled in public school after their release dropped out after approximately five months. Research has shown that obtaining a high school diploma or GED, or completing a vocational program, is critical to the future success of these youth, as juvenile offenders who obtain a GED or complete a vocational program have been found to be twice as likely to be employed six months following their release from a correctional setting as those who did not. Completing high school or obtaining a GED was also correlated with a decreased likelihood that a youth released from a juvenile correctional facility would be arrested again in the future.

Toward improving juvenile correctional Education programs

Several authors (Stephens & Arnette, 2000), utilizing the vast effective schools research literature, have suggested ways to improve delivery of appropriate educational programming to youth in juvenile correctional settings. One key component in ensuring that youth in juvenile correctional facilities receive the educational services they require is the implementation of a referral process by which all eligible youth with disabilities who enter a facility can be identified and assessed within a prescribed timeline. This process should include the identification of eligible youth with no prior history of special education, in addition to identification of youth who received special education services from previous school systems but who do not have a current individualized education plan (IEP). The first step in such a process would be for the juvenile correctional facility to obtain prior school records for all youth entering the facility, as prior school records provide information that is critical for individualized planning and educational service delivery. Therefore, juvenile correctional education programs need an effective and time-efficient administrative mechanism to request previous school records and to track school responses to the requests. Some states have already begun to move toward such a mechanism by implementing automated databases that provide information regarding a youth's history of special education services.

Another key step in ensuring that juvenile correctional education programs adequately address each youth's individual educational needs is the development of strategies that promote parent or guardian participation in IEP development. Currently, parent involvement in educational planning in the juvenile correctional setting is limited. Strategies that would promote parental involvement include use of speakerphones during IEP conferences when parents are unable to physically attend the conference, or the scheduling of IEP conferences to coincide with scheduled family visitation.

A final key step toward providing adequate educational services to all youth in the juvenile correctional setting, which must be considered, is the provision of uninterrupted access to appropriate instruction and instructional materials to all youth in the facility. Youth who have emotional or behavioral disabilities, learning disabilities, and developmental delays (all of whom are overrepresented within the juvenile correctional population) are particularly vulnerable to repeated disciplinary problems within the juvenile correctional setting. All too often, these youth may at times receive no educational services due to disciplinary segregation. Juvenile correctional facilities must design appropriate behavior management techniques in an effort to prevent disciplinary problems and to support youth in engaging in appropriate behaviors, which would in turn contribute to making educational programming more effective by decreasing the number of disruptions in a student's educational services.

Effective schools research has also shown that the provision of a continuum of options for the development of academic, vocational, social, and behavioral skills (e.g., literacy skills, GED preparation for youth unlikely to return to school) to all youth in juvenile correctional settings is an important component of successful educational programming. This is particularly important, as the provision of such a continuum of options begins to prepare these youth for their return to the community. However, because many juveniles released from juvenile correctional settings do not receive the supports needed to succeed once back in the community, outcomes (e.g., school dropout, recidivism) for these youth are often disheartening. Therefore, there is also great need for transition planning and aftercare for these youth to ensure their success after release. *Transition* refers to "a coordinated, outcome-based set of aftercare services for youth released from juvenile correctional settings" (National Center on Education, Disability, and Juvenile Justice, EDJJ, available online at www.edjj.org). Transition services should be in place to help youth adjust socially, gain employment, and succeed educationally. The ultimate goal of transition services is the reintegration of these youth into the community.

Several components of effective transition services have been identified, and these include inter-agency collaboration, team-based planning, and tracking and monitoring. With regard to inter-agency collaboration, transition services will only be effective if they are shared in collaboration between juvenile correctional educational staff, public schools, mental health, and social services agencies that work with individual youth. Team-based planning would entail the development and implementation of transition services by the IEP team in conjunction with correctional counselors and other staff, along with a youth's parent or guardian. This team would determine eligibility for special education services, plan for appropriate placement, develop IEPs that include transition services and goals, and provide appropriate educational and vocational services to juvenile offenders upon their release. Finally, the systematic monitoring of youth is essential, as it would allow for periodic evaluation of transition processes and outcomes.

In conclusion, youth in juvenile correctional settings face many educational challenges even prior to their arrest, including school behavior problems, school disengagement, multiple suspensions and expulsions, and low levels of academic achievement. Additionally, youth with learning disabilities, mild to moderate mental retardation, and developmental delays are overrepresented in juvenile correctional settings. For this particular population of youth, appropriate educational interventions, prior to incarceration, during incarceration, and following release, are critical to their future success. As school failure is linked to recidivism, it is crucial that these youth have the educational support they need to improve their academic achievement and obtain high school or equivalent diplomas. Currently, in most states, correctional educational programming is not adequately equipped to address the severe academic and social needs of youth within the juvenile justice system. However, much research has been done to delineate the characteristics of effective educational systems, and attempts are now being made to identify the key components necessary for the juvenile correctional educational system to provide adequate and individualized educational programming to incarcerated youth.

References

Balfanz, R., Spiridakis, K., Curran Neild, R. & Legters, N. (2003). High-poverty, secondary schools, and the juvenile justice system: how neither helps the other and how that could change. *New Directions for Youth Development*, **99**, 71–89.

Browne, J. A., Losen, D. J. & Wald, J. (2001). Zero tolerance: unfair, with little recourse. *New Directions for Youth Development*, **92**, 73–99.

Henke, R. R., Choy, S. C., Geis, S. & Broughman, S. P. (1996). *Schools and Staffing in the United States: A Statistical Profile, 1993–94*. Washington, DC: United States Department of Education, National Center for Education Statistics.

Khattri, N., Riley, K. W. & Kane, M. B. (1997). Students at risk in poor, rural areas: a review of the research. National Institute on the Education of At-Risk Students, Office of Educational Research and Improvement, US Department of Education.

Leone, P. E. *et al.* (2005). Youth with disabilities in juvenile corrections: a national survey. In *Exceptional Children*, Volume 71.

Marrison, G. M., Anthony, S., Storino, M. H. *et al.* (2001). School expulsion as a process and an event: before and after effects on children at risk for school discipline. *New Directions for Youth Development*, **92**, 45–71.

Meisel, S., Henderson, K., Cohen, M. & Leone, P. (1998). Collaborate to educate: special education in juvenile correctional facilities. The National Center of Education, Disability, and Juvenile Justice (EDJJ) website.

Miles, J. F. (1993). A Descriptive Analysis of Correctional Educational Funding in State Juvenile Agencies. Cited in Meisel, *et al.* (1998), Collaborate to Educate: Special Education in Juvenile Correctional Facilities, available online at www.edjj.org.

Office of Juvenile Justice and Delinquency Prevention (2006). *Juvenile Residential Facility Census, 2002: Selected Findings*.

Scahill, M. C. (2000). *Office of Juvenile Justice and Delinquency Prevention Fact Sheet, November 2000, #16, Female Delinquency Cases, 1997*. United States Department of Justice, Office of Justice Programs, Office of Juvenile Justice and Delinquency Prevention.

Sickmund, M. (2006). Juvenile residential facility census, 2002: selected findings, juvenile offenders and victims. National Report Series, June 2006, United States Department of Justice, Office of Justice Programs, Office of Juvenile Justice and Delinquency Prevention, available online at www.ojp.usdoj.gov/ojjdp.

Skiba, R. J. & Noam, G. G. (2001). Zero tolerance, zero evidence: an analysis of school discipli-nary practice. *New Directions for Youth Development*, **92**, 17–43.

Skiba, R. J. & Peterson, R. L. (1999). The dark side of zero tolerance: can punishment lead to safe schools? *Phi Delta Kappan*, **80**, 372–376, 381–382.

Snyder, H. N. & Sickmund, M. (2006). *Juvenile Offenders and Victims: 2006 National Report*. Washington, DC: United States Department of Justice, Office of Justice Programs, Office of Juvenile Justice and Delinquency Prevention.

Stenhjem, P. (2005). Youth with disabilities in the juvenile justice system: prevention and intervention strategies. In National Center on Secondary Education and Transition Issue Brief, February 2005, Volume 4, Issue 1, available online at www.ncset.org.

Stephens, R. D. & Arnette, J. L. (2000). From the courthouse to the schoolhouse: making successful transitions. *Juvenile Justice Bulletin*. Office of Juvenile Justice and Delinquency Prevention.

11

Science and the juvenile death penalty

David Fassler and Stephen K. Harper

Introduction

On March 1, 2005, the United States Supreme Court ruled that executing those who were under the age of 18, at the time of the crime, had become "cruel and unusual punishment" prohibited by the Eighth Amendment to the US Constitution (*Roper v. Simmons*, 125 S.Ct. 1183 [2005]). There has been criticism, by some, of the Court's legal reasoning in coming to that decision (e.g., so-called "judicial activism," incorrect Eighth Amendment analysis, improper consideration of foreign law). However, few have argued with Justice Kennedy's conclusion as to the "diminished culpability of juveniles." (*Simmons*, 2005, p. 1196). Adolescents are simply not as responsible as fully formed adults who commit similar crimes.

The Supreme Court's Eighth Amendment analysis in death penalty cases is based on two principles. The first, a fundamentally legal one, is whether "standards of decency" have evolved to the point where there is now national consensus that a particular form of punishment has become cruel and unusual. A second issue the Court has to address is whether the constitutionally legitimate purposes of the death penalty – retribution and deterrence – are applicable to this particular group of offenders. In coming to a conclusion regarding the level of culpability, and therefore the appropriate punishment, for 16- and 17-year-old offenders, the Court had to look outside the law and to science.

Pivotal to the ultimate outcome in *Simmons* was the involvement of the sciences and their instruction to the public, policy makers, and law makers prior to the Court taking up the case. Later, when making its decision, the Court considered the research and conclusions of – as well as the consensus in – the behavioral, medical, and neurological sciences. While there are many lessons to be learned from *Simmons*, the most important one for purposes here is the necessity of continued and increased interaction between the sciences and the law.

The Mental Health Needs of Young Offenders: Forging Paths toward Reintegration and Rehabilitation, eds. Carol L. Kessler and Louis J. Kraus. Published by Cambridge University Press. © Cambridge University Press 2007.

History of the juvenile death penalty and Eighth Amendment jurisprudence

According to the leading expert on the juvenile death penalty, Professor Victor Streib, at least 366 juveniles were executed in America – the first reportedly in 1642 (Streib, 2004, p. 3). Juvenile executions constituted "less than two percent of the total . . . executions since 1608" (Streib, 2004, p. 4). In 1972, the death penalty itself was found unconstitutional under the then existing sentencing schemes, *Furman v. Georgia*, 408 U.S. 238 (1972). After 1976, it was restored in 38 states and under federal law subsequent to that restoration, 228 juveniles were sentenced to death. While the vast majority of those sentences were reversed or commuted (86 percent), 22 juvenile offenders were actually executed (Streib, 2004, p. 5). At the time of the ruling in *Simmons*, of 38 states that permitted the death penalty, only 20 still had statutes permitting the execution of juvenile offenders. Of those 20 states, only 12 had juvenile offenders on their death rows. Of those 20 states, only 7 had carried out actual executions since 1976 (Texas, 13; Virginia, 3; Oklahoma, 2; South Carolina, 1; Louisiana, 1; Georgia, 1; Missouri, 1). There were 72 juvenile offenders on death row at the time of the ruling in *Simmons*.

The United States Supreme Court last considered the juvenile death penalty in two cases, *Thompson v. Oklahoma*, 487 U.S. 815 (1988) and *Stanford v. Kentucky*, 492 U.S. 361 (1989). Both cases were decided by the narrowest of majorities – five justices to four. Both cases involved strong and radically different views as to the Court's constitutional role in determining what is cruel and unusual punishment and as to the legal analysis to be employed.

In *Thompson*, four justices found that executing those who were under 16 at the time of the crime had become cruel and unusual punishment. Justice Stevens' plurality opinion (i.e., when a majority has concurred in the result only but not in the reasoning) focused both on the evidence that standards of decency had indeed evolved, and upon the fact that there was "broad agreement on the proposition that adolescents as a class are less mature and responsible than adults" (*Thompson*, 1988, p. 834). Stevens found that the legitimate purposes for the death penalty – retribution and deterrence – were inapplicable to 15-year-old offenders, given their "lesser culpability . . . the(ir) capacity for growth and society's fiduciary obligation to its children . . ." (*Thompson*, 1988, p. 836).

The fifth vote came from Justice Sandra Day O'Connor. She did not completely agree with Justice Stevens' analysis as to culpability, and she applied a far more narrow legal analysis as to how to measure evolving standards of decency. Nevertheless, she found that Oklahoma's statute lacked the kind of "careful consideration that we have required for other kinds of decisions leading to the death penalty" (*Thompson*, 1988, p. 857.) Her concurrence in *Thompson* effectively ended the death penalty for offenders who were under the age of 16 at the time of the crime.

The very next year, in *Stanford v. Kentucky*, the Court ruled that executing 16- and 17-year-old offenders was *not* cruel and unusual punishment. In another plurality opinion, Justice Scalia (joined by Rehnquist, White, and Kennedy) stated that "there was no degree of national consensus . . . to label (this) particular punishment cruel and unusual" (*Stanford*, 1989, p. 371). Justice Scalia also found that "it is not demonstrable that no 16-year-old is 'adequately responsible' or significantly deterred" (*Stanford*, 1989, p. 378). He went even further in rejecting the legal relevance of "socioscientific . . . or even purely scientific evidence" as to the issue of reduced culpability. According to his reasoning, the Supreme Court has "no power under the Eighth Amendment to substitute our belief in the scientific evidence for the society's apparent skepticism"(*Stanford*, 1989, p. 378). Thus, according to Justice Scalia, the Court was prohibited from making any independent determination as to the connection between the act and the blameworthiness of the actor.

While not joining the opinion as to the issue of culpability or the issue of how the Court must determine what has become cruel and unusual punishment, Justice O'Connor concurred in the result. She stated that "The day may come when there is such general legislative rejection of the execution of 16- or 17-year-old capital murders that a clear national consensus can be said to have developed . . . I do not believe that day has yet arrived" (*Stanford*, 1989, pp. 381–382). Again, O'Connor's focus was on state legislative action as the measure of national consensus.

Thompson and *Stanford* demonstrated that there was strong disagreement in the Court as to whether it had an independent constitutional obligation to determine whether "the nexus between the punishment imposed and the defendant's blameworthiness is proportional" *Enmund v. Florida*, 458 U.S. 410 (1982). However, in 2002, in the case of *Atkins v. Virginia*, 122 S.Ct. 2242 (2002), a six–three majority (including Justices O'Connor and now Kennedy) resolved this issue once and for all. In ruling that executing the mentally retarded had become "cruel and unusual punishment," the Court found: (1) that standards of decency had evolved into consensus, *and* (2) that its "own judgment will be brought to bear on the question of the acceptability of the death penalty under the Eighth Amendment" (*Atkins*, 2002, p. 2247). The Court went on to say that it was appropriate to exercise that judgment as to "criminal culpability . . . personal responsibility and moral guilt" (*Atkins*, 2002, p. 2247).

In considering the culpability of the mentally retarded, the Court found that "by definition they have diminished capacities to understand and process information, to communicate, to abstract from mistakes and learn from experience, to engage in logical reasoning, to control impulses, and to understand reactions of others" (*Atkins*, 2002, p. 2250). Because of "disabilities in areas of reasoning, judgment, and control of their impulses, ... they do not act with the level of moral culpability that characterizes the most serious *adult* criminal conduct" (*Atkins*, 2002, p. 2244) (emphasis added). The Court went on to find that imposition of the death penalty on a mentally retarded person would not "measurably advance the deterrent or the retributive purpose of the death penalty" (*Atkins*, 2002, p. 2252).

A year after *Atkins* and frequently citing *Atkins*, the Missouri Supreme Court ruled that executing 16- and 17-year-olds had indeed become cruel and unusual punishment as a matter of federal (not state) constitutional law (*State ex rel. Simmons v. Roper*, 112 S.W. 3rd, 397, 2003). The Attorney General of the State of Missouri petitioned the US Supreme Court for consideration of this federal issue. The Court agreed to hear the case of *Roper v. Simmons* and argument was held on October 13, 2004.

Evolving standards of decency

While there has been serious disagreement amongst the justices as to how to determine what is "cruel and unusual punishment," all agree that the Court cannot simply look to what was permissible at the time the Constitution was ratified in 1789. There were practices not considered cruel and unusual then that would simply be unacceptable today. For example, in Louisiana in 1867, "it was a capital crime to print or distribute material, to make a speech or display a sign, or even to have a private conversation, that might spread discontent among the free black population ... Virginia provided the death penalty for slaves who committed any crime for which free people would serve a sentence of three years or more" (Banner, 2002, pp. 112–113).

Thus, it was in *Trop v. Dulles*, 356 U.S. 86 (1958), that the Court adopted the measure of "evolving standards of decency that mark the progress of a maturing society" to interpret the Eighth Amendment (*Trop*, 1958 p. 100–101). As America evolved, practices once permitted could indeed become cruel and unusual punishment. In *Penry v. Lynaugh*, 492 U.S. 302 (1989), the Court went on to find that the "clearest and most reliable objective evidence of contemporary values is the legislation enacted by the country's legislatures" (*Penry*, 1989, p. 331). Thus, a "general legislative rejection" of the juvenile death penalty would confirm a national consensus, which would, in turn, require the Court to find it unconstitutional.

Subsequent to *Stanford*, legislatures in seven states did indeed pass laws that prevented the execution of juveniles: Kansas (1994), New York (1995), Montana (1999), Indiana (2002), South Dakota (2004), Wyoming (2004), and New Hampshire (2004, but vetoed by Governor). In 1988, when the federal death penalty was reinstated, and later in 1994 when it was further expanded, Congress specifically excluded offenders under the age of 18 from eligibility. In 1993, the

Washington state legislature made no response to the state's supreme court ruling that the juvenile death penalty was unconstitutional under state law. Similarly, in 1988, the Florida Supreme Court raised the age of eligibility from 16 to 17 in its state.

Between 2002–2005, the Florida Senate, the Nevada Assembly, and the Arkansas Senate all passed bills in legislative sessions. Legislators in Kentucky, Delaware, Pennsylvania, Arizona, and Virginia were also in the process of pushing legislation further and harder.

All of these legislative actions were indicators that standards had indeed evolved since the 1989 decision in *Stanford*. Moreover, this movement illustrated yet another indicator, *all* of the legislative changes were in a single direction. In *Simmons*, the Court termed this a "*consistency* in the trend toward abolition" (*Simmons*, 2003, p. 1193). It went on to say that the trend was even more telling because of the "the general popularity of anti-crime legislation . . . and in light of the particular trend in recent years toward cracking down on juvenile crime in other respects" (*Simmons*, 2003, p. 1193). This obviously refers to the more punitive juvenile programs and more juveniles being transferred to and sentenced in adult court.

The Court also acknowledged "the infrequency of its use even where it remains on the books . . ." (*Simmons*, 2003, p. 1194). Indicators were that fewer prosecutors were seeking the death penalty, and research concluded that fewer and fewer juries were imposing it. A study completed in 2004, found that there was "compelling evidence that, even in the states that theoretically permit the use of the juvenile death penalty, there is an emerging societal norm opposing the death penalty for juvenile offenders – which has, in the last several years, reduced the number of juveniles sentenced to death almost to zero" (Fagan & West, 2005). Indeed, in the entire United States, the numbers declined to only seven in 2000, seven in 2001, four in 2002, and two in 2003 (Streib, 2004, p. 10).

Other indicators of evolving standards of decency were mentioned by the Court in *Atkins v. Virginia*, (discussed more below). These include consistent "polling data," as well as consensus in the "widely diverse religious communities," in the "world community," and in those *professions with* "*germane expertise*" (emphasis added) (*Atkins*, 2002 footnote 21). In *Simmons*, the Court found that there was now a national consensus demonstrating that "standards of decency" had indeed evolved.

Evolution of science

It was long assumed that brain development was essentially completed in early childhood. However, beginning in the 1960s, researchers started to identify areas of the brain that appeared to show significant growth and change throughout adolescence and into early adulthood. The initial studies involved the physical examination of postmortem brain tissue. For example, Yakovlev and Lecours (1967) observed that different areas of the brain varied considerably in their rate of development. They noted that the limbic system appeared to mature during childhood, while the development of the cerebral cortex continued into early adulthood. Dekaban and Sadowsky (1978) demonstrated that overall brain weight did not peak until approximately age 20, and Huttenlocher (1979) observed a reduction in the density of synapses during adolescence, a process he called "pruning."

In the 1990s, researchers began to use the emerging technology of structural magnetic resonance imaging (MRI) to explore issues of brain development. Jernigan and Tallal (1990) published one of the first studies that used MRI to actually document the phenomenon of "pruning." These researchers demonstrated that children had significantly higher gray matter volumes than adults, findings which have since been replicated using more advanced techniques (e.g., Sowell, et al., 1999). In 1994, Pfefferbaum et al. (1994) demonstrated that the white matter continued to increase into the early 20s. These results have subsequently been replicated by numerous researchers (e.g., Geidd et al., 1999; Matsuzawa et al., 2001).

Another important aspect of brain development is the gradual increase in white matter, which represents the ongoing process of myelination. Myelin is a white fatty material that develops around the individual nerve cells forming a protective coating or "sheath." This myelin sheath acts as an insulator, enhancing the speed, accuracy and efficiency of impulse transmission throughout the brain. Research by Sowell et al. (1999) has demonstrated that myelination is not complete until the early 20s.

We also know that different parts of the brain undergo myelination at different rates. Specifically, the frontal lobes are one of the last areas to myelinate (Thatcher, 1991; Sowell et al., 1999). This observation is consistent with the fact that this is the region of the brain responsible for higher intellectual functioning, including planning, judgment, and impulse control.

The advent of functional magnetic resonance imaging (fMRI) allowed researchers to look at how people actually used their brains. Using this technology, Deborah Yurgelun-Todd and her colleagues (Baird et al., 1999; Yurgelun-Todd et al., 2000) presented adolescents and adults with a photograph depicting "emotional content." They reported two interesting findings. First, adolescents were more likely to misinterpret the emotion portrayed in the picture. Specifically, they were more likely to interpret the expression as anger or a threat, while most adults correctly identified the emotion as surprise. The second finding was that adolescents were more likely to use the more primitive parts of their brain, specifically the amygdala, when responding to this stimulus, while adults were more likely to use the more advanced and later developing parts of their brain, located in the frontal cortex.

Collectively, the above findings helped explain previous observations of adolescent development and behavior. Clinicians and researchers have long realized that adolescents are more likely to engage in impulsive, reckless, and potentially dangerous behavior, without fully considering the consequences of their actions. The evolving understanding of adolescent brain development provided a structural and functional explanation, consistent with earlier behavioral observations. Specifically, the research supported the theory that when confronted with emotional or ambiguous stimuli, adolescents are more likely to misinterpret information and respond using more primitive parts of their brain. The practical implication of these findings is that when confronted with an emotional or stressful situation, adolescents are more likely to react instinctually and impulsively. Based on their level of brain development, they are less able to stop, think, and modify their actions. In other words, from a biological perspective, a gun in the hand of an adolescent in a convenience store is more likely to go off than it is if held by an adult in exactly the same circumstance.

It's important to understand that our existing technology cannot be applied to specific individuals with any degree of reliability. In other words, at this point in time, we cannot say whether or not a specific person has or has not achieved "adult brain development." However, there is a growing consensus in the scientific community that as a group, adolescents are still developing and evolving and that the brain, in particular, continues to change and mature at least into the early 20s.

As summarized by Ruben C. Gur, Ph.D. (2002), Director of the Brain Behavior Laboratory at the University of Pennsylvania, "The evidence now is strong that the brain does not cease to mature until the early 20s in those relevant parts that govern impulsivity, judgment, planning for the future, foresight of consequences, and other characteristics that make people morally culpable." Dr. Gur went on to opine that "age 21 or 22 would be closer to the 'biological' age of maturity."

A number of studies in the behavioral sciences also demonstrate that juveniles process information, make decisions, and act differently than adults. The conclusion reached was that "an emerging understanding of the interactions among cognitive, psychosocial, and neurobiological development in adolescence supports the position that juveniles should not be held to the same standards of criminal responsibility as adults" (Steinberg *et al.*, 2003, p. 1018).

The role of science in the evolution of standards of decency

One of the reasons that state legislation is considered by the Court to be a good indicator of evolving standards is that passage of any bill almost always requires widespread support from the public, relevant interest groups, polling, the press, legislators, the legislative leadership, and the governor. There must be a willingness and a desire to pass it, particularly when it is competing with many other bills in a time-constrained legislative session. When it comes to legislation involving such an emotional and "loaded" issue as capital punishment, most legislatures and legislators support the sentence of death and, almost invariably, refuse to constrict its use.

Nevertheless, there were significant recent changes in states' death penalty legislation that resulted, in large part, because of the discoveries in the behavioral and neurological sciences that occurred subsequent to *Stanford*. Changes also occurred because of the involvement of those in the medical and scientific worlds in the legislative process. Informing policy and law makers is critical to their consideration of legislative change.

As a result of these discoveries, members of the American Society for Adolescent Psychiatry (ASAP), the American Academy of Child and Adolescent Psychiatry (AACAP), and the American Psychiatric Association (APA) agreed to provide testimony in states considering legislation to eliminate the juvenile death penalty. The research on brain development figured prominently in such testimony. For example, child and adolescent psychiatrists such as Dr. Fassler and Dr. Mark Wellek testified before legislative committees in South Dakota, Wyoming, Nevada, and New Hampshire. Neuro-researchers such as Ruben Gur from the University of Pennsylvania and Abigail Baird from Dartmouth's Laboratory for Adolescent Studies, prepared affidavits, briefed the press, or testified before legislatures. To many legislators, the discoveries helped to explain observations and experiences in their own families.

The research findings also attracted the interest of the popular media. Articles in *Newsweek, Time, U.S. News* and *World Report*, and the PBS show *Frontline* received considerable attention. The scientific data, the legislative testimony, and the popular media reports helped codify the growing consensus that the brains of adolescents function in fundamentally different ways than the brains of adults, and that these differences directly affect behavior.

Many psychiatrists and academics also wrote Op-Eds informing the public as to the policy implications of the science. Distinguished neuroscientists such as Ronald E. Dahl, Joseph Coyle, and Burce S. McEwan and former Surgeons General like Everett Koop joined the Physicians for Human Rights (PHR) "Call to Abolish the Juvenile Death Penalty." The Call was based on "our medical and scientific knowledge that these young people do not yet possess the maturity and mental capacities required to justify the imposition of the ultimate adult punishment" (PHR, 2004).

The recent and extensive research – and its implications – was presented to decision makers and legislators, not by lobbyists or advocates, rather by many of the M.D.s, Ph.D.s and researchers involved. Informing the public, policy makers, decision makers, and legislators was critical to legal practices, decision makers' policy, and legislative action. Professional consensus was a factor considered by the Supreme Court.

Science and legal culpability

Prior to oral argument before the Supreme Court in the *Simmons* case, a number of *amicus* briefs were filed in support of excluding juveniles from the death penalty. One brief was jointly filed by the American Medical Association (AMA), the American Psychiatric Association (APA), the American Society for Adolescent Psychiatry (ASAP), the American Academy of Child and Adolescent Psychiatry (AACAP), the American Academy of Psychiatry and the Law (AAPL), and the National Association of Social Workers (NASW). A separate *amicus* brief was filed by the American Psychological Association.

In terms of the scientific arguments, there was a clear preference to try to encourage the professional medical associations to join together on a single brief. It was felt that this would convey a strong statement regarding the scope and nature of the consensus on this issue. After extensive review, and several drafts, the final version was based on the science and the research findings. The APA, the AACAP, and the ASAP all agreed to sign up to this brief. The AMA also agreed to join in it. While the AMA did not have a specific policy regarding the juvenile death penalty, it did have policy supporting the UN Convention on the Rights of the Child, which has a provision prohibiting juvenile executions. As the AMA represents over 250 000 physicians, this was clearly an important statement.

The medical *amicus* brief focused on the recent discoveries in neuroscience and their behavioral implications. As the brief put it:

The adolescent's mind works differently from ours. Parents know it. This Court has said it. Legislatures have presumed it for decades or more. And now, new scientific evidence sheds light on the differences . . . Behavioral scientists have observed these differences for some time. Only recently, however, have studies yielded evidence of concrete differences that are anatomically based. Cutting-edge brain imaging technology reveals that regions of the adolescent brain do not reach a fully mature state until after the age of 18. These regions are precisely those associated with impulse control, regulation of emotions, risk assessment, and moral reasoning. Critical developmental changes in these regions occur only after late adolescence.

Science cannot, of course, gauge moral culpability. Scientists can, however, shed light on certain measurable attributes that the law has long treated as highly relevant to culpability. (ABA website, AMA *amicus*, pp. 2–3)

The APA's *amicus* focused on the behavioral science research that had taken place since *Stanford*. Agreeing with the brief filed by the AMA *et al.*, the APA stated that 16- and 17-year-olds:

as a group, are not yet mature in ways that affect their decision-making. Behavioral studies show that late adolescents are less likely to consider alternative courses of action, understand the perspective of others, and restrain impulses. Delinquent, even criminal, behavior is characteristic of many adolescents, often peaking around age 18. Heightened risk-taking is also common . . .

Adolescent risk-taking often represents a tentative expression of adolescent identity and not an enduring mark of behavior arising from a fully formed personality. Most delinquent adolescents do not engage in violent illegal conduct through adulthood. The unformed nature of adolescent character makes execution of 16- and 17-year-olds fall short of the purposes this Court has articulated for capital punishment. Developmentally immature decision-making, paralleled by immature neurological development, diminishes an adolescent's blameworthiness. With regard to deterrence, adolescents often lack an adult ability to control impulses and anticipate the consequences of their actions. Studies call into question the effect on juvenile recidivism of harsher criminal sanctions. (ABA website, APA *amicus,* p. 2)

Roper v. Simmons

In its opinion in *Roper v. Simmons,* the Court reaffirmed it's holding in *Atkins* that "Capital punishment must be limited to those offenders who commit 'a narrow category of the most serious crimes' and whose extreme culpability makes them the 'most deserving of execution'"(*Simmons,* 2005, p. 1193). The Court again acknowledged that there are certain classes of offenders, like the mentally retarded, who are not eligible for the death penalty, "no matter how heinous the crime" (*Simmons,* 2005, p. 1193). The question before the Court was whether 16- and 17-year-olds should be members of that class.

In addressing the issue of culpability, the *Simmons'* opinion tracks the findings of *amicus* briefs filed by the scientific and medical communities. The Court began by noting three basic differences between juveniles and adults. "First, . . . [a] lack of maturity and an underdeveloped sense of responsibility are found in youth more often than adults and are more understandable among the young" (*Simmons,* 2003, p. 1195). Second, juveniles are "more vulnerable or susceptible to negative influences and outside pressures, including peer pressure" (*Simmons,* 2003, p. 1195). Finally, "the character of a juvenile is not as well formed as that of an adult. The personality traits of juveniles are more transitory, less fixed" (*Simmons,* 2003, p. 1195).

The Court next concluded that the developmental differences between adults and adolescents were significant enough to make juvenile offenders ineligible for death. "Retribution is not proportional if the law's most severe penalty is imposed on one whose culpability or blameworthiness is diminished, to a *substantial degree,* by reason of youth and immaturity" (*Simmons,* 2003, p. 1196) (emphasis added). As to deterrence, the Court found that "the same characteristics that render juveniles less culpable than adults, suggests as well that juveniles will be less susceptible to deterrence" (*Simmons*, 2003, p. 1196).

After finding that standards of decency had evolved and that 16- and 17-year-olds were generally less culpable, the Court still had to deal with two troubling issues. The first was why juries could not, case by case, make "individualized" decisions based on weighing all of the aggravating and mitigating evidence (including youth). The second issue was the so called "bright line" rule. Opponents rejected the idea that an adolescent a day under 18 at the time would be ineligible for death, but a person a day over 18 would not. In resolving these challenging legal issues, the Court again turned to and relied upon the science.

The Court found that it was too "marked" a risk to permit a jury to decide which were the very few juveniles who were, in fact, fully developed and therefore as fully culpable as an adult. Recognizing that the DSM-IV-R prohibited diagnosing any-one under 18 with certain disorders, the Court went on to say, "If trained psychiatrists with the advantage of clinical testing and observation refrain, despite diagnostic expertise . . . we conclude that states should refrain from asking jurors to issue a far graver condemnation . . ." (*Simmons*, 2003, p. 1197). Indeed, the "diagnostic" bright line drawn by science guided the Court in drawing the "legal" bright line.

When articulating the reasons why adolescents are less culpable, the Court referred to *"the scientific and sociological studies respondent and his amici cite . . ."* (*Simmons*, 2003, p. 1195, emphasis added). Clearly, the Court had read, under-stood and incorporated the "science of culpability." This contribution of those with "germane expertise" was not only educational, it affected the outcome.

Reality

Although it is not clear how much it may have affected the Court's decision, the sciences made yet another contribution to the overall landscape – empirical research on the adolescents who had been sentenced to death. While the Court looks at the narrow legal issues, "actuality" can sometimes affect or even determine the outcome. For example, "separate but equal" treatment of the races was a principle that made logical sense in the legal "ivory tower." However, in *Brown v. The Board of Education*, 347 U.S. 483 (1954), which ended racial segregation, the Court simply could not ignore the empirical reality that separate was simply never equal.

Not surprisingly, research has found that most of the juveniles on death row suffered from serious abuse, mental illness, or neurological impairment – conditions that "substantially exacerbate the already existing vulnerabilities of youth" (AMA *amicus*, p 20). As noted in the *amicus* brief by Child Advocates:

In addition, the overwhelming majority have suffered from extreme childhood physical and/or sexual abuse. There is substantial evidence showing that a large proportion of the juvenile offenders who have been executed since 1973 and who currently sit on death row have suffered serious brain injuries, significant neurological deficits and serious psychiatric illnesses. Dorothy Otnow Lewis *et al.* Neuropsychiatric, Psychoeducational, and Family Characteristics of 14 Juveniles Condemned to Death in the United States, 145 Am. J. Psychiatry 584–589 (1988), found that twelve of fourteen subjects "had been brutally physically abused and five had been sodomized by relatives ... nine had major neurological impairment, seven suffered from psychotic disorders antedating incarceration, seven evidenced significant organic dysfunction ...." *Id* at 584. *See also* Chris Mallett, *Socio-Historical Analysis of Juvenile Offenders on Death Row*, 39 Criminal Law Bulletin, No. 4, at 445–448 (July–August 2003). Juvenile offenders on death row experienced "traumatic life determinant factors during their childhood or adolescence." (ABA website, Child Advocates *amicus*, p. 28.)

A subsequent study by Dr. Lewis *et al.* (2004) again found that nearly all juvenile offenders were indeed seriously impaired. The abstract of the study states:

Eighteen males condemned to death in Texas for homicides committed prior to the defendants' 18th birthdays received systematic psychiatric, neurologic, neuropsychological, and educational assessments, and all available medical, psychological, educational, social, and family data were reviewed. Six subjects began life with potentially compromised central nervous system (CNS) function (e.g., prematurity, respiratory distress syndrome). All but one experienced serious head traumas in childhood and adolescence. All subjects evaluated neurologically and neuropsychologically had signs of prefrontal cortical dysfunction. Neuropsychological testing was more sensitive to executive dysfunction than neurologic examination. Fifteen (83%) had signs, symptoms, and histories consistent with bipolar spectrum, schizoaffective spectrum, or hypomanic disorders. Two subjects were intellectually limited, and one suffered from parasomnias and dissociation. All but one came from extremely violent and/or abusive families in which mental illness was prevalent in multiple generations ... (Lewis *et al.*, 2004)

While these findings were not directly "on point" with the legal issue before the Court, they do provide a richer, if not powerful, context in which to understand the adolescents who actually committed homicides. Such research also results in more informed and objective decision-making on the part of legislators and those in the executive branch as well as policy makers, prosecutors, and law enforcement.

Conclusions

The Supreme Court has now clearly recognized that people who lack fully developed and functioning adult brains should not be eligible for the death penalty. The scientific basis for this evolving legal standard has clear implications for people who suffer from mental illness. Accordingly, in December 2004, the APA board adopted a position on "Diminished responsibility in capital sentencing" (APA, 2004).

The emerging data on adolescent brain development also has significant implications within the broader field of juvenile justice. We no longer execute people for crimes committed as juveniles. Do we also need to reconsider the imposition of life sentences for adolescents convicted of serious crimes? Will the growing body of scientific data slow the tendency to transfer younger and younger defendants into the adult court system? Will the science evolve to a point where we are able to accurately assess the brain development of a specific individual? Clearly, the answers to these questions will have a significant impact on the future of our justice system. Justice itself is dependent upon the discoveries, implications, and the teachings of science.

References

ABA website. AMA *amicus*. www.abanet.org/crimjust/juvjus/simmons/ama.pdf.

ABA website. APA *amicus*. www.abanet.org/crimjust/juvjus/simmons/apa.pdf.

ABA website. Child Advocates *amicus*. www.abanet.org/crimjust/juvjus/simmons/childad.pdf.

APA (2004). Diminished responsibility in capital sentencing. Position statement. Arlington, VA: American Psychiatric Association.

Atkins v. Virginia, 122 S.Ct. 2242 (2002).

Baird, A. A., Gruber, S., Fein, D. *et al.* (1999). Functional magnetic resonance imaging of facial affect recognition in children and adolescents. *Journal of the American Academy of Child & Adolescent Psychiatry*, **38**(2), 195–199.

Banner, S. (2002) *The Death Penalty: An American History*. Harvard University Press.

Brown v. The Board of Education, 347 U.S. 483 (1954).

Debakan, A. S. & Sadowsky, D. (1978). Changes in brain weight during the span of human life. *Annals of Neurology*, **4**, 345–356.

Enmund v. Florida, 458 U.S. 410 (1982).

Fagan, J. & West, V. (2005). The decline of the juvenile death penalty: scientific evidence of evolving norms. *Journal of Criminal Law and Criminology*, **95**, 427–501.

Furman v. Georgia, 408 U.S. 238 (1972).

Giedd, J. N., Blumenthal, J., Jeffries, N. O. *et al.* (1999). Brain development during childhood and adolescence: a longitudinal MRI study. *Nature Neuroscience*, **2**, 861–863.

Gur, R. C. (2002). Declaration of Ruben C. Gur, Ph. D., *Patterson v. Texas*. Petition for Writ of Certiorari to US Supreme Court, J. Gary Hart, Counsel. (Online at http://www/abanet.org/crimjust/juvjus/Gur%20affidavit.pdf).

Huttenlocher, P. R. (1979). Synaptic density in human frontal cortex: developmental changes and effects of age. *Brain Research*, **163**, 195–205.

Jernigan, T. L. & Tallal, P. (1990). Late childhood changes in brain morphology observable with MRI. *Developmental Medicine & Child Neurology*, **32**, 379–385.

Lewis, D., Yeager, C., Blake, P., Bard, B. & Strenzoik, M. (2004). Neuropsychiatric, neuropsychological, educational, and family characteristics of 18 juvenile offenders awaiting execution in Texas. *Journal of the American Academy of Psychiatry and the Law*, **32**, 408–429.

Matsuzawa, J., Matsui, M., Konishi, T. *et al.* (2001). Age-related volumetric changes of brain gray and white matter in healthy infants and children. *Cerebral Cortex*, **11**(4), 335–342.

Penry v. Lynaugh, 492 U.S. 302 (1989).

Pfefferbaum, A., Mathalon, D. H., Sullivan, E. V. *et al.* (1994). A quantitative magnetic resonance imaging study of changes in brain morphology from infancy to late adulthood. *Archives of Neurology*, **51**, 874–887.

PHR website (2004). Former US Surgeons General and more than 400 child health professionals call for an end to the juvenile death penalty. www.physiciansforhumanrights.org/library/news-2004-07-19.html. July 19, 2004.

Roper v. Simmons, 125 S.Ct. 1183 (2005).

Sowell, E. R., Thompson, P. M., Holmes, C. J. *et al.* (1999) In vivo evidence for post-adolescent brain maturation in frontal and striatal regions. *Nature Neuroscience*, **2**(10): 859–861.

Stanford v. Kentucky, 492 U.S. 361 (1989).

State ex rel. Simmons v. Roper, 112 S. W. 3rd, 397 (2003).

Steinberg, L. & Scott, E. (2003). Less guilty by reason of adolescence: developmental immaturity, diminished responsibility, and the juvenile death penalty. *American Psychologist*, **58**(12), 1009–1018.

Streib, V. (2004). *Death Penalty Today: Death Sentences and Executions for Juvenile Crimes.* www.law.onu.eud/faculty/streib/documents/JuvDeathDec2004.pdf

Thatcher, R. W. (1991). Maturation of the human frontal lobes: physiological evidence for staging. *Developmental Neuropsychology*, **7**, 397–419.

Thompson v. Oklahoma, 487 U.S. 815 (1988).

Trop v. Dulles, 356 U.S. 86 (1958).

Yakovlev, P. I. & Lecours, A. R. (1967). The myelogenetic cycles of regional maturation if the brain. In: *Regional Development of the Brain in Early Life*, Minowski A., ed. Oxford, England: Blackwell, pp. 3–65.

Yurgelun-Todd, D., Gruber, S., Kanayama, G. *et al.* (2000). fMRI during affect discrimination in bipolar affective disorder, *Bipolar Disorders*, **2**(3.2), 237–248.

12

Medical issues regarding incarcerated adolescents

Robert E. Morris

Introduction

Adolescence is commonly viewed as a healthy time of life with little need for medical care. Although there is some truth to this belief, individual adolescents may suffer from a wide variety of illnesses and injuries (Council on Scientific Affairs, 1990; Feinstein et al., 1998), which can have immediate and, in many cases, lifetime effects. Many teenagers coming to detention also have deferred medical needs because of barriers to access (Council on Scientific Affairs, 1990), including absent or limited insurance, lack of parental involvement (Hein et al., 1980), chaotic lives and limited understanding of medical care requirements. Incarceration provides the best chance to meet the medical and dental needs of this particularly vulnerable group (Hein et al., 1980; American Academy of Pediatrics, 1989; Society for Adolescent Medicine, 2000). In addition, the act of detaining citizens removes their ability to seek care voluntarily thus placing a legal and moral imperative on the detaining authority to provide care that meets community standards (Costello & Jameson, 1987). Resources expended on youth provide a cost-effective intervention because this prevents more serious sequellae requiring greater expenditures in the future. Lastly, rehabilitation of delinquent youth proceeds most smoothly when the youth is free of disease, pain, and disability.

This review is divided into four sections: medical problems that may predispose to delinquent behavior; medical illness and injury likely to result from delinquent behavior; health concerns for all adolescents; and health maintenance issues.

Medical/organic issues that may predispose to delinquency

In recent years a number of studies have pointed to genetic, hormonal, neurotransmitter, and structural causes of violent and delinquent behavior (Brunner et al., 1993; Saudou et al., 1994; Chen et al., 1994; Cases et al., 1995; Stones & Kelner,

The Mental Health Needs of Young Offenders: Forging Paths toward Reintegration and Rehabilitation, eds. Carol L. Kessler and Louis J. Kraus. Published by Cambridge University Press. © Cambridge University Press 2007.

2000; de Waal, 2000; Davidson *et al.*, 2000). Discussion of these molecular mechanisms is beyond the scope of this chapter and can be found in *Neurobiology of Violence* by Jan Volavka, M. D., Ph.D (Volavka, 2002).

Head trauma resulting in brain injury may be somewhat more common in delinquent teens compared to non-delinquents (Shanok & Lewis, 1981; Lewis *et al.*, 1985; Lewis *et al.*, 1988; Hux *et al.*, 1998; Otnow-Lewis, 1998). However, the differences between these two groups are not always great (Hux *et al.*, 1998). Confounding the issue of cause and effect is the likelihood that hyperactivity and delinquent acts such as fighting may result in head trauma, thus increasing the incidence of brain injury subsequent to the development of violent behavior.

A history of physical child abuse is also found in some juvenile delinquents (Shanok & Lewis, 1981; Lewis *et al.*, 1988). In addition to the direct effect of head trauma caused by the assault, there may also be subtle neurobiological effects on the developing brain leading to a lifetime of social maladjustment (Otnow-Lewis, 1998; Perry *et al.*, 1995). Here, too, separating the effect of physical, anatomic damage from "emotional" and "neuroendocrine" effects may be very difficult. Careful neurological examinations may identify adolescents with more severe and diagnostically accessible lesions, but more subtle lesions limited to behavioral effects would be missed. Patients with histories of significant and/or repetitive head injuries may benefit from imaging studies such as computed tomography, magnetic resonance imaging or positron emission tomography of the brain (Tonkonogy, 1991; Tonkonogy & Geller, 1992; Volkow & Tancredi, 1987). An electroencephalogram (EEG) study may also uncover abnormal brain function and point to a structural lesion or seizure disorder, but the study is rarely helpful (Hsu *et al.*, 1985).

Temporal-limbic epilepsy involves complex neurologic, behavioral, and psychiatric symptoms usually, but not always seen, in adolescents with *developmental disorders* (Kastner, 1998). In Holmes and Mikati's review of the subject, they report that one third of patients had pre-existing brain injury, one third had generalized status epilepticus before the onset of temporal lobe seizures, and one third had no preceding history (Holmes & Mikati, 1991). Most often the epileptic behavior is non-specific and involves tic-like behavior, body jerks, or occasionally self-injury (Gedye, 1989). *Rarely* there may be explosive or undirected aggression. If temporal lobe epilepsy is suspected, nasopharyngeal or anterior temporal leads may be necessary to detect the seizure focus on the EEG (Goodin *et al.*, 1990). It should be stressed that this seizure disorder is mostly limited to patients with developmental disorders or other significant psychiatric or neurologic history (Kastner, 1998; Gedye, 1989).

At least two genetic disorders may be associated with juvenile offenders. Boys with Klinefelter's Syndrome, karyotype of 47 XXY, can be mildly intellectually impaired, socially withdrawn (Jones, 1983b), and occasionally engage in delinquent behavior such as fire setting (Miller & Sulkes, 1988, 1989; Kaller *et al.*, 1989). It is important to realize that the phenotypic expression of Klinefelter's Syndrome varies widely and the *great majority* of boys do not offend. Small, very firm testicles about the size of a peanut provide the most reliable physical finding. Patients may have variable degrees of under-virulization, with some boys appearing normal. A karyotype will make the diagnosis. Generally testosterone levels are low (but may be normal in the early teen years), while follicle stimulating hormone and lutenizing hormone levels are elevated. Treatment with testosterone can improve virulization and social functioning (Nielsen *et al.*, 1988). These boys are usually sterile, information that is presented best in a setting less threatening than confinement after testosterone treatment has begun and in older, more mature teens and young adults.

Exposure of fetuses to alcohol during gestation results in a wide range of physical, psychological, and behavioral problems, which are partially dose dependent. These children have characteristic facial features including short palpebral fissures, short nose, and smooth philtrum. The intelligence quotient (IQ) averages 63 with hyperactivity, poor social judgment, and difficulty recognizing social cues, causing problems interacting with society (Jones, 1983a). Occasionally these children may offend and become detained (Streissguth *et al.*, 1991; Fast *et al.*, 1999).

Exposure to illicit drugs, especially cocaine, during pregnancy may result in subtle effects on IQ and behavior (Volpe, 1992; Martin, 1993; Lester *et al.*, 1998). The short duration of follow-up for most studies of illicit drug effects on the fetus limits our understanding of the long-term problems that may surface years later in teenagers.

Low levels of lead exposure have been associated with neurobehavioral problems (Needleman *et al.*, 1990) and mild reduction in intelligence (Needleman & Gastonis, 1990) with one study reporting a four to five percent drop in IQ for a blood lead concentration of 40 μg per deciliter (Baghurst *et al.*, 1992). Needleman reported a correlation between elevated bone lead levels, as measured by K x-ray fluorescence spectroscopy, and delinquent behavior measured in boys chosen to be at risk for antisocial behavior (Needleman *et al.*, 1996). On the other hand, Huscroft found no elevated blood levels in 1000 teenagers without retained bullets consecutively admitted to a juvenile hall (Huscroft *et al.*, 1994). Further work on the contribution of lead exposure should be carried out to determine if exposure to lead has a significant impact on delinquent behavior.

Health problems resulting from delinquent behavior

Recently, in 2004, a study of 26 000 adult volunteers seeking comprehensive medical evaluation at Kaiser Permanente, a health maintenance organization, found child maltreatment to be associated with compulsive behaviors of smoking, alcoholism, and injection drug use. Adverse experiences included are: recurrent and severe physical abuse, recurrent and severe emotional abuse, contact sexual abuse, and growing up in a household with: an alcoholic or drug-user, a family member being imprisoned, a mentally ill, chronically depressed or institutionalized member, the mother being treated violently, and both biological parents not being present. The more adverse the experiences, the greater the tendency to engage in compulsive behaviors (Feletti, 2004).

Violence surrounds delinquents and often causes injury to them. Some detained teens will enter detention soon after they are injured, and in some cases they are transferred from hospital to the institution. Automobile accidents, falls, blunt trauma caused by objects during fights, knife wounds, and gunshot wounds, inflict acute trauma and in some cases permanent injury. Brain injury, bowel resection and later obstruction, as well as paraplegia are a few of the serious long-term problems. Juvenile facilities should have an appropriate physical plant to accommodate handicapped patients and their equipment such as wheelchairs. The medical expertise to handle complicated posttraumatic injuries must also be available.

Retained bullets can cause lead poisoning acutely or years later (Huscroft et al., 1994; Linden et al., 1982; Selbst et al., 1986; Huscroft, 1994; Woolf & Funk, 1985; Feletti, 2004; Ellis, 1874). Bullets in bone, joints, or lung tissue are at high risk for lead absorption. Patients with symptomatic elevations of lead, usually between 60–90 µg per deciliter, will require chelation therapy followed by surgical removal of the lead material. Chelation without removal of the bullet will not reduce the long-term lead burden (Huscroft, 1994).

Many orthopedic and sports type injuries happen to delinquent youth both before and during incarceration (Woolf & Funk, 1985). Metacarpal and scaphoid fractures occur during punching, as can tooth lacerations of knuckles, causing serious infections of bone, joint, and tendons in the hand. Hyperextension of the thumb results in skier's thumb, a torn medial collateral ligament. Knee and ankle sprains resulting in torn ligaments occur during contact sports.

Delinquents engage in multiple-risk behaviors (Morris, 1995; Morris et al., 1998) including sexual activity with multiple partners resulting in acquisition of sexually transmissible infections (Shafer et al., 1993; Oh et al., 1994; Alexander-Rodriguez & Vermund, 1987; Centers for Disease Control and Prevention, 1999; Bell et al., 1985), and pregnancy (Morris, 1995; Breuner & Farrow, 1995; Nesmith et al., 1997). Illicit drug use is common (Morris, 1995; National Institute of Justice, 1996; Crowe, 1998). Therefore, some youths will be intoxicated by street drugs upon admission and should be sent to an emergency department for physiological monitoring until they are medically stable. Occasionally youths may require support during drug withdrawal, especially from narcotics. A combination of clonidine, a non-steroidal anti-inflammatory drug, and an antispasmotic medication for intestinal cramps, will greatly reduce the suffering related to withdrawal from narcotics (Seymour & Smith, 1987; Schwartz, 1998).

The risk of HIV infection remains a concern, although in most cities relatively few teenagers are known to be infected (MacKay et al., 2000; Centers for Disease Control and Prevention, 2006). Certain populations, including men who have sex with men (Lemp et al., 1994; Osmond et al., 1994; Rosenberg & Biggar, 1998), people who use injection drugs, and women, especially women whose sex partners use injection drugs, remain at higher risk (Rosenberg & Biggar, 1998). It is important to realize that a number of youth engage in sexual activity with both genders and may be a particularly vulnerable group for HIV infection (Morris et al., 1998). In Los Angeles, California, USA through 1990, the rate of identified positive serologic tests for HIV in detained juveniles ranged from one–three per year (Morris et al., 1998). This rate appears to be stable in Los Angeles through 2005.

General adolescent medical problems

Initial screening upon arrival in detention should include questions and simple tests to rule out infectious diseases such as tuberculosis (TB) (Ozuah et al., 2001), sexually transmitted infections, hepatitis, or contagious viral infections causing a rash, such as chicken pox or herpes zoster.

A tuberculosis skin test (PPD) should be considered for all children residing in high-risk areas or exposed to travelers from endemic areas. Many cities with large immigrant populations are at risk for TB and their youth should be tested (AAP, 2006). Those with positive tests should have a chest radiograph. After obtaining cultures, patients with active TB found in chest radiographs should begin three-or four-drug therapy after consultation with the local public health department. These patients should be in respiratory isolation and reverse-flow rooms until they are non-infectious. Prophylaxis for dormant TB to prevent reactivation may be considered in facilities where youth will remain for at least six–nine months.

Gonorrhea and chlamydia genital infections are common (Robertson et al., 2005) and diagnosed best using the new nucleic acid amplification tests (NAATS) of urine for both males and females. Alternatively, a pelvic exam with collections of secretions for NAATS testing from sexually active girls can be used. A papanicolaou (PAP) smear should be done, beginning three years after onset of sexual activity (Saslow et al., 2002). Most cases of gonorrhea and chlamydia (66–90 percent) are currently asymptomatic, thus ruling out any utility of waiting for symptoms to indicate the presence of infection. It is particularly important to find these infections, because untreated they result in serious disseminated infections such as pelvic inflammatory disease (PID), that can result in lifetime complications including ectopic pregnancies (Chow *et al.*, 1990), infertility (Cates *et al.*, 1994), and chronic pelvic pain (Westrom *et al.*, 1992). Recently, the long-term burden of *asymptomatic* PID (Wolner-Hanssen *et al.*, 1990) caused by undiagnosed chlamydia infection has increased interest in case finding in order to prevent complications by providing timely treatment. Treatment of asymptomatic chlamydia infection in young women reduces the incidence of subsequent PID (Scholes *et al.*, 1996).

Pregnancy should be diagnosed using a urine test. Pregnant adolescent females in many states of the USA have the right to consent for pre-natal care and pregnancy termination if they desire. Pregnant females require appropriate pre-natal care, vitamins, food, snacks, and limited activity as the pregnancy progresses. In addition, a number of psychosocial services should be provided to these girls including dealing with pregnancy in detention, separation from the baby post partum, and parenting skills. Programs allowing frequent contact with their babies and children are vitally important to helping preserve a nurturing relationship between mothers and their children.

Headaches caused by temporomandibular joint pain, impacted wisdom teeth, sinusitis, allergic rhinitis, as well as migraine processes will be encountered in detained teens.

Likewise, chest pain secondary to costochondritis and chest-wall trauma brings concerned adolescents to seek care. When these pains trigger a hyperventilation spell with lightheadedness, tingling extremities (often described as weakness), and sometimes syncope or seizure-like behavior, both the youth and staff may become frightened. Nonetheless, this is a benign, self-limited process. A spontaneous pneumothorax will cause dyspnea and chest pain and requires urgent intervention. Cardiac disease rarely causes chest pain in teenagers who have no preceding history of congenital heart disease. Occasionally hyperthyroidism may cause tachycardia and/or palpitations. Individuals who pass out or have severe chest pain during exercise should have a careful cardiac examination, electrocardiogram, and echocardiograph. Exercise-induced asthma may also cause shortness of breath or chest pain during running or vigorous exercise and may preclude participation in boot or wilderness camp experiences, and contraindicates assignment to forest fire fighting.

Abdominal pain has many causes. Peptic ulcers (caused by infection with *H. pylori*) may have an increased incidence in crowded living circumstances (Drumm *et al.*, 1990; Blecker *et al.*, 1994; Tompkins & Falkow, 1995; Parsonnet *et al.*, 1999), thus targeting lower socioeconomic groups. A positive stool antigen test makes this diagnosis, and is the test of choice in children (Graham & Qureshi, 2001; Suerbaum & Michetti, 2002).

Hepatitis in children and adolescents does not always result in jaundice, i.e., anecteric cases. Therefore the diagnosis is often obscured. Any teen who vomits for more than two or three days should have liver enzymes measured. Four drugs commonly used in adolescents, especially if two or more are used together, have caused liver enzyme elevations and on occasion, fulminant liver failure and death. Isoniazid (Black *et al.*, 1975; Snider & Caras, 1992), acetaminophen (Saslow *et al.*, 2002), isotretinoin acid and the azole antifungals should be used singly, never two or more simultaneously. Because the symptoms of serious toxicity can be subtle, any adolescent with protracted vomiting should have liver enzymes measured and, if elevated, the medication stopped and the patient referred to a liver specialist. If the laboratory results will be delayed for more than one–two days, the medication should be stopped until the results are obtained. Constipation may appear in teens whose natural schedule is disrupted by the regimentation of life in detention. The incidence of appendicitis peaks in teen years and will be diagnosed fairly frequently in larger juvenile halls.

Pelvic inflammatory disease and ectopic pregnancies must be considered for all females with lower quadrant pain. Cyclic or chronic pelvic pain may be secondary to endometriosis. Dysmenorrhea can be quite debilitating. If it does not respond to non-steroidal anti-inflammatory medication (NSAIDs) started at the very beginning of the menstrual period, the clinician should consider prescribing oral contraceptives or depomedroxyprogesterone acetate after a complete work-up to rule out pathology. Studies measuring the degree of osteoporosis caused by depomedroxyprogesterone acetate will soon determine the risk of this method of contraception for adolescents.

Painful urination in boys may be caused by urethritis, urethral stricture either congenital or acquired (skateboard injuries), meatal stenosis, or urethral condyloma. Occasionally urinary tract infections will occur but almost always in the clinical setting of previous urologic abnormalities. Testicular pain most often results from epididymitis and more rarely from torsion of the testis or appendix testis. Torsion of the testis must be corrected within six hours to avoid death of the testis.

A complete discussion of sexually transmissible infections is beyond the scope of this chapter, but it should be mentioned that secondary syphilis can cause a rash with varying morphology that resembles many other rashes. Condyloma-like (condyloma lata), viral exanthem-like, pittoriasis rosea, and psoriosis can all be mimicked by syphilis. The management of human papilloma virus infections and abnormal PAP smears in girls is complex and constantly changing (Moscicki *et al.*, 2004; Murphy *et al.*, 1990). The reader should consult recent consensus publications.

Other dermatologic problems in teens include acne (which can cause scarring and/ or pain), tinea (fungus infection) in various locations; impetigo, atopic dermatitis, and dysplastic moles are just a few of the skin conditions that may require treatment.

Prisons and detention facilities have high rates of skin infections with methicillin-resistant staphylococcus aureus (MRSA) that can cause abscesses, osteomylitis, and deep infections. Patients with MRSA should be isolated until they are not infectious (Center for Disease Control and Prevention, 2003; Pan *et al.*, 2003). Medical personnel in prisons and detention facilities should not attempt to eradicate nasal colonization in their population, as this will add to drug resistance in the community.

A variety of benign and malignant tumors occur during adolescence. Osteochondromas develop at the ends of long bones, especially in the femur and tibia. These are asymptomatic hard, bony swellings that only cause pain if they impinge on other structures. Osteoid osteomas cause pain, especially at night. The pain responds dramatically to NSAIDS. Pain just below the knee after exercise may be due to Osgood-Schlatter's disease. Malignant bone tumors cause pain, especially at night, and/or pathologic fractures and should be considered in any teen with bone pain unrelated to trauma or exercise. Leukemia also peaks during adolescence and may cause confusing symptoms such as tiredness and "failure to follow the program."

All organs can become diseased during adolescence. Renal failure, hypertension, and rheumatic problems will all occur occasionally.

Many intracity youth (Mitchell *et al.*, 2003) and incarcerated youth (Richmond, 1978; Anderson & Farrow, 1998) have significant unmet dental care needs. Juvenile facilities should provide all dental services, and not offer solely extractions for relief of pain.

Deafness and decreased visual acuity are insidious and can be misinterpreted by custody and medical staff as failure to follow directions or malingering.

Male gay (homosexual) teens with high-risk partners, or teens with multiple sexual partners, who engage in sex for money, drugs, survival, or who have an STI, should be offered voluntary HIV testing. Girls whose sexual partners have used injection drugs represent a particularly susceptible group and ought to be offered testing.

Adolescent obesity, an emerging problem in developed countries, looms on the horizon as the next major public health problem challenge for juvenile incarceration facilities. A multidisciplinary approach involving kitchen staff, correctional officers, and healthcare providers, requires coordination and cooperation at all levels of the facility. The continuous effort that is needed from the staff for this work means substantial resources for training, and motivation will be needed in order for the staff to remain committed to youth weight stabilization over the long term.

Malingering

Teens in detention are a natural target for staff's belief that complex or confusing medical presentations must be secondary to malingering. In reality, incarcerated teens very rarely malinger. When the clinician is unable to make a diagnosis, consultation should be sought. In rare instances when the patient's symptoms are fabricated, the clinician will be rewarded by looking into the circumstances leading to the fabrication. Fear of other inmates or a correctional officer might be at the root of the problem. In these circumstances, the medical staff should intervene on the adolescent's behalf. Failure to determine a convincing reason for suspected malingering should rekindle the interest in finding a clinical pathophysiological cause of the symptoms.

Health maintenance

A complete physical examination, recommended immunizations, and health counseling should be provided for each adolescent upon entry into detention. With the emergence of meningococcal meningitis as a threat to college students (Richmond, 1978), consideration should be given to adding meningococcal immunizations to those already provided to detained youth (Harrison *et al.*, 1999; Rosenstein *et al.*, 1998; Tappero *et al.*, 1996). A pertussis vaccine is now available for use in adolescents and should be provided, as this tactic will reduce the societal burden of pertussis and protect vulnerable infants. Vaccination for human papilloma virus is now available and is particularly important for detained youth, many of whom engage in high-risk sexual behavior. Referrals for chronic illness, follow-up planning, and case management after release from detention assures appropriate diagnoses and treatment of chronic medical problems.

Research

Grossly inappropriate research involving incarcerated populations has resulted in stringent limits on studies involving prisoners in the United States of America. However, prisoners have many legitimate medical and psychological research needs. Infections such as STIs, hepatitis C, and mental health problems including anxiety, impulsiveness, borderline personality traits, and depression can be addressed by studies designed to reduce the incidence of disease or improve its detection and treatment for those in confinement. Rigorous evaluation of rehabilitative programs is also in the best interests of imprisoned persons and society in general. Any attempt to study prisoners and their specific problems must be balanced so the welfare of individuals is not compromised. Governmental agencies advocate for appropriate research and have built-in safeguards for all research involving prisoners, including stipulating the types of permissible research (United States Department of Health and Human Services, 1991). Medical personnel at large facilities should be involved as primary investigators or as collaborators with other investigators. The significant problems of our youthful offenders cannot be solved unless and until we have made systematic efforts to study their treatments. Consent laws and regulation for participation in studies vary from jurisdiction to jurisdiction. Parental permission for youth participation in minimal risk studies (studies with risk equal to everyday life, such as drawing blood for medical evaluation and answering questionnaires) can be expensive and difficult to obtain. A judicial or governmental agency may be vested with authority to give permission for these types of studies. Conducting sound ethical, targeted research will greatly aid progress in reducing the burden of crime and illnesses for juvenile delinquents. Cooperation is necessary among medical, custody, and judicial personnel to obtain funding for studies and to facilitate the conduct of research.

Conclusion

Incarcerated teens are at risk for a wide variety of injuries and illnesses. Careful screening and follow-up assures the teen will medically benefit from incarceration and improve their chances of rehabilitation.

References

Alexander-Rodriguez, T. & Vermund, S. H. (1987). Gonorrhea and syphilis in incarcerated urban adolescents: prevalence and physical signs. *Pediatrics*, **80**(4), 561–564.

American Academy of Pediatrics, Committee on Adolescence (1989). Health care for children and adolescents in detention centers, jails, lock-ups, and other court-sponsored residential facilities. *Pediatrics*, **84**(6), 1118–1120.

American Academy of Pediatrics (2006). In L. K. Pickening, C. J. Baker, S. S. Long and J. A. McMillan, eds., *Red Book: 2006 Report of the Committee on Infectious Diseases*, 27th edn. Elk Grove Village, IL: American Academy of Pediatrics, p. 683, Table 3.70.

Anderson, B. & Farrow, J. A. (1998). Incarcerated adolescents in Washington state. *Journal of Adolescent Health*, **22**, 363–367.

Baghurst, P. A., McMichael, A. J., Wigg, N. R. *et al.* (1992). Environmental exposure to lead and children's intelligence at the age of seven years. *New England Journal of Medicine*, **327**(18), 1279–1284.

Bell, T. A., Farrow, J. A., Stamm, W. E. *et al.* (1985). Sexually transmitted diseases in females in a juvenile detention center. *Sexually Transmitted Diseases*, **12**(3), 140–144.

Black, M., Mitchell, J. R. & Zimmerman, H. J. (1975). Isoniazid associated with hepatitis in 114 patients. *Gastroenterology*, **69**, 289–302.

Blecker, U., Lanciers, S. & Vandenplas, Y. (1994). Epidemiology of *Helicobacter pylori* seropositivity in Belgium. *International Pediatrics*, **9**(4), 230–233.

Breuner, C. C. & Farrow, J. A. (1995). Pregnant teens in prison: prevalence, management, and consequences. *Western Journal of Medicine*, **162**, 328–330.

Brunner, H. G., Nelen, M., Breakefield, X. O., Ropers, H. H. & vanOost, B. A. (1993). Abnormal behavior associated with a point mutation in the structural gene for monoamine oxidase A. *Science*, **262**, 578–580.

Cases, O., Seif, I., Grimsby, J. *et al.* (1995). Aggressive behavior and altered amounts of brain serotonin and norepinephrine in mice lacking MAOA. *Science*, **268**, 1763–1766.

Cates, W. Jr., Wasserheit, J. N. & Marchbanks, P. A. (1994). Pelvic inflammatory disease and tubal infertility: the preventable conditions. *Annals of the New York Academy of Sciences*, **709**, 179–195.

Centers for Disease Control and Prevention (1999). High prevalence of chlamydial and gonococcal infection in women entering jails and juvenile detention centers: Chicago, Birmingham, and San Francisco, 1998. *Morbidity and Mortality Weekly Report*, **48**, 793–796.

Centers for Disease Control and Prevention (2003). Methicillin-resistant *Staphylococcus aureus* infections in correctional facilities – Georgia, California, and Texas, 2001–2003. *Morbidity and Mortality Weekly Report*, **52**(41), 992–996.

Centers for Disease Control and Prevention (2006). *HIV/AIDS Surveillance Report, 2005*, Vol.17, Atlanta, US: Department of Health and Human Services, p. 18. (www.cdc.gov/hiv/topics/surveillance/resources/reports)

Chen, C., Rainnie, D. G., Greene, R. W. & Tonegawa, S. (1994). Abnormal fear response and aggressive behavior in mutant mice deficient for α – calcium-calmodulin kinase II. *Science*, **266**, 291–300.

Chow, J. M., Yonekura, M. L., Richwald, G. A. *et al.* (1900). The association between *Chlamydia tracomatis* and ectopic pregnancy. *Journal of the American Medical Association*, **263**(23), 3164–3167.

Costello, J. C. & Jameson, E. J. (1987). Legal and ethical duties of health care professionals to incarcerated children. *Journal of Legal Medicine*, **8**, 191–263.

Council on Scientific Affairs (1990). Health status of detained and incarcerated youths. *Journal of the American Medical Association*, **263**(7), 987–991.

Crowe, A. H. (1998). *Drug Identification and Testing in the Juvenile Justice System*. Washington, DC: Department of Justice, Office of Justice Programs, Office of Juvenile Justice and Delinquency Prevention.

Davidson, R. J., Putnam, K. M. & Larson, C. L. (2000). Dysfunction in the neural circuitry of emotion regulation – a possible prelude to violence. *Science*, **289**, 591–594.

de Waal, F. B. M. (2000). Primates – a natural heritage of conflict resolution. *Science*, **289**, 586–590.

Drumm, B., Perez-Perez, G. I., Blaser, M. J. & Sherman, P. M. (1990). Intrafamilial clustering of *Helicobaster pylori* infection. *New England Journal of Medicine*, **322**(6), 359–363.

Ellis (1874). A case of probable lead poisoning resulting fatally, from a bullet lodged in the knee-joint twelve years previously. *Boston Medical & Surgical Journal*, **91**, 472–473.

Fast, D. K., Conry, J. & Loock, C. A. (1999). Identifying fetal alcohol syndrome among youth in the criminal justice system. *Journal of Developmental and Behavioral Pediatrics*, **29**(5), 370–372.

Feinstein, R. A., Lampkin, A., Lorish, C. D. *et al.* (1998). Medical status of adolescents at time of admission to a juvenile detention center. *Journal of Adolescent Health*, **22**, 190–196.

Feletti, V. J. (2004). *The Origins of Addiction: Evidence from the Adverse Childhood Experiences Study*. San Diego, CA: Department of Preventive Medicine, Kaiser Permanente Medical Care Program.

Gedye, A. (1989). Extreme self-injury attributed to frontal lobe seizures. *American Journal of Mental Retardation*, **94**, 20–26.

Goodin, D. S., Aminoff, M. J. & Laxer, K. D. (1990). Detection of epileptiform activity by different noninvasive EEG methods in complex partial seizures. *Annals of Neurology*, **27**, 330–334.

Graham, D. Y. & Qureshi, W. A. (2001). Markers of infection. In H. L. T. Mobley, G. L. Mendz and S. L. Hazell, eds., *Helicobacter pylori; Physiology and Genetics*. Washington, DC: ASM Press, pp. 499–510.

Harrison, L. H., Dwyer, D. M., Maples, C. T. & Billmann, L.(1999). Risk of meningococcal infection in college students. *Journal of the American Medical Association*, **281**(20), 1906–1910.

Hein, K., Cohen, M. I., Litt, I. F. *et al.* (1980). Juvenile detention: another boundary issue for physicians. *Pediatrics*, **66**(2), 239–245.

Holmes, G. L. & Mikati, M. (1991). Temporal lobe epilepsy in children. *International Pediatrics*, **6**(2), 201–213.

Hsu, L. K. G., Wisner, K., Richey, E. T. & Goldstein, C. (1985). Is juvenile delinquency related to an abnormal EEG? A study of EEG abnormalities in juvenile delinquents and adolescent psychiatric inpatients. *Journal of the American Academy of Child Psychology*, **24**(3), 310–315.

Huscroft, S. (1994). Lead poisoning from retained bullets: health threat to inmates? *Correctional Health Care and Management*, February 1994, 27–31.

Huscroft, S., Morris, R. E., Baker, C. J. & Evans, C. A. (1994). Retained bullets: A cause of lead poisoning in teenagers. Presented at the 122nd annual meeting of the American Public Health Association, Washington, DC, October 30–November 3, 1994. Abstract.

Hux, K., Bond, V., Skinner, S., Belau, D. & Sanger, D. (1998). Parental report of occurrences and consequences of traumatic brain injury among delinquent and non-delinquent youth. *Brain Injury*, **12**(8), 667–681.

Jones, K. L. (1983a). Fetal alcohol syndrome. In *Smith's Recognizable Patterns of Human Malformation*, 5th edn. Philadelphia, PA: W.B. Saunders Company, pp. 555–558.

Jones, K. L. (1983b). XXY Syndrome, Klinefelter Syndrome. In *Smith's Recognizable Patterns of Human Malformation*, 5th edn. Philadelphia, PA: W.B. Saunders Company, pp. 72–75.

Kaller, S. G., White, B. J. & Kruesi, M. J. P. (1989). Fire setting and Klinefelter Syndrome. Letters to the editor. *Pediatrics*, **84**(4), 749.

Kastner, T. (1998). Developmental disabilities. In S. B. Friedman, M. Fisher, S. K. Schonberg, and E. M. Alderman, eds., *Comprehensive Adolescent Health Care*, 2nd edn. St. Louis, MO: Mosby – Year Book, Inc., pp. 885–886.

Lemp, G. F., Hirozawa, A. M., Givertz, D. *et al.* (1994). Seroprevalence of HIV and risk behaviors among young homosexual and bisexual men. The San Francisco/Berkeley young men's survey. *Journal of the American Medical Association*, **272**(6), 449–454.

Lester, B. M., LaGasse, L. L. & Seifer, R. (1998). Cocaine exposure and children: the meaning of subtle effects. *Science*, **282**, 633–644.

Lewis, D. O., Moy, E., Jackson, L. D. *et al.* (1985). Biopsychosocial characteristics of children who later murder: a prospective study. *American Journal of Psychiatry*, **142**(10), 1161–1167.

Lewis, D. O., Pincus, J. H., Bard, B. *et al.* (1988). Neuropsychiatric, psychoeducational, and family characteristics of 14 juveniles condemned to death in the United States. *American Journal of Psychiatry*, **145**(5), 584–589.

Linden, M. A., Manton, W. I., Stewart, M. R. *et al.* (1982). Lead poisoning from retained bullets – pathogenesis, diagnosis, and management. *Annals of Surgery*, **195**, 305–313.

MacKay, A. P., Fingerhut, L. A. & Druan, C. R. (2000). *Adolescent Health Chartbook. Health, United States, 2000*. Hyattsville, MD: National Center for Health Statistics.

Martin, B. R. (1993). What are the long-term consequences for the child of in utero exposure to drugs? In L. N. Robins and J. L. Mills (eds). Effects of in utero exposure to street drugs. *American Journal of Public Health*, Suppl **83**, 18–20.

Miller, M. E. & Sulkes, S. (1988). Fire-setting behavior in individuals with Klinefelter Syndrome. *Pediatrics*, **82**(1), 115–117.

Miller, M. E. & Sulkes, S. (1989). Klinefelter Syndrome and fire-setting behavior. Letters to the editor. *Pediatrics*, **83**(4), 649–650.

Mitchell, D. A., Abluwalia, K. P., Albert, D. A. *et al.* (2003). Dental caries experience in northern Manhattan adolescents. *Journal of Public Health Dentistry*, **63**(3), 189–194.

Morris, R. E. (1995). Health risk behavior survey from thirty-nine juvenile correctional facilities in the United States. *Journal of Adolescent Health*, **17**, 334–344.

Morris, R. E., Baker, C. J., Valentine, M. & Pennisi, A. (1998). Variations in HIV risk behaviors of incarcerated juveniles during a four year period: 1989–1992. *Journal of Adolescent Health*, **23**(1), 39–48.

Moscicki, A., Shiboski, S. Hills, N. K. *et al.* (2004). Regression of low-grade squamous intra-epithelial lesions in young women. *Lancet*, **364**, 1678–1683.

Murphy, R., Swartz, R. & Watkins, P. B. (1990). Severe acetaminophen toxicity in a patient receiving isoniazid. *Annals of International Medicine*, **113**, 799–900.

National Institute of Justice (1996). *1995 Drug Use Forecasting: Annual Report on Adult and Juvenile Arrestees*. Washington, DC: Department of Justice, Office of Justice Programs, National Institute of Justice.

Needleman, H. L. & Gastonis, C. A. (1990). Low-level lead exposure and the IQ of children. A meta-analysis of modern studies. *Journal of the American Medical Association*, **263**(5), 673–678.

Needleman, H. L., Schell, A., Bellinger, D., Leviton, A. & Allred, E. N. (1990). The long-term effects of exposure to low doses of lead in childhood. An 11-year follow-up report. *New England Journal of Medicine*, **322**(2), 83–88.

Needleman, H. L., Riess, J. A., Tobin, M. J., Biesecker, G. E. & Greenhouse, J. B. (1996). Bone lead levels and delinquent behavior. *Journal of the American Medical Association*, **275**(5), 363–369.

Nesmith, J. D., Klerman, L. V., Oh, M. K. & Feinstein, R. A. (1997). Procreative experiences and orientations toward paternity held by incarcerated males. *Journal of Adolescent Health*, **20**, 198–203.

Nielsen, J., Pelsen, B. & Sorensen, K. (1988). Follow-up of 30 Klinefelter males treated with testosterone. *Clinical Genetics*, **33**, 262–269.

Oh, M. K., Cloud, G. A., Wallace, L. S. *et al.* (1994). Sexual behavior and sexually transmitted diseases among male adolescents in detention. *Sexually Transmitted Diseases*, **21**, 127–132.

Osmond, D. H., Page, K., Wiley, J. *et al.* (1994). HIV infection in homosexual and bisexual men 18 to 29 years of age: the San Francisco young men's health study. *American Journal of Public Health*, **84**(12), 1933–1937.

Otnow-Lewis, D. (1998). *Guilty by Reason of Insanity: A Psychiatrist Probes the Minds of Killers.* New York, NY: Fawcett Columbine.

Ozuah, P. O., Ozuah, T. P., Stein, R. E., Burton, W. & Mulvihill, M. (2001). Evaluation of a risk assessment questionnaire used to target tuberculin skin testing in children. *Journal of the American Medical Association*, **285**(4), 451–453.

Pan, E. S., Diep, B. A., Carleton, H. A. *et al.* (2003). Increasing prevalence of methicillin-resistant *Staphylococcus aureus* infection in California jails. *Clinical Infectious Diseases*, **37**(10), 1384–1388.

Parsonnet, J., Shmuely, H. & Haggerty, T. (1999). Fecal and oral shedding of *Helicobacter pylori* from healthy infected adults. *Journal of the American Medical Association*, **282**(23), 2240–2245.

Perry, B., Pollard, R., Blakley, T., Baker, W. & Vigilante, E. (1995). Childhood trauma, the neurobiology of adaption and "use-dependent" development of the brain: how "states" become "traits". *Infant Mental Health Journal*, **16**, 271–289.

Richmond, N. L. (1978). The dental clinic at Indiana girls' school. *Alumni Bulletin School of Dentistry Indiana Univ* 1978 Fall, 17–8, 104.

Robertson A. A., Thomas, C. B., St. Lawrence, J. S. & Pack, R. (2005). Predictors of infection with chlamydia and gonorrhea in incarcerated adolescents. *Sexually Transmitted Diseases*, **32**(2), 115–122.

Rosenberg, P. S. & Biggar, R. J. (1998). Trends in HIV incidence among young adults in the United States. *Journal of the American Medical Association*, **279**(23), 1894–1899.

Rosenstein, N., Levine, O., Taylor, J. P. *et al.* (1998). Efficacy of meningococcal vaccine and barriers to vaccination. *Journal of the American Medical Association*, **279**(6), 435–439.

Saslow, D., Runowicz, C. D., Solomon, D. *et al.*(2002). American Cancer Society guideline for the early detection of cervical neoplasia and cancer. *CA: Cancer Journal for Clinicians*, **52**(6), 342–362.

Saudou, F., Amara, D. A., Dierich, A. *et al.* (1994). Enhanced aggressive behavior in mice lacking 5-HT$_{1B}$ receptor. *Science*, **265**, 1875–1878.

Scholes, D., Stergachis, A., Heidrich, F. E. *et al.* (1996). Prevention of pelvic inflammatory disease by screening for cervical chlamydial infection. *New England Journal of Medicine*, **334**, 1362–1366.

Schwartz, R. H. (1998). Adolescent heroin use: a review. *Pediatrics*, **102**(6), 1461–1466.

Selbst, S. M., Henretig, F., Fee, M. A., Levy, S. E. & Kitts, A. W.(1986). Lead poisoning in a child with a gunshot wound. *Pediatrics*, **77**(3), 413–416.

Seymour, R. B. & Smith, D. E. (1987). *Guide to Psychoactive Drugs: An Up-to-the-Minute Reference to Mind-Altering Substances.* New York, NY: Harrington Park Press, p. 9.

Shafer, M. S., Hilton, J. F., Elkstrand, M. *et al.* (1993). Relationship between drug use and sexual behaviors and the occurrence of sexually transmitted diseases among high-risk male youth. *Sexually Transmitted Diseases*, **20**, 307–313.

Shanok, S. S. & Lewis, D. O. (1981). Medical histories of abused delinquents. *Child Psychiatry and Human Development*, **11**(4), 222–231.

Snider, D. E. & Caras, G. J. (1992). Isoniazid-associated hepatitis deaths: a review of available information. *American Review of Respiratory Disease*, **145**, 494–497.

Society for Adolescent Medicine (2000). Position paper. Health care for incarcerated youth. *Journal of Adolescent Health*, **27**, 73–75.

Stone, R. & Kelner, K. (eds) (2000). Violence: no silver bullet. *Science*, **289**, 569–585.

Streissguth, A. P., Aase, J. M., Clarren, S. K. *et al.* (1991). Fetal alcohol syndrome in adolescents and adults. *Journal of the American Medical Association*, **265**(15), 1961–1967.

Suerbaum, S. & Michetti, P. (2002). *Helicobacter pylori* infection. *New England Journal of Medicine*, **347**(15), 1175–1186.

Tappero, J. W., Reporter, R., Wenger, J. D. *et al.* (1996). Meningococcal disease in Los Angeles County, California, and among men in the county jails. *New England Journal of Medicine*, **335**(17), 833–840.

Tompkins, L. S. & Falkow, S. (1995). The new path to preventing ulcers. *Science*, **267**, 1621–1622.

Tonkonogy, J. M. (1991). Violence and temporal lobe lesion: head CT and MRI data. *Journal of Neuropsychiatry*, **3**, 189–196.

Tonkonogy, J. M. & Geller, J. L. (1992). Hypothalamic lesions and intermittent explosive disorder. *Journal of Neuropsychiatry*, **4**, 45–50.

US Department of Health and Human Services (1991). Protection of human subjects, part 46, subpart c46.301–46.306. In *Code of Federal Regulations, Title 45, Public Welfare*. Bethesda, MD: Department of Health and Human Services, National Institutes of Health, Office for Protection from Research Risks.

Volavka, J. (2002). *Neurobiology of Violence*, 2nd edn. Washington, DC: American Psychiatric Publishing, Inc.

Volkow, N. D. & Tancredi, L. (1987). Neural substrates of violent behavior: a preliminary study with positron emission tomography. *British Journal of Psychiatry*, **151**, 668–673.

Volpe, J. J. (1992). Effect of cocaine use on the fetus. *New England Journal of Medicine*, **327**(6), 399–407.

Westrom, L., Josesoef, R., Reynolds, G., Hagdu, A. & Thompson, S. E. (1992). Pelvic inflammatory disease and fertility: a cohort of 1844 women with laparoscopically verified disease and 657 control women with normal laparoscopy. *Sexually Transmitted Diseases*, **19**, 185–192.

Wolner-Hanssen, P., Kiviat, N. B. & Holmes, K. K. (1990). Atypical pelvic inflammatory disease: subacute, chronic, or subclinical upper genital tract infection in women. In K. K. Holmes, P. A. March, P. F. Sparling and P. J. Wiesner, eds., *Sexually Transmitted Diseases*, 2nd edn. New York, NY: McGraw-Hill Information Services, pp. 615–20.

Woolf, A. & Funk, S. G. (1985). Epidemiology of trauma in a population of incarcerated youth. *Pediatrics*, **75**(3), 463–468.

13

Mental health screening and assessment in juvenile justice

Gina M. Vincent, Thomas Grisso, and Anna Terry

Mental health screening in juvenile justice

Over 106 000 youths are in the custody of juvenile justice facilities in the US daily (Synder & Sickmund, 1999). Recent estimates suggest that nearly 60 percent of boys and over two-thirds of girls involved with the juvenile justice system meet criteria for one or more psychiatric disorders, even after controlling for conduct disorder (Teplin et al., 2002). These prevalence rates are higher than those found in youth in the general population (around 14–22 percent; e.g., Kazdin, 2000; Rutter, 1989) and substantially higher than adult prisoners in areas where such comparisons can be made. For example, 13 percent of male delinquents (Teplin et al., 2002) would meet criteria for major depression in contrast to only 4 percent of male adult offenders (Teplin, 1994).

In light of these statistics, accurate identification of mental, behavioral, and emotional disturbances that require immediate attention; namely, risk of suicide or self-harm, risk of aggression, or a pressing mental disorder, is essential as youths enter the juvenile justice system. State juvenile justice facilities have a legal and moral responsibility to respond to the mental health needs of adolescents in their custody (Grisso, 2004). When youths are identified as having a high potential for serious mental health issues, it allows staff to respond immediately to these needs by making appropriate placement decisions in the institution or by referring the youth for a clinical evaluation.

This chapter provides a brief description of the benefits and procedures of mental health screening and assessment in juvenile justice settings. The chapter begins with a discussion of the reasons for and benefits of identification of mental health problems in juvenile justice settings, and the developmental complications involved in this undertaking. The next section defines and differentiates mental health screening versus assessment by describing the characteristics of both. Finally, we provide a brief review of the current mental health screening tools, which are in the public domain and have been validated for use in juvenile justice

The Mental Health Needs of Young Offenders: Forging Paths toward Reintegration and Rehabilitation, eds. Carol L. Kessler and Louis J. Kraus. Published by Cambridge University Press. © Cambridge University Press 2007.

settings. This chapter does not include a similar review of assessment tools. Given the wide availability of assessment tools for delinquent youth, such a review could be a chapter in itself.

Several scholarly works have described the benefits and procedures of mental health screening and assessment in juvenile justice, the process of implementation of these procedures, and screening and assessment instruments available for these purposes (e.g., Bailey, Doreleijers & Tarbuck, 2006; Grisso, 2004; Grisso & Underwood, 2004; Grisso, Vincent & Seagrave, 2005; Wasserman, Jensen & Ko, 2003). As such, this chapter should be seen as a brief review of an area of mental health that has been described previously in considerable detail (particularly by Grisso *et al.*, 2005). The reader is referred to these pieces for greater detail about specific screening and assessment instruments and recommendations for implementing procedures for the identification of mental health problems in juvenile justice settings.

Reasons for identifying youths' mental health problems in juvenile justice

There are several important benefits to the identification of youths' mental health problems in the juvenile justice system. One benefit is *safety* from harm to self or others. Accurate identification reduces the likelihood of youths hurting themselves, for example, by signaling staff to place a youth with serious suicide ideation on suicide watch or some other special placement. Likewise, identification can reduce the likelihood of harm to others by targeting youth at risk for aggressive or violent behavior, which permits staff to make an informed placement decision (segregation for example) commensurate with the risk.

Another benefit of identification is to maintain the *health and welfare* of youths involved in the juvenile justice system, particularly those with serious mental disorders. It is crucial for staff to be aware of youths with serious mental disorders in order to respond appropriately to their treatment needs. For example, youths with psychotic disorders need psychiatric medication, monitoring from clinical staff, and in some cases, placement in a facility or on a unit designated for juveniles with mental health needs. Many disorders can put youths at higher risk for harm to self or others, especially when these go undetected and untreated.

Another potential benefit of the identification of youths' mental health problems is *delinquency prevention and rehabilitation*. Early identification of mental health needs increases the likelihood of interventions that may reduce risk for future crime and violence, and prevent the development of serious mental disorders down the road, several of which are tied to crime and violence (Grisso, 2004; Mash & Dozois, 2003). Finally, identification is a benefit because it provides a means for facilities to *document the need* for mental health services. Awareness of the extent of mental health concerns is critical in order for facilities and local juvenile justice systems as a whole to allocate resources and develop appropriate policy and management plans.

Developmental complications to identification

Clinicians and designated juvenile justice personnel should evaluate the process of identification of mental disorders in light of several complications involved when dealing with youth. Identification of any mental disorders prior to adulthood is complicated by several factors that, for the purposes of this review, may fall within one of two categories: definitional problems and developmental influences. With regards to definitional problems, it is unclear whether childhood disorders should be defined according to categorical or dimensional syndromes, individual symptoms, or significant departures from normality (Mash & Dozios, 2003). There are complications with each of these strategies, such as evidence that most children will express behavioral or emotional symptoms characteristic of psychopathology at some point (Achenbach & Edelbrock, 1984), normal childhood development is hard to define, and no categorical classification scheme has achieved adequate reliability and validity (Mash & Terdal, 1997). Current nosological frameworks have produced abnormally high *co-morbidity* among various childhood disorders (see Mash & Dozois, 2003, for a review) and high *heterogeneity* within diagnostic subgroups (e.g., Kazdin, 1993). To complicate matters further, variability in the manifestation, prevalence, and etiology of childhood disorders can occur as a function of demographic characteristics such as, gender, culture, and socioeconomic status (Mash & Dozois, 2003).

Identification of serious childhood disorders is further hampered by *discontinuity* in the expression and presence of symptoms. Childhood psychopathology appears to continue into adulthood for some, but not all, children (Mash & Dozois, 2003). Though the study of developmental stability is in its infancy, three main hurdles to targeting chronic psychopathology have been elucidated (e.g., Cicchetti & Cohen, 1995; Cicchetti & Rogosch, 1996). First, different developmental pathways can lead to the same adult psychopathology. Second, similar pathways of abnormal development can lead to different outcomes in adulthood, including normal psychological processes. Finally, *heterotypic discontinuity* (instability in the expression of symptoms over time) is common.

Distinguishing screening from assessment

One method for identifying youths with mental health needs would involve having psychologists on staff in probation offices and detention facilities to conduct extensive interviews and testing with every youth, resulting in a detailed assessment of the risk for aggression and suicide, and potential psychiatric diagnoses. The problem with this approach is that it would be extremely costly given about

1.7 million youths are arrested and 320 000 youths are admitted to pre-trial detention facilities per year in the US (Synder & Sickmund, 1999). Instead, a more efficient way of handling the problem is to implement a two-tiered process that involves "screening" and "assessment." As Grisso (2005) described, screening provides a form of economical identification that can be applied to all youths entering the juvenile justice system, whereas assessment provides more extensive and individualized identification of mental health needs for only those youths whose screening results suggest it is warranted.

In the recent book by Grisso *et al.* (2005), *Mental Health Screening and Assessment for Juvenile Justice*, Grisso provided a detailed explanation of the differences between screening and assessment in the juvenile justice system, and the areas of potential confusion around distinguishing the two. Grisso noted that the field's choice of these terms is confusing, because the term "assessment" is often used to refer to *any* type of measurement of psychological characteristics. A second source of potential confusion is the lack of consensual definitions of "screening" and "assessment" in the current juvenile justice literature (Grisso & Underwood, 2004; Trupin & Boesky, 1999; Wasserman *et al.*, 2003). One author's screening might be another author's assessment. Another source of confusion is in test authors' labeling of instruments as screening or assessment tools. Regardless of an instrument's name, some tools may work better for one process or the other. In other words, the simple fact that an instrument is called a "screening" tool does not guarantee that it will serve all juvenile justice programs' needs for a screening process. A final source of confusion is that screening and assessment tools do not necessarily differ in the mental health conditions they attempt to identify. Both may seek to learn about the presence and severity of symptoms often associated with mental disorders (e.g., anxiety), the potential for problem behaviors (e.g., suicide, aggression), psychiatric diagnoses (e.g., generalized anxiety disorder), or problems in functional areas (e.g., school problems, peer relations). Typically, however, screening will identify these conditions more tentatively than assessment, its results will be valid for a shorter period of time, and it will provide a less individualized perspective on the nature of the youth's mental health needs.

The nature of mental health screening

Grisso *et al.* (2005) described *screening* as having two main purposes. The first purpose of screening is to identify youths at contact who might require an *immediate response to mental health needs* – for example, those with an immediate need for psychoactive medication or consideration of placement on suicide watch. Second, screening is intended to "sift" through the total number of youths in order to *identify a subset with the higher likelihood of having mental health needs* requiring special attention. In this sense, the results of a screening tool are used to signal the need for a more thorough assessment of mental health symptoms and potential psychiatric diagnoses.

The process for mental health screening has several characteristics. First, it is applied with every youth at entry into some part of the juvenile justice system, the first day after entrance to a pre-trial detention center for example. Second, at these points, the purpose of screening is to sort youths into at least two groups: one group that is very unlikely to have the characteristics in question (e.g., risk of harm to self) and one group that is more likely to have the characteristics in question. As Grisso (2005) described, "the objective is similar to triage in medical settings, where incoming patients are initially classified (in triage, into three categories) indicating their level of urgency. Like triage, screening is useful in systems that have limited resources and therefore cannot respond comprehensively or immediately to every individual's particular needs." (p. 13). In other words, the value of a screening method is in its ability to identify a group of youths who are more greatly at risk of mental health problems than the group of youths that was "screened out." For the group of youths that was "screened in," only a proportion actually will have mental health problems. That proportion will be significant, but will vary based on the quality of the screening tool and its sensitivity.

Results of screening can lead to any of four responses by juvenile justice personnel. First, results can lead to decisions to place youths in *special custody placements* or to take special precautions, such as placement in segregation, specification of any level of suicide watch, or placement on a specialized unit or in a specialized facility where staff may be trained to handle mental health needs. Another response would be to *respond to emerging crises*, by fulfilling psychiatric medication needs for example. Other potential responses would be a clinical referral to *seek more information from the youth* in specific problem areas or to *conduct a detailed assessment* that may result in some sort of psychiatric diagnosis.

In sum, the purpose of mental health screening is to identify youths' short-term mental and emotional needs at the time of intake in order to signal the need for an immediate response or comprehensive psychological assessment. It is important to be clear about what mental screening *does not do*. Mental health screening *is not* designed to provide clinically valid diagnoses of mental disorders. This is the task of assessment procedures. Screening does not provide clinicians or staff with the causes or etiology of mental health problems, it only identifies current symptomatology. Finally, mental health screening is not appropriate for long-range treatment or rehabilitation planning. Scores or ratings on mental health screening tools are intended to fluctuate by definition because they target acute symptoms or problem areas. A good rule of thumb would be to consider these scores as valid for only two–four weeks. Put simply, they have a short shelf-life.

The nature of assessment

In contrast to screening, the purpose of *assessment* is to gather a more comprehensive and individualized profile of a youth. Thus, assessment is performed selectively with those youths "screened in" from the screening process as requiring a more thorough identification of mental health needs. The intent of assessment is to verify the presence or absence of mental health needs, determine how disorders manifest for a particular youth, and provide recommendations for longer-range interventions. Interventions may include diversion, referral to community mental health services for treatment, or special programming within juvenile justice detention or correctional facilities. Assessment can take many forms, including a more detailed interview by trained juvenile justice staff, a clinical interview by a professional, clinical consultation by on-call professionals outside the facility, or comprehensive evaluation involving psychological testing. In this sense, the process often relies less on standardized approaches and more on individualized inquiry into the needs of the particular youth.

There are several other characteristics of assessment that distinguish it from screening. First, the timing of assessment methods is more variable than it is for screening. Assessment may occur soon after first contact in response to screening information to determine whether an emergency situation truly exists, the specific nature of the emergency, and how best to handle it. Or, assessment may be delayed, focusing instead on comprehensive collection of data aimed at developing longer-range treatment planning or meeting legal needs by responding to a forensic question. Second, assessment tools typically involve longer administration times (more than 30 minutes), comprehensive psychological testing, clinical interviews, and/or gathering of past records. Third, assessment tools often require administration by a clinician (psychiatrists, psychologists, or social workers) and definitely require considerable training and expertise.

Another characteristic of assessment is that, with some exceptions, the procedures and tools rely less on standardized methods because they will be tailored to the needs of the youth. For example, a youth with problems with aggression and irritability may receive an assessment of their future risk for violence whereas a youth with symptoms of thought disturbance may receive an assessment of prior substance abuse problems and/or a diagnostic assessment of the presence of psychotic disorders. Finally, the conclusions generated from assessment procedures are intended to be more stable than findings from screening tools, because they tend to examine both the duration (lifetime) and severity of symptoms and level of impairment.

Selecting screening tools

There are several factors involved in the selection of a screening tool for use in a particular juvenile justice setting or facility. These factors were described in depth by Grisso *et al.* (2005) and will be reviewed only briefly here. First, administrators should consider the *feasibility* of conducting the screening with every youth. Generally, tools that will be favored are those that require no more than 10–30 minutes of administration time. Second, for economical reasons, tools capable of being *administered by existing staff* that do not have advanced training or credentials in mental health are probably preferable. Third, tools that work best will be *standardized* and highly structured in the sense that the same process can be used for every youth.

Juvenile justice administrators also will want to select a screening tool that is *relevant* and suited to their particular needs. There is fair variability across instruments in terms of the mental health concerns and types of behaviors that they are designed to identify. Though most legal directives do not prescribe the types of mental health needs for which a system must screen, several sources provide guidance as to the intentions of regulations in this area (e.g., Grisso, 2004; Grisso & Underwood, 2004; Wasserman *et al.*, 2003). As summarized by Grisso and Vincent (2005), screening tools that fulfill legal obligations are those that include at a minimum:

- one or more scales aimed at current affective and anxiety symptoms
- some indication of the short-term likelihood of aggression
- some indicator of risk for suicide or self-harm, and
- an indicator geared toward alcohol and drug abuse and dependence.

Another factor in the selection of screening tools is whether or not there is research evidence of its *reliability and validity* for use with juvenile justice samples. In other words, will the tool produce consistent results across administration regardless of the trained individual rating the tool, and does the tool measure what it purports to measure? Finally, the most effective screening tools will be those that are *amenable to providing clear decision rules*. The test manuals of some tools define standardized cut-off scores that prescribe specific actions. For example, a youth scoring in a particular range should receive a diagnostic assessment, or a youth scoring in a particular range should be seen as having a high risk for suicide requiring immediate action. Other tools provide guidelines for the use of scores but require administrators to create the decision-making rules that are best suited to their needs and availability of resources.

Screening tools available for juvenile justice settings

This section reviews most of the instruments in the public domain that have been either designed for mental health screening within juvenile justice settings or validated for use within juvenile justice settings. We did not include a review of assessment tools available for use in juvenile justice because it is outside of the scope of this chapter. For more detailed information about the screening tools reviewed here, their research evidence and validity data, and for assessment tools available for juvenile justice, the reader is referred to Grisso *et al.* (2005). For a more comprehensive list of tools available for mental health screening and assessment of youth with potential for use in the juvenile justice system, readers are referred to Grisso and Underwood (2004). Finally, this review covers only tools in distribution within the US. For information about additional screening and assessment instruments currently used by other countries see Bailey *et al.* (2006). For the purposes of this review, we defined screening tools along three categories: (1) multidimensional brief screening tools, (2) problem or needs-oriented interview schedules, and (3) multidimensional scales identifying clinical disorder.

Multidimensional brief screening tools

Screening tools vary considerably in their specifics. Some focus on symptoms, others social problem areas, others on dimensions of psychopathology or diagnoses, and still others on the risk of suicidal or aggressive behaviors. The tools in this section are defined as "multidimensional" because they target each of these areas, and are defined as "brief" because they require 15 minutes or less to complete. These tools are in contrast to "single-focused" brief screening tools, which also exist but are not reviewed here. Single-focused or unidimensional screening tools available for juvenile justice include the Substance Abuse Subtle Screening Instrument (SASSI; Miller & Lazowski, 2001), the Trauma Symptom Checklist for Children (TSCC; Briere, 1996), the Suicide Ideation Scale (SIS; Rudd, 1989), and several brief tools that screen for attention-deficit/hyperactivity disorder (see Loney & Counts, 2005). Again, for a description of these measures, readers are referred to Grisso *et al.* (2005) and/or Grisso and Underwood (2004).

Massachusetts Youth Screening Instrument – Version 2 (MAYSI-2)

The Massachusetts Youth Screening Instrument-Version 2 (MAYSI-2; Grisso & Barnum, 2006) is a 52-item self-report scale that screens for symptoms of mental and emotional disturbance, as well as potential crisis areas, of all youths aged 12–17 upon entry into any juvenile justice program or facility (e.g., probation intake, pre-trial detention, or correctional programs). The MAYSI-2 requires 10–15 minutes to complete and can be administered by clinical or non-clinical staff in one of three ways: (1) youths can read the items themselves and circle their answers; (2) juvenile justice staff can read the items to youths who cannot read the form, while the youths circle their answers; or (3) youths can complete the MAYSI-2 through an audio computer administration called MAYSIWARE. Both the computer and paper-and-pencil versions of the test can be administered in Spanish or English. The MAYSI-2 is typically administered to youths at their first intake probation interview or in the first few days (usually within 24 hours) of admission to a juvenile justice facility.

The MAYSI-2 was developed during a six-year project (1994–2000), including conceptual development, piloting, and development of reliability and validity on large samples of youths in juvenile justice settings in two states. First manualized in 2000, the project continued with an aggressive program of dissemination designed to place the MAYSI-2 at the front door of juvenile justice facilities nationwide. Within five years, the MAYSI-2 has come to be used to screen every youth at admission in probation, detention, or juvenile corrections systems statewide in 35 states. The widespread use allowed the test authors to develop national norms for the MAYSI-2, which were reported in the updated test manual published in 2006.

Yes/no responses to the 52 items are summed to create scores on seven scales. The six primary scales are alcohol/drug use, angry–irritable, depressed–anxious, somatic complaints, suicide ideation, and thought disturbance (this scale is for boys only). The seventh scale, traumatic experiences, is not a primary measure of a potential mental health problem but instead identifies potential recent traumas that may have contributed to mental health problems. Scores on each scale are compared to cut-off scores suggested in the manual. There are two types of cut-off scores for each scale: (1) the "caution" cut-offs signify a "clinical level of significance," and (2) the "warning" cut-offs indicate that the youth has scored higher than 90 percent of the normative sample. The procedure does not require specific staff responses to specific scores. How a program responds to scores at or above the two cut-off levels, as manifested on particular scales or combinations of scales, is left to each program's discretion (Grisso & Quinlan, 2005).

Global Appraisal of Individual Need – Short Screener (GAIN-SS)

The Global Appraisal of Individual Need – Short Screener (GAIN-SS; Dennis *et al.*, 2005) is a 20-item behavioral health screening tool designed to identify adolescents in need of more detailed assessment because they may qualify as having a provisional diagnoses on the GAIN. The GAIN-SS is a self-report tool that youths can take by paper-and-pencil or by computer and complete in 3–5 minutes. Responses are given in terms of the recency of the problem. There are two versions of the GAIN-SS, one that asks about the recency of problems and one that asks about the past year.

The GAIN instruments were developed through a ten-year collaboration between clinicians, researchers, and policy makers from various organizations around the US. The GAIN-SS was designed for use in the general population but can be used in a variety of service contexts, such as residential substance abuse programs, therapy settings, and juvenile justice programs. According to the GAIN website, it has been adopted by over four dozen systems of care and agencies around the US and is being used in a number of large-scale research projects.

The GAIN-SS' 20-items comprise four subscales: (1) internal disorders, (2) behavioral disorders, (3) substance use disorders, and (4) crime/violence. The subscales were derived via factor analyses of symptoms among clinical samples. Research with adolescents has demonstrated that total scores on the GAIN-SS have high sensitivity and specificity for identifying youth with a high likelihood of having or not having a mental disorder.

Problem or needs-oriented interview schedules

The "problem-oriented" approach is another alternative for defining psychopathology among adolescents. Instruments designed based on this approach identify areas of strengths and impairments in practical, everyday functioning. These tools are often organized according to common areas of activity for adolescents, such as school, peer relations, family problems, work, leisure activities, and so forth. Generally, the level of functioning is expressed on scales according to the degree of impairment relative to same age peers. These instruments tend to be longer than the brief, multidimensional tools described previously, generally requiring about 30 minutes to administer. This section describes three commonly used instruments designed according to the problem or needs-oriented approach that have some validity data from juvenile justice samples.

Problem-Oriented Screening Instrument for Teenagers (POSIT)

The Problem-Oriented Screening Instrument for Teenagers (POSIT; Rahdert, 1991) is a 139-item self-report screening tool designed for use with youths aged 12–19 years to identify psychosocial functioning in ten areas requiring more thorough assessment. The POSIT requires approximately 20–30 minutes to complete, it is available in both English and Spanish, and in both a paper-and-pencil version and CD-ROM. It can be administered by staff without special training. Test administrators should be available to answer questions or to read the questions to youths with reading difficulties, and should verify youth responses with collateral information. According to Dembo and Anderson (2005), the POSIT is most helpful to juvenile justice facilities when it is used during intake where it may be followed by a referral for more comprehensive assessment when indicated.

The POSIT was developed as a part of the Adolescent Assessment/Referral System (AARS), funded by the National Institute on Drug Abuse (NIDA) in 1987. It was not designed specifically for use in juvenile justice. The POSIT can be used in a variety of adolescent environments, including drug treatment programs, schools, and medical and mental health service providers. This widespread implementation has enabled studies supporting the POSIT as valid for use with juvenile delinquents.

The instrument probes ten areas of psychosocial functioning: (1) substance use/abuse, (2) physical health status, (3) mental health status, (4) family relationships,

(5) peer relations, (6) educational status, (7) vocational status, (8) social skills, (9) leisure and recreation, and (10) aggressive behavior and delinquency. The raw score in each problem area determines the level of risk (low, medium, or high) in that functional area. There is a follow-up version of the POSIT that screens for change on seven of the ten scales.

Child and Adolescent Functional Assessment Scale (CAFAS)

The Child and Adolescent Functional Assessment Scale (CAFAS; Hodges, 2000) is a behavioral rating scale that assesses impairment in functioning across different settings (e.g., school, work, social interactions) and indicates whether or not functioning is affected by problems that may require specialized interventions (e.g., self-harming behavior, substance use). The CAFAS can be used to determine the need for evaluation or services, and for reassessment to track changes in functioning among school-aged youth (kindergarten through Grade 12). Behavioral descriptors are rated based on a trained rater's observations, the youth's reports, and informants' reports of the youth's behavior over the past three months. According to Hodges (2005), the CAFAS requires about 10 minutes to complete and can be administered by trained non-clinical or clinical juvenile justice staff. A self-training manual is available for this purpose. There are several different forms of the CAFAS, including a parent report version and both paper-and-pencil and software versions (see Hodges, 2005, for a detailed description).

As described by Hodges (2005), the precursor to the CAFAS (the Child Assessment Schedule) was developed in 1978. The CAFAS was developed in 1989 for use in the Fort Bragg Evaluation Study and was revised based on these findings in 1994. Although it was originally intended for use in the mental health field, some studies have shown the CAFAS to be valid for use with juvenile delinquents. In fact, in the Fort Bragg study it was the strongest predictor of more restrictive care and indicators of high treatment costs (Hodges & Wong, 1997). Over 25 states use the CAFAS today, but only a portion of these use it within the juvenile justice system.

The behavioral descriptor items are categorized according to eight subscales that assess the youth (school/work, home, community, behavior toward others, moods/emotions, self-harmful behavior, substance use, and thinking) and two optional subscales that assess caregivers' ability to care for the youth (material needs, and family/social). The behavioral descriptors within each scale are organized in terms of the severity of impairment indicated (severe, moderate, mild, or minimal). There is also the option to endorse a youth's strengths in each area. Levels of impairment on the various scales are used to make decisions about security, level of care, need for further evaluation, and prioritization of levels of intervention.

Child and Adolescent Needs and Strengths – Juvenile Justice (CANS-JJ)

The Child and Adolescent Needs and Strengths – Juvenile Justice (CANS-JJ; Lyons *et al.*, 1999) is a descriptive tool that identifies needs or strengths in a variety of areas to guide service delivery for children and adolescents with mental, emotional, and behavioral health needs and juvenile justice involvement. The CANS-JJ approach encourages information integration from multiple sources, including the child or youth, parents and families, and all involved professionals. Completion of the CANS-JJ requires ratings from trained staff based on interviews with the youth and appropriate collaterals. It is unclear how long the CANS-JJ requires for administration, but given its comprehensive nature, it is unlikely that this could be completed in less than 30 minutes.

The CANS was developed to provide a system for communicating care needs. According to the authors, it can be used either as a *prospective information integration* tool for decision support by providing a structured profile of youth in various areas related to service planning; or as a *retrospective decision support* tool based on the review of existing information for use in the design of high quality systems of services; or care coordinators and supervisors can use the CANS as a *quality assurance/monitoring* device. A review of the case record in light of the CANS tool will provide information as to the appropriateness of the individual plan of care and whether individual goals and outcomes are achieved.

The CANS-JJ has eight scales: (1) functional status, (2) delinquent behavior, (3) substance abuse complications, (4) other youth risk behaviors, (5) mental health needs, (6) child safety, (7) family/caregiver needs and strengths, and (8) strengths. Each of the scales is rated on a four-point scale (0 = no evidence, 1 = mild, 2 = moderate, 3 = severe). The ratings prescribe the level of action required: a 0 indicates no need for action, a 1 indicates a need for watchful waiting to see whether action is warranted, a 2 indicates a need for action, and a 3 indicates the need for either immediate or intensive action.

Multidimensional scales identifying clinical disorder

The screening tools described up to this point value brevity. They were designed to be efficient by "sorting" youths into groups, but were not intended to provide sufficient detail about a youth's condition to allow for an individualized decision about diagnoses or the need for specific services. In contrast, the lengthier screening tools described in this section provide a better basis for deciding on certain types of responses like hospitalization, by sorting youths into probable diagnostic categories and various levels of impairment. The cost is greater time and resources. Thus there is a trade-off to the use of these tools. They provide more information and identify a narrower group of youths for further assessment than the brief screening tools; however, they are more costly and time-consuming (over 30 minutes).

Diagnostic Interview Schedule for Children – Present State Voice Version (DISC)

The Present State Voice Version of the Diagnostic Interview Schedule for Children (Voice DISC; Shaffer *et al.*, 2000) is a self-administered, computerized test, which aims to provide an accurate and efficient assessment of child and adolescent mental health problems. The Voice DISC screens for more than 30 current DSM-IV diagnoses and conditions warranting further evaluation, in modules that correspond to diagnostic groupings. The Voice DISC also provides detailed information about the current level of impairment based on responses to six sets of questions regarding the effect of symptoms on relationships with caretakers, family, and peers and on school functioning. The Voice DISC does not require any special clinical expertise for administration; it is readily scored by a computer; and it requires about 60 minutes for youths to complete. Because the Voice DISC requires a minimal reading ability, caution should be exercised before administering the tool to very young or cognitively limited juveniles (Wasserman *et al.*, 2005).

The DISC was developed in response to a National Institute of Mental Health (NIMH) request to develop a highly structured and standardized psychiatric interview for children (Shaffer *et al.*, 1996). Since that time, there have been three major revisions (DISC-R, DISC-2 [2.1 and 2.3] and DISC-IV), and each has been extensively tested in both clinical and community settings.

Each youth administered the Voice DISC receives a unique interview produced by interactive software, dependent upon the pattern of his or her responses. Therefore, administrations are somewhat individualized. Youth meet diagnostic criteria for a particular disorder on the Voice DISC based on the type and severity of symptoms (onset, frequency, and duration). For those who meet diagnostic criteria for a given disorder, the Voice DISC will ask additional questions about impairment attributed to symptoms of the specific disorder. The questions are categorized into disorder modules including anxiety, mood, disruptive behavior, substance use, and miscellaneous. Scores can be used to provide a provisional diagnosis and plan of action.

Practical Adolescent Dual Diagnosis Interview (PADDI)

The Practical Adolescent Dual Diagnosis Interview (PADDI; Estroff & Hoffmann, 2001) is a comprehensive diagnostic interview developed for use with adolescents. It helps identify both DSM-IV substance abuse/dependence diagnoses and the most important and prevalent major mental health disorders. It can be useful in mental health clinics, private practices, courts, and juvenile justice facilities. The interview was based on the following criteria: it had to be easy to administer, easy to score, and had to not require expertise in both substance abuse and mental health. Furthermore, the PADDI had to be adaptable to a variety of settings and applications. The PADDI may be administered by a professional, trained technician, or juvenile justice personnel during an outpatient or intake interview and can take anywhere from 20–40 minutes, depending on the problems identified. Special training is not needed to administer or score the PADDI; however, final interpretation of the interview should be done by a professional.

Questions directly address DSM-IV diagnostic criteria. In addition to substance abuse disorders, the PADDI helps identify major depressive episodes, anxiety disorders, posttraumatic stress disorders, behavioral disorders, and obsessions and compulsions. The questions also address dangerousness to self and others, as well as neglect, and physical and sexual abuse. When the PADDI captures an adequate amount of information, algorithms are used to suggest a provisional diagnosis. Scores place individuals into one of five categories: no symptoms, subdiagnostic, meeting minimal criteria, exceeding minimal criteria, and far exceeding minimal criteria. For those individuals who meet diagnostic criteria, indications of severity are identified by the extent of symptoms endorsed. A clear distinction between an adolescent who manifests a particular disorder and one who does not tends to be made from the clinical profiles provided by the PADDI or in a comprehensive assessment by a trained mental health clinician.

Global Appraisal of Individual Needs (GAIN-Q)

The Global Appraisal of Individual Needs – Quick (GAIN-Q; Dennis *et al.*, 2002) is an instrument used to assess various life problems in both adolescents and adults in a variety of settings, including health clinics, juvenile justice facilities, and student assistance programs. While the GAIN-Q does not provide diagnostic information, it may be helpful with identifying those individuals who would benefit from more in-depth assessment, assist staff in placement decisions, and identify individuals who may need a brief intervention. The GAIN-Q screening instrument can be self-administered or given by a trained staff member during the interview process. It takes over 30 minutes (if completing the "full" version) and is available both in pencil-and-paper and computer format.

The GAIN-Q is available in two forms: the "core" instrument and the "full" instrument. The GAIN-Q core instrument has ten sections including: background, general factors, sources of stress, physical health, emotional health, behavioral health, substance-related issues, service utilization, end, and case disposition. The sections aim to provide background information on factors that may be related to the behavioral health problems, assess the severity and prevalence of the problems, and question an individual's desire for help. The GAIN-Q full instrument incorporates the GAIN-Q core instrument and one or more additional scales, which are tailored to an individual's needs.

The GAIN-Q has five scales that are necessary to score. These are the general life problem index (GLPI), the internal behavior scale (IBS), the external behavior scale (EBS), and the substance problem scale (SPS). A number of subscales make up each of these scales. However, the total symptom severity scale (TSSS) comprises all of the scales and subscales and includes every item on the GAIN-Q. After the scales and subscales have been scored, the individual's raw scores are converted to percentages of symptoms and mapped onto three levels of urgency: no/minimal (0–24 percent), moderate (25–74 percent), and high (75–100 percent). These levels help to indicate the severity of the symptoms, as well as the immediacy with which each scale and subscale area should be addressed.

Conclusions

This chapter has described the importance of implementing routine mental health screening and assessment procedures in juvenile justice settings, defined the characteristics of both these processes, and reviewed the most common instruments available for screening purposes. Screening is a cost-effective method used to determine which subset of youths is most likely to require a more comprehensive and costly assessment. The comparative advantages and costs of screening and assessment methods have resulted in their use in many juvenile justice programs. Indeed, most states have implemented a standardized procedure for mental health screening in their juvenile justice system.

The goal of this chapter was to provide enough information about the screening and assessment process to assist administrators in their understanding of the importance of establishing these procedures, the difference between the two procedures, and the selection of appropriate screening tools. This chapter does not describe the various stages necessary for implementation of these procedures, however. As noted by Grisso *et al.* (2005), this involves "context-instrument" considerations. The selection of tools must be commensurate with the purposes, demands, and constraints of the situations in which they will be used. For example, a system with limited resources and a high volume of intakes would probably want to select the MAYSI-2 or GAIN-SS for screening given the brevity of these instruments and the fact that they can be administered by a wide variety of staff without special credentials. Administrators are referred to Grisso *et al.* (2005) for the stages involved in implementation, which include preparing and training staff, establishing specific screening procedures, establishing procedures for how data will and will not be used, and developing a policy for decision-making based on screening results.

References

Achenbach, T. & Edelbrock, C. (1984). Psychopathology of childhood. *Annual Review of Psychology*, **35**, 227–256.

Bailey, S., Doreleijers, T. & Tarbuck, P. (2006). Recent developments in mental health screening and assessment in juvenile justice systems. *Child and Adolescent Psychiatric Clinics of North America*, **15**, 391–406.

Briere, J. (1996). *Trauma Symptom Checklist for Children (TSCC): Professional Manual*. Odessa, FL: Psychological Assessment Resources.

Cicchetti, D. & Cohen, D. J. (1995). *Developmental Psychopathology: Theory and Methods*, Vol. 1. New York, NY: Wiley.

Cicchetti, D. & Rogosch, F. A. (1996). Equifinality and multifinality in developmental psychopathology. *Development and Psychopathology*, **8**, 597–600.

Dembo, R. & Anderson, A. (2005). Problem-oriented screening instrument for children. In T. Grisso, G. Vincent and D. Seagrave, eds., *Mental Health Screening and Assessment in Juvenile Justice*. Guilford Press, pp. 112–122.

Dennis, M., Titus, J., White, M., Unsicker, J. & Hodgkins, D. (2002). *Global Appraisal of Individual Needs: Administration Guide for the GAIN and Related Measures*. Bloomington, IL: Chestnut Health Systems.

Dennis, M. L., Scott, C. K., Funk, R. R. & Foss, M. A. (2005). The duration and correlates of addiction and treatment. *Journal of Substance Abuse Treatment*, **28**(Supplement 1), S51–S62.

Estroff, T. W. & Hoffmann, N. G. (2001). *PADDI: Practical Adolescent Dual Diagnosis Interview*. Smithfield, RI: Evince Clinical Assessments.

Grisso, T. (2004). *Double Jeopardy: Adolescent Offenders with Mental Disorders*. Chicago: University of Chicago Press.

Grisso, T. (2005). Why we need mental health screening and assessment in juvenile justice programs. In T. Grisso, G. Vincent and D. Seagrave, eds., *Mental Health Screening and Assessment in Juvenile Justice*. New York, NY: Guildford Press, pp. 3–21.

Grisso, T. & Barnum, R. (2006). *Massachusetts Youth Screening Instrument – Version 2: User's Manual and Technical Report*. Sarasota, FL: Professional Resource Press.

Grisso, T. & Quinlan, J. C. (2005). Massachusetts Youth Screening Instrument – Version 2. In T. Grisso, G. Vincent and D. Seagrave, eds., *Mental Health Screening and Assessment in Juvenile Justice*. Guilford Press, pp. 99–111.

Grisso, T. & Underwood, L. (2004). *Screening and Assessing Mental Health and Substance Use Disorders Among Youth in the Juvenile Justice System: A Resource Guide for Practitioners*. Washington, DC: US Department of Justice, Office of Juvenile Justice and Delinquency Prevention.

Grisso, T. & Vincent, G. (2005). The context for mental health screening and assessment. In T. Grisso, G. Vincent and D. Seagrave, eds., *Mental Health Screening and Assessment in Juvenile Justice*. New York, NY: Guildford Press, pp. 44–70.

Grisso, T., Vincent, G. & Seagrave, D. (eds.) (2005). *Mental Health Screening and Assessment in Juvenile Justice*. New York, NY: Guildford Press.

Hodges, K. (2000). *Child and Adolescent Functional Assessment Scale*, 3rd edn. Ypsilanti: Eastern Michigan University.

Hodges, K. (2005). Child and adolescent functional assessment scale. In T. Grisso, G. Vincent and D. Seagrave, eds., *Mental Health Screening and Assessment in Juvenile Justice*. New York, NY: Guildford Press, pp. 123–136.

Hodges, K. & Wong, M. (1997). Use of the child and adolescent functional assessment scale to predict service utilization and cost. *Journal of Mental Health Administration*, **24**, 278–290.

Kazdin, A. E. (1993). Adolescent mental health: prevention and treatment programs. *American Psychologist*, **48**, 127–141.

Kazdin, A. E. (2000). *Psychotherapy for Children and Adolescents: Directions for Research and Practice*. New York, NY: Oxford University Press.

Loney, B. & Counts, C. (2005). Scales for assessing attention-deficit/hyperactivity disorder. In T. Grisso, G. Vincent and D. Seagrave, eds., *Mental Health Screening and Assessment in Juvenile Justice*. New York, NY: Guildford Press, pp. 166–184.

Lyons, J., Griffin, E., Fazio, M. & Lyons, B. (1999). *Child and Adolescent Needs and Strengths: An Information Integration Tool for Children and Adolescents with Mental Health Challenges (CANS-MH), Manual*. Chicago: Buddin Praed Foundation.

Mash, E. J. & Dozois, D. J. (2003). Child psychopathology: A developmental-systems perspective. In E. J. Mash and R. A. Barkley eds., *Child Psychopathology*, 2nd edn. New York, NY: Guilford Press, pp. 3–74.

Mash, E. J. & Terdal, L. G. (eds.) (1997). *Assessment of Childhood Disorders*, 3rd edn. New York, NY: Guilford Press.

Miller, F. & Lazowski, L. (2001). *The Adolescent Substance Abuse Subtle Screening Inventory-A2 (SASSI-A2) Manual*. Springville, IN: SASSI Institute.

Rahdert, E. (1991). *The Adolescent Assessment/Referral System*. Rockville, MD: National Institute on Drug Abuse.

Rudd, P. (1989). The prevalence of suicidal ideation among college students. *Suicide and Life-Threatening Behavior*, **19**, 173–183.

Rutter, M. (1989). Isle of Wight revisited: twenty-five years of child psychiatric epidemiology. *Journal of the American Academy of Child and Adolescent Psychiatry*, **28**, 633–653.

Shaffer, D., Fisher, P., Dulcan, M. *et al.* (1996). NIMH Diagnostic Interview Schedule for Children (DISC-2.3): description, differences from previous versions, and reliability of some common diagnoses. *Journal of the American Academy of Child and Adolescent Psychiatry*, **35**, 865–877.

Shaffer, D., Fisher, P., Lucas, C., Dulcan, M. & Schwab-Stone, M. (2000). NIMH Diagnostic Interview Schedule for Children Version IV (DISC-IV): description, differences from previous versions, and reliability on some common diagnoses. *Journal of the American Academy of Child and Adolescent Psychiatry*, **39**, 28–38.

Synder, H. & Sickmund, M. (1999). *Juvenile Offenders and Victims: 1999 National Report*. Washington, DC: Office of Juvenile Justice and Delinquency Prevention.

Teplin, L. A. (1994). Psychiatric and substance abuse disorders among male urban detainees. *American Journal of Public Health*, **84**, 290–293.

Teplin, L. A., Abram, K. M., McClelland, G. M., Dulcan, M. K. & Mericle, A. A. (2002). Psychiatric disorders in youth in juvenile detention. *Archives of General Psychiatry*, **59**, 1133–1143.

Trupin, E. & Boesky, L. (1999). *Working Together for Change: Co-occurring Mental Health and Substance Use Disorders Among Youth Involved in the Juvenile Justice System (Curriculum)*. Delmar, NY: The National GAINS Center.

Wasserman, G., Jensen, P. & Ko, S. (2003). Mental health assessments in juvenile justice: report on the Consensus Conference. *Journal of the American Academy of Child and Adolescent Psychiatry*, **42**, 751–761.

Wasserman, G., McReynolds, L., Fisher, P. & Lucas, C. (2005). Diagnostic Interview Schedule for Children: present state voice version. In T. Grisso, G. Vincent and D. Seagrave, eds., *Mental Health Screening and Assessment in Juvenile Justice*. New York, NY: Guildford Press, pp. 224–239.

14

Psychological testing in juvenile justice settings

Ruth Kraus and Julie Wolf

Introduction

Children and adolescents generally enter the juvenile justice system as a result of externalizing behavior problems. Yet the majority of these youths have difficulties in other areas that contribute to their presentation as delinquents. Specifically, risk factors for juvenile delinquency include poor academic performance, school failure, low educational aspiration, and low school motivation (Loeber & Farrington, 2000), suggesting possible underlying deficits in cognition and learning. Indeed, delinquent youth have been shown to have intelligence quotient (IQ) scores ranging from 8–17 points lower than controls, and 11–61 percent of adolescents with conduct disorders have co-morbid learning problems (Vermeiren *et al.*, 2002b; Vermeiren *et al.*, 2002a). Neuropsychological deficits in general have been found to occur in 60–80 percent of delinquent youths (Teichner & Golden, 2000). Although a causal relationship between neuropsychological deficits and delinquency has not been identified, it is important to understand and address the neuropsychological deficits associated with delinquency, as doing so may contribute to the prevention of future delinquent behavior.

Several areas of neuropsychological function have been the focus of studies of adolescent delinquency, and deficits in two areas, namely, executive functioning and verbal ability, have been associated with delinquency. Executive function involves the ability to regulate behaviors, as well as the ability to think about one's own thought processes, also termed metacognition. Examples of behavior regulation skills include controlling impulsivity and emotional responses, and maintaining a stable set of behaviors across different contexts. Metacognition involves the ability to initiate, plan, and organize goal-directed activities, to use environmental feedback to monitor and change behaviors, to sustain and shift attention as needed, to think flexibly and generate different strategies to solve problems, to formulate concepts, and to maintain information in working memory long enough to act on it. The frontal lobes of the brain, which are some of the

The Mental Health Needs of Young Offenders: Forging Paths toward Reintegration and Rehabilitation, eds. Carol L. Kessler and Louis J. Kraus. Published by Cambridge University Press. © Cambridge University Press 2007.

latest-developing brain structures, are associated with executive function skills. Teichner and Golden (2000) noted that adolescents with frontal lobe damage show patterns of behavior similar to those seen in delinquency, including behavioral disinhibition, particularly for aggression, impulsivity, poor insight into behavior, and rage reactions. With regard to executive functioning, delinquents have been found to exhibit deficits in cognitive flexibility, and sustaining and shifting attention appropriately, as evidenced by their poor performance on executive functioning measures (Teichner & Golden, 2000).

Longstanding deficits in verbal ability are also associated with delinquency, regardless of executive functioning skills (Dery et al., 1999). In terms of intellectual functioning, delinquent adolescents have lower overall IQ scores. Within IQ scores, however, verbal scores are significantly lower than non-verbal scores, suggesting pronounced deficits in the verbal domain. A study by Speltz et al. (1999) investigated neuropsychological profiles in pre-school boys with oppositional defiant disorder (ODD) to examine whether the verbal deficits typical of youths with conduct problems were evident early on. Delinquency in adolescents is often preceded by a diagnosis of ODD earlier in childhood. Speltz et al. found that, when compared to controls, pre-schoolers with ODD had lower full scale IQ scores and lower scores on measures of overall verbal ability and verbal fluency. In general, pre-schoolers with ODD displayed a significant split in their scores on verbal and visual–perceptual tasks, with lower verbal scores. Furthermore, preschoolers with co-morbid attention-deficit/hyperactivity disorder (ADHD) and ODD were more likely to have verbal deficits than those with ODD alone.

In their study of delinquent Flemish adolescents, Vermeiren et al. (2002a) describe a number of theories that have been posited to explain the relationship between verbal deficits and externalizing behavior problems. One theory suggests that verbal deficits affect the development of self-control strategies. Typically, in the face of frustration or other negative emotions, individuals rely on verbal skills to modulate their emotional state and control impulsive responses. Verbal skills are fundamental to the processes of seeking help and resolving conflict. The ability to mediate emotions and behaviors verbally develops gradually throughout childhood and adolescence. Adolescents with verbal deficits, therefore, may have a limited range of behavioral responses to perceived threats and emotional distress, thus increasing their reliance upon aggressive responses. An alternate theory suggests that verbal deficits limit a child's ability to learn the range of acceptable and unacceptable behaviors. Parents and teachers typically use verbal strategies to teach children appropriate responses to negative emotions. A child with verbal deficits will have difficulty learning these strategies, and will tend to exhibit more inappropriate, externalizing behaviors in response to negative emotions. Finally, verbal ability has been associated with both social skills and academic success.

Thus, children with verbal impairments may experience greater social difficulties and less academic success than their peers. A child who receives frequent negative feedback from the environment, such as criticism from teachers or social rejection, is at a higher risk to develop externalizing behavior problems.

While the neuropsychological deficits associated with delinquency have consistently been found in the verbal and executive domains, there is some variability in presentation even among those delinquents who demonstrate neuropsychological impairment. Attempts to describe different subgroups of delinquents based on their neuropsychological or cognitive profiles have had mixed success (Teichner *et al.*, 2000; Moffit, 1990; Vermeiren *et al.*, 2002a), suggesting that neuropsychological profiles of youths with conduct problems are quite heterogeneous. While deficits in verbal functioning remain a fairly robust finding in adolescents with conduct problems, deficits in other areas of cognitive or executive function are less clearly associated with conduct problems alone, but rather associated with co-morbid learning disorders and ADHD. The heterogeneity of profiles further confirms the need to obtain individual assessments of all young offenders to determine interventions that will be effective for their particular pattern of abilities.

Relationship of conduct problems to ADHD

The co-morbidity of conduct disorder with ADHD is extremely high, with estimated rates ranging from 43 percent up to 93 percent (Smith *et al.*, 2000). The neuropsychological profiles of children with ADHD have been widely studied, and core deficits in executive functioning have been identified in boys (Seidman, *et al.*, 1997) and girls (Hinshaw *et al.*, 2002). The similarity in neuropsychological profiles seen in ADHD and conduct disorder (CD) has led to an exploration of the relationship between CD/ODD and ADHD, with somewhat equivocal results. Moffitt and Henry (1989) investigated whether ADHD mediates the relationship between delinquency and executive functioning deficits. They found that executive functioning deficits did not discriminate pure cases of either ADHD or delinquency from non-disordered controls. However, executive function deficits did differentiate participants with co-morbid ADHD and delinquency from controls, even when controlling for cognitive ability. Thus, they conclude that executive function deficits are related to neither ADHD nor delinquency in a univariate fashion, but are rather related to the co-morbidity between the two.

In a separate study of the same participants, Moffitt (1990) found that non-delinquent individuals with ADHD had mild (non-significant) reading problems, but no deficits in verbal IQ or motor ability, and only mild antisocial behaviors. Delinquents without ADHD similarly displayed no significant verbal or reading deficits and no motor problems. They had a later onset of delinquent behaviors (around age 13) and were less aggressive than individuals with co-morbid ADHD and delinquency. Those with co-morbid ADHD and delinquency were found to have significant motor skills deficits, IQ deficits emerging by age five, reading failure and other academic difficulties, and persistent antisocial behavior. Thus, as with executive functioning deficits, other neuropsychological deficits appear to be related to the co-morbidity between ADHD and delinquency.

Nigg *et al.* (1998) investigated whether neuropsychological deficits in an ADHD sample could be accounted for by co-morbid symptoms of oppositional defiant disorder (ODD), conduct disorder (CD), or reading disorder. They found that core neuropsychological deficits associated with ADHD, particularly those requiring controlled processing, continued to be evident after controlling for the co-morbid disorders. Co-morbid CD, but not ODD, was associated with lower verbal ability, whereas verbal deficits were not found in the ADHD-only group. Based on these findings, the authors conclude that, with regard to executive functioning skills, children with co-morbid ADHD and CD may be more similar to children with ADHD alone than to children with CD alone. With regard to verbal deficits, however, the opposite pattern emerges: children with co-morbid ADHD and CD may be more similar to children with CD alone than to those with ADHD alone.

Frick *et al.* (1991) have found that ADHD and CD are each associated with academic problems. However, when controlling for the co-morbidity between the two disorders, they found that only ADHD was associated with academic underachievement, suggesting that CD is related to underachievement only through its association with ADHD. The authors identify several possible causal mechanisms to account for the relationship between ADHD and underachievement. It may be that having ADHD prevents children from achieving their full potential, due to both the behavioral manifestations and cognitive processing deficits associated with ADHD. Likewise, it may be that children with academic underachievement are more likely to be identified as having ADHD.

Finally, Hinshaw (1992) noted that the relationship between externalizing behaviors and underachievement is extremely complex and most likely multiply determined. He identified a developmental progression in this relationship. Specifically, in early and middle childhood, the association between aggression and underachievement can be accounted for by the ADHD, and specifically the impulsivity, that often accompanies aggression. However, by adolescence, a direct link emerges between antisocial behavior and underachievement/verbal deficits. From a developmental perspective, young children are not expected to use verbal strategies to regulate behaviors very adeptly; they are just developing this skill. By adolescence, however, there is an expectation that behaviors can be more successfully managed through verbal mediation. Thus, it makes sense that the direct link and skill deficit emerges at a later developmental time point.

Deficits associated with recidivism

Some researchers have identified neuropsychological profiles associated with patterns of recidivism among adolescent delinquents. Vermeiren *et al.* (2002b) investigated predictors of recidivism in adolescents referred to juvenile court. The authors hypothesized that future recidivists would have greater psychopathology and neuropsychological impairments than non-recidivists. Their findings revealed that 44 percent of the variance between recidivists and non-recidivists was explained by a combination of low verbal IQ, diagnosis of conduct disorder, and absence of major depressive disorder (MDD). Adolescents with ADHD had slightly (non-significantly) higher rates of recidivism; however, most adolescents with ADHD also had CD, so the additional influence of ADHD on recidivism rate is unclear. Co-morbid MDD, on the other hand, was found to have a protective influence on future recidivism. The authors proposed several possible mechanisms by which this protective influence occurs: (1) feelings of guilt and shame associated with depression may result in greater reflection upon one's actions, and thus less impulsive aggressive acts; (2) apathy and decreased energy resulting from depression may reduce criminal involvement; and (3) adolescents with co-morbid CD and depression may reflect a distinct subgroup with unique patterns of functioning.

Life-course persistent vs. adolescent onset conduct disorder

The DSM-IV differentiates between childhood-onset type (also called life-course persistent) conduct disorder, in which the onset of symptoms occurs prior to age ten, and adolescent-onset type conduct disorder, which is characterized by symptoms presenting after age ten. McMahan and Estes (1997) describe different pathways leading to the two different types of CD.

Vermeiren *et al.* (2002a) investigated neuropsychological profiles associated with recidivism in early and late offending adolescents. Their findings revealed that early-onset CD recidivists had lower full scale IQ, and both lower verbal and performance IQ scores, as well as greater deficits in memory and self-control than non-recidivists. Late-onset CD recidivists, on the other hand, differed from non-recidivists only on verbal IQ. The early-onset and late-onset recidivists differed from one another in IQ, verbal IQ, and long-term memory. The authors note that many of the participants had academic difficulties prior to age 12, but that this was particularly true of the early-onset recidivists. Thus, overall, the recidivists with an early history of offenses had greater neuropsychological deficits than those with no early offenses, consistent with other studies suggesting that adolescent-limited delinquency is associated with fewer deficits than life-course persistent delinquency.

Assessment tools

Externalizing behavior disorders, specifically ADHD, ODD, and CD, are diagnosed primarily through behavior and symptom checklists, collected from parents and teachers, as well as self-report measures. There are no specific psychological tests that can reliably diagnose these disorders. However, the checklists do not provide information about an individual's cognitive functioning, which has a significant impact on education as well as response to interventions. In addition, as noted above, certain cognitive profiles are more typical of youths with CD (lowered verbal ability relative to other skills), or with co-morbid CD and ADHD (deficits in executive functioning, particularly in working memory). A comprehensive psychological assessment can identify an individual's pattern of cognitive strengths and weaknesses, thereby allowing more efficient, targeted behavioral, psychiatric, and educational interventions. This section will present an overview of some of the most common instruments used to assess intelligence, cognition, executive function, academic achievement, personality, and behavior. All of the measures described have normative data based on national samples, and are published measures. It should be noted that the intent here is not to provide a comprehensive description of available and published assessment tools, but rather, this section will present a few examples of each type of measure.

General intelligence tests

A variety of measures (IQ tests) have been developed based on different theories of the nature and structure of human intelligence, as well as empirical research, to assess overall intelligence. These measures have been thoroughly described elsewhere (e.g., Flanagan & Harrison, 2005), and will only be briefly summarized here. In general, measures of overall intelligence involve the assessment of abilities in discrete domains, which become factored into an overall IQ score. The specific domains measured depend on the theory of intelligence underlying test construction. Most intelligence tests measure a number of factors, including crystallized intelligence, which refers to learned, primarily verbal information, and fluid intelligence, which refers to reasoning and novel problem-solving skills, memory functions, and processing speed. In general, measures of crystallized intelligence are much more sensitive to environmental and cultural factors than measures of fluid intelligence, memory, and processing speed. IQ scores are predictive of academic achievement, and are necessary to make the diagnosis of learning disabilities, mental retardation, and giftedness. In addition, certain psychiatric and neurological disorders, such as ADHD, are associated with specific patterns of cognitive functioning, and so IQ profiles are also useful in making differential diagnoses.

The most widely-used and most researched instruments to measure general intelligence are the Wechsler scales (Wechsler, 1997a, 2002b, 2003), which include the Wechsler Adult Intelligence Scale, 3rd edn. (WAIS-III), for ages 16–89, the Wechsler Intelligence Scale for Children, 4th edn. (WISC-IV) for ages 7–16, and the Wechsler Pre-school and Primary Scale of Intelligence, 3rd edn. (WPPSI-III) for ages 2–7. The Wechsler scales yield four index scores that are averaged together to generate an overall IQ score, the Full Scale IQ. The index and full scale scores are normally distributed, standard scores that have a mean of 100 and a standard deviation of 15. That is, 68 percent of all individuals have scores ranging between 85–115 in all domains measured.

The four factors assessed by the Wechsler scales include verbal comprehension, perceptual reasoning, working memory, and processing speed. The Verbal Comprehension Index measures verbal concept formation, inductive reasoning, acquired knowledge, and comprehension. It is highly correlated to school performance, and, as a measure of crystallized intelligence, is also sensitive to environmental factors such as a lack of early cognitive stimulation or inadequate schooling, or to cultural factors. The Perceptual Reasoning Index provides measures of visual–motor integration, non-verbal problem-solving, and spatial processing. It measures skills more associated with fluid intelligence and, as such, is less sensitive than the Verbal Comprehension Index to environmental or cultural factors. Therefore, in instances where there are suspected environmental insults that may impact verbal skills – common in youths with disruptive behavior disorders – the Perceptual Reasoning Index may yield a more valid estimate of intellectual functioning than the Full Scale IQ score. The Working Memory Index assesses short-term auditory memory and the capacity to store verbal information temporarily so that it can be manipulated mentally. Working memory is considered to be a key component of learning, and deficits in working memory are often associated with learning disorders or ADHD. Finally, the Processing Speed Index measures an individual's ability to process and respond to simple visual stimuli rapidly and accurately. Performance on the processing speed tasks may also be impacted by learning or attention deficits, as well as by visual–motor weaknesses.

Each Wechsler index score comprises scores on separate subtests, which have a mean of 10, a standard deviation of 3, and a range from 1–19. The indices and subtests of the WISC-IV are described in Table 14.1. The majority of people, regardless of age, have a fairly even profile of scores across subtests and across domains. Therefore, significantly discrepant scores between domains can be indicative of specific processing deficits.

In addition to the Wechsler scales, other commonly used tests of general intelligence include the Woodcock-Johnson-III, Tests of Cognitive Ability (WJ-III) (Woodcock *et al.*, 2001) the Stanford-Binet, 5th edn. (SB5) (Roid, 2003),

Table 14.1. Indices and subtests of the WISC-IV

Verbal Comprehension Index	Perceptual Reasoning Index
Similarities	Block design
Vocabulary	Picture concepts
Comprehension	Matrix reasoning
Information (optional)	Picture completion (optional)
Word reasoning (optional)	
Working Memory Index	**Processing Speed Index**
Digit span	Coding
Letter–number sequencing	Symbol search
Arithmetic (optional)	Cancellation (optional)

the Differential Ability Scales (DAS) (Elliot, 1990), the Cognitive Assessment System (CAS) (Naglieri & Das, 1997), and the Kaufman Assessment Battery for Children, 2nd edn. (K-ABC-II) (Kaufman & Kaufman, 2004). The WJ-III is based on a theory of intelligence that posits eight broad cognitive abilities contributing to a general intelligence factor. Seven of the eight factors are measured by the WJ-III, and include comprehension–knowledge (crystallized intelligence), fluid reasoning (fluid intelligence), long-term retrieval, visual–spatial thinking, auditory processing, processing speed, and short-term memory. The WJ-III is normed for ages 2–90.

Similar to the WJ-III, the SB5 is normed for a wide range of ages (2–85 years), making it possible to monitor intelligence with greater validity over the course of development. The SB5 is based on a five-factor model of intelligence. Cognitive factors that constitute intelligence, according to SB5 test design, include fluid reasoning, knowledge (crystallized intelligence), quantitative reasoning, visual–spatial processing, and working memory. The SB5 assesses all abilities in both verbal and non-verbal modalities, an advantage when testing youths with verbal deficits.

The DAS is based on a theory of intelligence similar to the SB5 and WJ-III, but is designed to measure discrete cognitive functions that can be interpreted individually, as well as in terms of factors. The DAS is normed for ages 2 years 6 months to 17 years 11 months. In addition to a general cognitive ability (GCA) score, which is comparable to the full scale IQ score, the DAS provides a special non-verbal composite score, which is helpful when evaluating youths with verbal deficits. The DAS also breaks down into three clusters, assessing verbal ability, non-verbal reasoning ability, and spatial ability. The distinction between non-verbal reasoning and spatial ability allow for the assessment of specific visual–motor or spatial processing deficits with intact non-verbal reasoning.

Two general intelligence tests, the CAS and the K-ABC-II, were developed according to a somewhat different theory of the construct of human intelligence. The K-ABC-II, normed for ages 2 years 0 months to 18 year 11 months, yields a mental processing index that measures sequential processing, simultaneous processing, learning ability, and planning ability. The CAS, normed for ages 5–17, consists of four scales that measure basic psychological processes rather than scales based on the verbal–non-verbal or crystallized–fluid theories of intelligence. These scales, similar to the K-ABC-II scales, include planning, attention, simultaneous processing, and successive processing. Planning is considered to be a process involving the selection and use of a strategy to solve a problem efficiently. Impulse control is also involved in planning. Attention is the process of focusing and sustaining selective cognitive effort over time while inhibiting impulses and avoiding distractions. Simultaneous processing involves the integration of separate stimuli into a whole or groups, understanding logic, and grammatical relationships. Finally, successive processing is the activity of working with sequences of information or stimuli in a serial order. Since the CAS and, to a lesser extent, the K-ABC-II avoid measures of crystallized intelligence, they are useful in cases in which cultural or environmental factors are thought to impact test scores.

Tests of non-verbal intelligence

Individuals with language deficits do not typically do well on general intelligence tests, which tend to be skewed toward verbal reasoning, even on perceptual tasks. Therefore, when language deficits are present, it is often advisable to use non-verbal tests to obtain a measure of general intelligence. Non-verbal IQ tests measure a variety of skills, including inductive and deductive reasoning, concept formation, analogic reasoning, and spatial ability. Most are designed to be administered in a completely non-verbal format, thereby eliminating all demands on receptive or expressive language. The most comprehensive non-verbal intelligence test is the Leiter International Performance Scale – Revised (Leiter-R) (Roid & Miller, 1997), which can be used for individuals between the ages of 2–21. In addition to scales measuring reasoning and visualization, which make up the general IQ score, the Leiter-R also has scales measuring attention and memory. Other tests of non-verbal intelligence include the Universal Non-verbal Intelligence Test (UNIT) (Bracken & McCallum, 1998), which provides measures of symbolic and non-symbolic memory and reasoning, the Test of Non-verbal Intelligence – 3 (TONI-3) (Brown, Sherbenou & Johnsen, 1997), and the Comprehensive Test of Non-verbal Intelligence (C-TONI) (Hammill, Pearson & Wiederholt, 1997).

Tests of language functioning

Domain-specific tests of language functioning not only provide measures of expressive and receptive language and pragmatics, but are also useful in determining effective treatment approaches for an individual. Specifically, language skills and cognitive levels impact an individual's ability to take advantage of certain forms of language-based treatment, such as individual or group psychotherapy. In addition, since school is a highly language-based activity, students with language deficits are at a great risk of developing significant academic difficulties. Understanding the nature of a student's language deficit will allow for targeted interventions. Several test batteries include broad measures of language functioning across specific domains, while other tests measure discrete language skills, such as vocabulary. The Clinical Evaluation of Language Fundamentals – 4 (CELF-4) (Semel, Wiig & Secord, 2003) is widely used, and includes indices measuring receptive and expressive language, language content (semantic language), and language memory. It also includes a parent or teacher interview about a student's pragmatics skills. The Comprehensive Assessment of Spoken Language (CASL) (Carrow-Woolfolk, 1999), another broad measure of language skills, parses language domains somewhat differently. It provides scales measuring lexical/semantic knowledge, syntactic knowledge, and supralinguistic knowledge, as well as expressive and receptive language. Supralinguistic knowledge includes tasks measuring a student's understanding of non-literal language and inferential thinking. Language pragmatics is measured on the CASL through an actual test of a student's knowledge about appropriate linguistic behaviors, rather than observational reports.

Expressive and receptive vocabulary tests measure single aspects of language functioning. Vocabulary knowledge is highly correlated with academic success, and is mediated by reading; children who read more tend to have stronger vocabulary skills, and academically at-risk youths tend to be poor readers and/or do not choose reading as an activity of choice in their free time. Expressive vocabulary tests also provide information about a student's ability to retrieve information from memory. Therefore, discrete measures of vocabulary skills can serve as quick and simple screening tools for other domains as well.

In addition to the vocabulary tests, other tests of language functioning measure higher-order linguistic skills. For example, the Adolescent Test of Problem-Solving (TOPS-A) (Zachman *et al.*) assesses the ability to use language as a critical thinking tool in problem-solving. It involves reading a series of short vignettes about social situations and factual information, and then asking the student questions that require the student to make inferences, draw conclusions, evaluate situations, and explore implications and consequences. The TOPS-A also provides information about a student's understanding of interpersonal relationships, and ability to infer motivations for the actions of others. In doing so, the TOPS-A can also be used as a rough measure of an individual's interpretation of social situations.

Tests of visual–motor and visual–spatial processing

While youths with conduct problems do not generally exhibit difficulties with visual–motor or visual–spatial functioning, deficits in these areas are associated with certain types of learning disabilities. For example, difficulties with visual–motor skills can lead to problems with written language, as writing is a visual–motor task. In addition, non-verbal learning disabilities are associated with visual–spatial and motor deficits. Many test batteries include non-motor tests of visual–spatial skills. The Woodcock-Johnson-III, Test of Cognitive Abilities, has a visual–spatial cluster, and the Differential Ability Scale divides the non-verbal composite score into two different scales, one measuring non-verbal reasoning and the other measuring spatial skills. Spatial functions include skills such as object identification, spatial memory, mental rotation or displacement of images, and visual discrimination. In contrast to non-motor spatial tasks, tests of visual–motor functioning involve spatial construction, such as drawing and building. One widely used measure of visual–motor skills, the Beery–Buktenica Developmental Test of Visual–Motor Integration (Beery, Buktenica & Beery, 2004) includes measures of design copying – which integrates the visual and motor systems – and also purely visual and purely motor tasks. When more significant visual–motor and/or fine motor deficits are suspected, a specialized evaluation by an occupational therapist is warranted.

Tests of executive functioning ability

As noted above, children with conduct problems often display impairments in executive functioning, and so obtaining objective measures of executive functioning is vital in gaining a full understanding of an individual's cognitive abilities. A number of standardized tests are available to assess the various executive functions, including sustaining attention, inhibiting impulsive responding, planning, mental flexibility, and working memory. One overall battery, the Delis–Kaplan Executive Function System (D-KEFS) (Delis, Kaplan & Kramer, 2001), assesses most of these areas. In addition, several neuropsychological test batteries also measure executive functions as one aspect of neuropsychological processes (other domains measured by neuropsychological test batteries include memory and learning, language, motor, and visual–spatial skills). Other test batteries may contain subtests or scales that measure discrete executive functioning skills. For example, the CAS includes scales assessing attention and planning, two aspects of executive functioning. The WJ-III contains an executive processing scale, and the Working Memory Index (WMI) on the Wechsler scales also provides a measure of one area of executive processing.

In addition to the batteries, several individual tests measure elements of executive function. Specifically, continuous performance tests (CPTs), tests of sustained attention and impulse inhibition, typically require the individual to attend to a stimulus for an extended period of time and inhibit an automatic response. For example, an individual may be required to attend to a computer screen that rapidly displays a series of letters, and must hit a key in response to all letters except "X," and then only when it is followed by "A." Errors of omission, not noting the stimuli, are associated with attention, while errors of commission, hitting the key at the wrong time, are associated with impulsivity. The Stroop Color-Word test is another task that requires inhibition of an automatic response. In this task, the individual is presented with color names printed in an opposing colored ink (e.g., the word "red" printed in blue ink), and the task is to state the color of the ink rapidly and errorlessly. For most people, reading the color name occurs automatically, and therefore naming the color of the ink requires inhibition of this automatic response. Individuals with executive functioning deficits have more difficulty with this task than individuals without such deficits.

Another measure of executive functioning, Trails B, requires the individual to connect numbered and lettered dots with a pencil, and alternate between numbers and letters (1–A–2–B, etc.). Trails B exerts demands on working memory, in that the individual must mentally store their positions in both the number and letter sequence simultaneously. A number of measures assess the ability to plan one's actions. Tower tasks (e.g., Tower of Hanoi, Tower of London), and maze tasks require careful advanced planning of one's sequence of moves, and the ability to think flexibly when moves do not work. Sorting and categorization tasks (e.g., Wisconsin Card Sorting Test, Grant & Berg, 1993; Children's Category Test, Boll, 1993) also provide information about cognitive flexibility, as well as the ability to use feedback to guide problem-solving behavior.

Tests of memory and learning

Memory and learning could be considered a subdomain of executive functioning. There are a number of tests, however, that specifically assess verbal and visual memory and learning separate from other executive function tasks. The Children's Memory Scale (CMS) (Cohen, 1997) or, for older youths, the Wechsler Memory Scale – III (WMS-III) (Wechsler, 1997b) assess visual and verbal memory, both immediately after presentation and then again after a delay, as well as learning, attention, and cued recall (delayed recognition). The CMS and WMS scores can be compared directly to Wechsler IQ scores, allowing for the identification of specific deficits in memory. In a youth with significantly low scores on measures of working memory, performance on the CMS or WMS-III can also help differentiate between a general memory deficit, of which working memory is one aspect, and a more specific deficit in working memory only, which is more associated with attentional deficits. The Wide Range Assessment of Memory and Learning-2 (WRAML-2)(Adams & Sheslow, 2003), similar to the CMS, provides measures of verbal and visual immediate and delayed recall, as well as learning. More narrow tests of verbal learning, such as the California Verbal Learning Test – Children (CVLT-C) (Delis *et al.*, 1994) provide valuable information about the strategies an individual uses to learn and remember verbal information.

Tests of academic achievement

As noted above, there is a high rate of co-morbidity between conduct problems and learning disabilities, so any psychological assessment should include tests to rule out the presence of a specific learning disability. Under the current revision of the Individuals with Disabilities Education Act (IDEA Revision 2004), a learning disability may be defined as a significant discrepancy between an individual's cognitive potential and academic achievement levels in one or more areas, with a concomitant processing deficit. The discrepancy must not be due to factors such as health, cultural, or environmental concerns. While some school districts have begun to adopt alternative methods to diagnose learning disabilities (e.g., response to intervention), many districts continue to use the discrepancy model. Nationally-normed tests of academic achievement are used to determine discrepancies between potential and achievement. These tests are often tied to a specific IQ test, making a direct comparison possible. For example, the Wechsler Individual Achievement Test – II (Wechsler, 2002a) can be compared directly to the Wechsler IQ scales; the Woodcock-Johnson-III, Tests of Achievement are directly comparable to the Woodcock-Johnson-III, Tests of Cognitive Ability, (Woodcock *et al.*, 2001), and so forth.

Nationally-normed achievement tests generally measure basic academic skills, such as individual word decoding, spelling, and written mathematical calculations, as well as an individual's ability to apply those basic skills to higher-order academic tasks, such as reading comprehension, written expression, and mathematical reasoning. Since a learning disability may appear in any of these domains, obtaining measures of both basic and applied academic skills is necessary to diagnose a learning disability. Therefore, tests that measure only basic academic skills, such as the Wide Range Achievement Test – Third Edition (Wilkinson, 1993), or that measure single domains, such as individual tests of reading comprehension or word decoding, are of questionable use in the diagnosis of a learning disability, although they are useful in measuring certain discrete abilities.

Tests of adaptive functioning

The formal definition of mental retardation from the DSM-IV (APA, 1994) includes impairments in both cognitive and adaptive functioning. There is a subset of individuals, some of whom display conduct problems, who have cognitive impairments but do not exhibit impairments in adaptive functioning. Since individuals with mental retardation have a different legal status than individuals without mental retardation, obtaining a measure of adaptive functioning when IQ scores are below 70 is necessary. Measures of adaptive functioning tend to be questionnaires, administered by an examiner or completed independently by the respondent, who is usually a parent, guardian, or primary caregiver. Adaptive functioning refers to an individual's ability to function in an age-appropriate manner across a number of domains.

There are several published adaptive functioning scales. One widely-used measure, the Vineland – II Adaptive Behavior Scales (Sparrow & Cicchetti, 2005), provides measures of adaptive functioning across the broad domains of communication, daily living skills, and socialization. Each broad domain is divided into subdomains, making possible more specific identification of adaptive strengths and weaknesses. The communication domain includes scales measuring receptive, expressive, and written language. The daily living skills domain includes measures of personal, domestic, and community daily living skills. Finally, the socialization domain measures interpersonal relationships, coping skills, and an individual's ability to manage play and leisure time. Identifying strengths and weaknesses in specific domains helps in designing interventions for specific individuals. For example, an individual with impaired adaptive functioning and specific weaknesses in personal and community daily living skills would require a different set of interventions from an individual with deficits in the domain of interpersonal relationships and coping skills.

Personality questionnaires

Personality questionnaires specific to psychopathy and delinquency are discussed elsewhere in this volume (see chapters by Kraus & Sobel, and Vincent, Grisso & Terry), and so will not be covered here. There are a number of personality inventories, however, that provide important information about psychopathy as well as other personality and affective disorders. While measuring psychopathy as an independent construct is important, the high co-morbidity rates in individuals with delinquent behaviors require a broader assessment of personality and social-emotional functioning. Broad-bandwidth personality inventories specifically for adolescents include self-report measures such as the Minnesota Multiphasic Personality Inventory – Adolescent (MMPI-A) (Butcher *et al.*, 1992), the Millon Adolescent Clinical Inventory (MACI) (Millon, Millon & Davis, 1993), and the Adolescent Psychopathology Scale (APS) (Reynolds, 1999). These questionnaires yield normative information about an individual's functioning across a wide range of psychiatric and personality domains, and are useful in making diagnoses and treatment recommendations. The measures all include validity scales, making it possible to ascertain whether the respondent approached the test in an honest manner.

The MMPI-A, used for adolescents between the ages of 14–18, consists of ten clinical scales, six supplementary scales, and fifteen content scales, which provide a great deal of information about an individual. While the clinical scales cannot be directly correlated to any particular psychiatric diagnosis, and therefore are referred to by number rather than by name, the scales do tap into different personality characteristics. For example, a significantly high score on scale four can be indicative of externalizing and delinquent behaviors, academic problems, difficulty with authority, family conflict, drug and/or alcohol problems, impulsivity, and aggression, while a high score on scale six is also associated with academic and externalizing behavioral problems, but is more characteristic of adolescents who display labile, unpredictable moods and are suspicious, guarded, and withdrawn. MMPI-A content scales reflect more specific areas of concern, and can be used to help interpret the clinical scales. For instance, content scales provide information about an individual's level of anxiety, depression, self-esteem, anger, sense of alienation, social discomfort, family conflict, and school problems. MMPI-A supplementary scales can provide information about an individual's substance use or risk of using substances.

The MACI is divided into indices measuring personality patterns (e.g., conforming, inhibited, unruly, forceful), expressed concerns (e.g., peer insecurity, self-devaluation, family discord) and clinical syndromes (e.g., anxiety, depression, delinquent predisposition). There is some evidence to suggest that the MACI can differentiate delinquent youths with psychopathic traits from those delinquents without psychopathic traits. Murrie and Cornell (2000) found that adolescents who score high on psychopathy scales tend to have lower scores on the MACI scales measuring conformity, submission, anxiety, and sexual discomfort. They scored higher than non-psychopathic adolescents on scales of unruly, delinquent, and impulsive behaviors, as well as being more prone to substance abuse. In addition to information about psychopathy, the MACI provides information about general personality functioning and clinical syndromes, making it useful in diagnosing co-morbidities in youth with conduct problems.

The APS, unlike the MMPI-A and the MACI, was designed to link symptoms reported by adolescents to DSM-IV diagnoses. The APS can be used with adolescents as young as 12, while the MMPI-A and the MACI are only normed on older youths. The APS contains 20 clinical scales, roughly divided in externalizing and internalizing disorders, 5 personality disorder scales, 11 psychosocial problem scales, and 4 validity scales. The APS also lists severity ratings of significant elevations, from subclinical symptom range to severe clinical symptom range. The conduct disorder scale on the APS includes items that map onto the DSM-IV criteria for conduct disorder, while the aggression scale evaluates only aggressive acts, although it overlaps with the conduct disorder scale. The APS also contains specific scales measuring substance use and suicidality. Given that many of the items on the APS map directly onto DSM-IV diagnoses, the APS can be used as more of a diagnostic tool than a measure of personality traits, as the MMPI-A and the MACI.

Behavioral questionnaires

While self-report data from personality inventories are essential in the evaluation, gathering information from collateral sources, and in particular from caregivers and teachers, is crucial in obtaining a description of behaviors across different contexts. Most behavioral questionnaires have different forms for parents or caregivers and teachers, and many also have self-report forms. Two widely used questionnaires, the Achenbach Child Behavior Checklist (CBCL) (Achenbach & Rescorla, 2000) and the Behavior Assessment System for Children, Second Edition (BASC-II) (Reynolds & Kamphaus, 2004), provide broad information about a range of internalizing and externalizing behaviors across contexts in children ages 2–18. Clinical scales on the CBCL include measures of anxiety and depression, somatic complaints, withdrawal, social problems, thought problems, attention problems, delinquent behavior, and aggressive behavior. The BASC contains similar scales, as well as scales measuring hyperactivity, learning problems (on the teacher form), and adaptive functioning. In the subset of delinquent youth who present with internalizing disorders (e.g., depression, anxiety), obtaining measures of these behaviors is critical in planning interventions and determining prognoses.

Given the high propensity of youth with conduct problems to exhibit deficits in executive function, obtaining collateral data about the behavioral manifestations of executive function deficits is critical. One measure, the Behavior Rating

Inventory of Executive Functioning (BRIEF) (Gioia *et al.*, 2000), offers parent, teacher, and self-reports of executive functioning. The BRIEF is divided into two separate indices, one of which assesses behavioral regulation, while the other assesses metacognition. In addition, the BRIEF yields a composite score that encompasses both indices, as well as individual subdomain scores. The Behavior Regulation Index comprises subscales measuring the ability to inhibit impulsive responses, to shift attention, topic, and activity, and to exert control over emotional responses. The Metacognition Index includes subscales measuring the ability to initiate goal-directed tasks, working memory, planning and organization skills, organization of materials, the ability to monitor the environment for feedback about one's behaviors and, on the self-report version, task completion. The BRIEF is useful in conjunction with the cognitive measures of executive functioning described above, to provide a complete picture of an individual's strengths and weaknesses in this area.

Conclusion

Youths with conduct problems and delinquency who become involved with the juvenile justice system overwhelmingly present with co-morbid disorders, ranging from internalizing disorders such as depression and anxiety, to disorders of learning and attention. In particular, deficits in the domains of learning, attention, executive functioning, and verbal ability have been shown to be associated with conduct problems in youth. Impairments in these domains impact school functioning in particular, and academic/school problems are a risk factor for juvenile delinquency. Patterns of strengths and weaknesses in many of these domains can only be determined through a comprehensive, individualized psychological evaluation that includes measures of cognitive, academic, and personality functioning. While the externalizing behaviors must be addressed through interventions targeting those specific behaviors, being aware of co-morbid issues allows for a more comprehensive and focused treatment plan.

References

Achenbach, T. M. & Rescorla, L. A. (2000). *Child Behavior Checklist*. Vermont: ASEBA.

Adams, W. & Sheslow, D. (2003). *Wide Range Assessment of Memory and Learning*. San Antonio, TX: The Psychological Corporation.

American Psychiatric Association (1994). *Diagnostic and Statistical Manual of Mental Disorders*, 4th edn. Washington, DC: American Psychiatric Association.

Beery, K. E., Buktenica, N. A. & Beery, N. A. (2004). *Beery–Buktenica Developmental Test of Visual–Motor Integration*, 5th edn. Lutz, FL: Psychological Assessment Resources, Inc.

Boll, T. (1993). *Children's Category Test*. San Antonio, TX: PsychCorp.

Bracken, B. A. & McCallum, R. S. (1998). *The Universal Nonverbal Intelligence Test*. Itasca, IL: Riverside.

Brown, L., Sherbenou, R. J. & Johnsen, S. K. (1997). *Test of Nonverbal Intelligence – 3*. San Antonio, TX: Harcourt Assessment, Inc.

Butcher, J. N., Williams, C. L., Graham, J. R. *et al.* (1992). *Minnesota Multiphasic Personality Inventory – Adolescent*. Bloomington, MN: Pearson Assessments.

Carrow-Woolfolk, E. (1999). *Comprehensive Assessment of Spoken Language*. Circle Pines, MN: American Guidance Service, Inc.

Cohen, M. (1997). *Children's Memory Scale*. San Antonio, TX: The Psychological Corporation.

Delis, D. C., Kramer, J. H., Kaplan, E. & Ober, B. A. (1994). *California Verbal Learning Test – Children's Version*. San Antonio, TX: The Psychological Corporation.

Delis, D., Kaplan, E. & Kramer, J. (2001). *Delis–Kaplan Executive Function System*. San Antonio, TX: Harcourt Assessment, Inc.

Dery, M., Toupin, J., Pauze, R., Mercier, H. & Fortin, L. (1999). Neuropsychological character-istics of adolescents with conduct disorder: association with attention-deficit-hyperactivity and aggression. *Journal of Abnormal Child Psychology*, **27**, 225–236.

Elliot, C. (1990). *Differential Ability Scales*. San Antonio, TX: PsychCorp.

Flanagan, D. & Harrison, P., eds. (2005). *Contemporary Intellectual Assessment: Theories, Tests, and Issues*. New York: The Guilford Press.

Frick, P. J., Kamphaus, R. W., Lahey, B. B. & Loeber, R. (1991). Academic underachievement and the disruptive behavior disorders. *Journal of Consulting and Clinical Psychology*, **59**, 289–294.

Gioia, G. A., Isquith, P. K., Guy, S. C. & Kenworthy, L. (2000). *Behavior Rating Inventory of Executive Function*. San Antonio, TX: The Psychological Corporation.

Grant, D. & Berg, E. (1993). *Wisconsin Card Sorting Test*. Odessa, FLA: Psychological Assessment Resources Inc.

Hammill, D. D., Pearson, N. A. & Wiederholt, J. L. (1997). *Comprehensive Test of Nonverbal Intelligence*. San Antonio, TX: Harcourt Assessment, Inc.

Hinshaw, S. P. (1992). Externalizing behavior problems and academic underachievement in childhood and adolescence: causal relationships and underlying mechanisms. *Psychological Bulletin*, **111**, 127–155.

Hinshaw, S. P., Carte, E. T., Sami, N., Treuting, J. J. & Zupan, B. A. (2002). Preadolescent girls with attention-deficit/hyperactivity disorder: II. Neuropsychological performance in relation to subtypes and individual classification. *Journal of Consulting and Clinical Psychology*, **70**, 1099–1111.

Individual with Disabilities Education Act, Revision (2004). Pub. L. 108–446.

Kaufman, A. S. & Kaufman, N. L. (2004). *Kaufman Assessment Battery for Children – Second Edition*. Circle Pines, MN: American Guidance Service.

Loeber, R. & Farrington, D. P. (2000). Young children who commit crime: epidemiology, developmental origins, risk factors, early interventions, and policy implications. *Development and Psychopathology*, **12**, 737–762.

McMahon, R. J. & Estes, A. M. (1997). Conduct problems. In E. J. Mash and L. G. Terdal, eds., *Assessment of Childhood Disorders*, 3rd edn. New York, NY: Guilford pp. 130–193.

Millon, T., Millon, C. & Davis, R. (1993). *Millon Adolescent Clinical Inventory.* Bloomington, MN: Pearson Assessments.

Moffitt, T. E. (1990). Juvenile delinquency and attention deficit disorder: boys' developmental trajectories from age 3 to age 15. *Child Development*, **61**, 893–910.

Moffitt, T. E. & Henry, B. (1989). Neuropsychological assessment of executive functions in self-reported delinquents. *Development and Psychopathology*, **1**, 105–118.

Murrie, D. C. & Cornell, D. G. (2000). The Millon Adolescent Clinical Inventory and Psychopathy. *Journal of Personality Assessment*, **75** (1), 110–125.

Naglieri, J. A. & Das, J. P. (1997). *Das–Naglieri Cognitive Assessment System (CAS).* Itasca, IL: Riverside.

Nigg, J. T., Hinshaw, S. P., Carte, E. T. & Treuting, J. J. (1998). Neuropsychological correlates of childhood attention-deficit/hyperactivity disorder: explainable by comorbid disruptive behavior or reading problems? *Journal of Abnormal Psychology*, **107**, 468–480.

Reynolds, C. R. & Kamphaus, R. W. (2004). *BASC-II: Behavior Assessment System for Children*, 2nd edn. Circle Pines, MN: American Guidance Service.

Reynolds, W. M. (1999). *Adolescent Psychopathology Scale.* San Antonio, TX: The Psychological Corporation.

Roid, G. H. (2003). *Stanford-Binet Intelligence Scales, Fifth Edition.* Itasca, IL: Riverside.

Roid, G. H. & Miller, L. J. (1997). *Leiter International Performance Scale – Revised.* Wood Dale, IL: Stoelting Co.

Seidman, L. J., Biederman, J., Faraone, S. V. & Weber, W. (1997). Toward defining a neuropsychology of attention deficit-hyperactivity disorder: performance of children and adolescents from a large clinically referred sample. *Journal of Consulting and Clinical Psychology*, **65**, 150–160.

Semel, E., Wiig, E. & Secord, W. A. (2003). *Clinical Evaluation of Language Fundamentals*, 4th edn. San Antonio, TX: The Psychological Corporation.

Smith, S. R., Wingenfeld, S. A., Hilsenroth, M. J., Reddy, L. A. & LeBuffe, P. A. (2000). The use of the Devereux Scales of Mental Disorders in the assessment of attention-deficit/hyperactivity disorder and conduct disorder. *Journal of Psychopathology and Behavioral Assessment*, **22**(3), 237–255.

Sparrow, S. & Cicchetti, D. (2005). *Vineland Adaptive Behavior Scales*, 2nd edn. Circle Pines, MN: American Guidance Service.

Speltz, M. L., DeKlyen, M., Calderon, R., Greenberg, M. T. & Fisher, P. A. (1999). Neuropsychological characteristics and test behaviors of boys with early onset conduct problems. *Journal of Abnormal Psychology*, **108**, 315–325.

Teichner, G. & Golden, C. J. (2000). The relationship of neuropsychological impairment to conduct disorder in adolescence: a conceptual review. *Aggression and Violent Behavior*, **5**, 509–528.

Teichner, G., Golden, C. J., Crum, T. A. *et al.* (2000). Identification of neuropsychological subtypes in a sample of delinquent adolescents. *Journal of Psychiatric Research*, **34**, 129–132.

Vermeiren, R., De Clippele, A., Schwab-Stone, M., Ruchkin, V. & Deboutte, D. (2002a). Neuropsychological characteristics of three subgroups of Flemish delinquent adolescents. *Neuropsychology*, **16**, 49–55.

Vermeiren, R., Schwab-Stone, M., Ruchkin, V., De Clippele, A. & Deboutte, D. (2002b). Predicting recidivism in delinquent adolescents from psychological and psychiatric assessment. *Comprehensive Psychiatry*, **43**, 142–149.

Wechsler, D. (1997a). *Wechsler Adult Intelligence Scale*, 3nd edn. San Antonio: The Psychological Corporation.

Wechsler, D. (1997b). *Wechsler Memory Scale*, 3rd edn. San Antonio: The Psychological Corporation.

Wechsler, D. (2002a). *Wechsler Individual Achievement Test*, 2nd edn. San Antonio: The Psychological Corporation.

Wechsler, D. (2002b). *Wechsler Preschool and Primary Scale of Intelligence*, 3rd edn. San Antonio: The Psychological Corporation.

Wechsler, D. (2003). *Wechsler Intelligence Scale for Children*, 4th edn. San Antonio: The Psychological Corporation.

Wilkinson, G. (1993). *Wide Range Achievement Test 3*. San Antonio, TX: PsychCorp.

Woodcock, R. W., McGrew, K. S. & Mather, N. (2001). *Woodcock-Johnson-III*. Itasca, IL: Riverside.

Zachman, L., Barrett, M., Huisingh, R., Orman, J. & Blagden, C. (1991). *Adolescent Test of Problem Solving*. East Moline, IL: LinguiSystems, Inc.

15

Psychopharmacology and juvenile delinquency

Niranjan S. Karnik, Marie V. Soller, and Hans Steiner

The miserable have no other medicine, but only hope.

William Shakespeare, *Measure for Measure*, Act III, Scene I.

Introduction

Psychopathology among juvenile offenders is widely considered to be a significant problem and has been examined in recent, broad psycho-epidemiological studies (Teplin *et al.*, 2002; Vermeiren, 2003; Wasserman *et al.*, 2003; Vermeiren *et al.*, 2006). These estimates of psychiatric illness may partially overestimate the prevalence of psychopathology among all offenders due to the fact that incarcerated juveniles are more likely to have illness and to have greater morbidity than first-time offenders or those in diversion programs. Nevertheless, the high prevalence rates for psychopathology among juvenile offenders should be a cause of concern. The best approach to this population entails taking a developmental perspective which takes into account that despite their crimes these children continue to mature, grow, and change in profound ways (Frick, 2006; Karnik *et al.*, 2006).

Treatment of confined juveniles has certain ethical and moral problems due to the unique consent and assent issues at play for this potentially vulnerable group of patients. A recent consensus report recommends behavioral management and psychotherapy be used where clinical indications clearly allow these as first-line interventions (Pappadopulos *et al.*, 2003). Only after these approaches have failed should psychopharmacological interventions be considered (Pappadopulos *et al.*, 2003; Schur *et al.*, 2003). For example, an acutely manic offender who presents with pressured speech, aggressive behavior, and delusional thoughts would merit anti-psychotic medications for stabilization followed by psychotherapy and medications if needed, whereas a youth offender presenting with mild anxiety

The Mental Health Needs of Young Offenders: Forging Paths toward Reintegration and Rehabilitation, eds. Carol L. Kessler and Louis J. Kraus. Published by Cambridge University Press. © Cambridge University Press 2007.

symptoms might merit psychotherapy as initial treatment. Similarly, acute aggression should first be managed with non-pharmacological interventions, such as stimulus reduction (Pappadopulos *et al.*, 2003; Schur *et al.*, 2003). When these fail, or when physical restraints are needed, medications may be warranted.

Acute aggression poses a particularly challenging treatment dilemma because a complete diagnostic assessment is often not possible before the need becomes urgent to intervene in order to protect the safety of the patient and those around him or her. Particularly difficult is discerning adaptive from maladaptive aggression; the former perhaps protecting the youth in a high risk and high trauma setting, and the latter posing serious threat. Daniel Connor defines maladaptive aggression as that which occurs independent of an expectable social context; in the absence of expectable antecedent social cues; disproportionate to its causes in intensity, severity, duration, or frequency; or without appropriate termination (Connor, 2002; Steiner *et al.*, 2003b). While it may not always be possible to make this distinction, it is essential that an attempt is always made.

Several controlled clinical trials of medications in youth make it clear that psychopharmacology can significantly contribute to rehabilitation and possibly recovery. Thus to deprive youths of these interventions is as fraught with difficulties as discerning the appropriateness of using medications can be. This is increasingly true as the development of new classes of medications and the rational expanded use of older medications now provide practitioners with new choices for the provision of sound and integrated treatment planning.

In this brief chapter, we aim to summarize the clinical indications for pharmacological interventions that may help in reducing pathology in this population. Our combined knowledge of clinical care, clinical trials, and the recommendations generated by consensus in practice guidelines suggests that the most appropriate approach to using medications in juvenile offenders requires employing a cautious and supportive attitude, and always weighing risks and benefits. We propose that clinicians should use the integrated provision of services, including medication when necessary, to attempt to target the subtype of aggression that may be underpinning the delinquent behaviors of the juvenile. This is a symptom-based approach, which is useful in this population because providers often must act quickly to intervene in situations where much harm may come to many as a result of the severe and sustained aggression commonly found in youth offenders. A primary disorder-oriented approach is also useful when a less acute situation allows time to perform a more extensive diagnostic assessment. The goal of this approach is to identify a treatable disorder, treat this disorder as specifically as possible, and then expect that the aggressive behavior will recede. Because delinquent youth often present with extensive co-morbidity (Teplin *et al.*, 2002;

Vermeiren, 2003; Wasserman *et al.*, 2003; Vermeiren *et al.*, 2006), it may not always be possible to proceed in this fashion. However, a diagnosis-based approach should always be considered if at all possible.

Aggression and juvenile delinquency

There are two forms of aggression – acute and chronic. Juvenile delinquents often present acutely aggressive or can be made so by interactions in institutional environments. Behavioral techniques should be used, if possible, to reduce or deescalate violence. These include contingency management programs, specific training in social skills and anger management, and behavioral therapy (Pappadopulos *et al.*, 2003). In the event that these prove ineffective, and the juvenile poses a risk of harm to themselves or others, acute pharmacological strategies can be employed as one component of an overall treatment plan.

If the juvenile is cooperative, then oral medication can be given. Fast-acting benzodiazepines like lorazepam or atypical antipsychotics like olanzapine or risperidone can be used. Both olanzapine and risperidone come in formulations specifically designed for rapid oral delivery. Caution should be used when dosing benzodiazepines as some children have paradoxical, disinhibited reactions to this class of medications.

In the case of emergent situations where the risks of harm are significant, and the juvenile cannot be redirected to use oral medications, then intramuscular (IM) preparations may be indicated. It is always better to have the juvenile in a secure environment when dosing with these formulations; placing the juvenile in physical restraints may be necessary to avoid the possibility of harm during the delivery of the medication. In these circumstances, haloperidol and lorazepam are often used for acute management and combined with diphenhydramine or benztropine given for prophylaxis against extra-pyramidal symptoms (EPS). Thorazine has also historically been used, but due to its high potential for significant cardiac prolongation and neuroleptic malignant syndrome, has lost some of its appeal. More recently, IM preparations are available of atypical antipsychotics like olanzapine and ziprasidone. Both of these are far less likely to cause EPS than the typical antipsychotics and tend to be less acutely sedating. One advantage of using less sedating medications for juveniles is that behavioral control can be obtained while allowing communication with staff during the incident, and therefore better management from a behavioral perspective. Consideration should also be given to the fact that all antipsychotics have the potential to cause QTc prolongation; careful monitoring should be given to children who are emergently medicated, with regular checks and vital signs when their safety can be ensured. Another reason to use these medications in juveniles, is that they are easily converted from the IM form to an oral form of the same agent. Children who are placed in restraints for safety and medication delivery should be released as soon as they are able to contract with staff for safety, or after enough time has passed for the medications to take effect. Dosing schedules have recently been published in the TRAAY consensus report (Pappadopulos *et al.*, 2003).

Subtyping of aggression: aiming at causal processes

One of the challenging aspects of dealing with juvenile offenders is addressing the nature of long-term control of chronic, repetitive aggression. Recent evidence from multiple lines of research in the neurobiology and psychology of aggression increasingly demonstrates that there are two major subtypes of aggressive behavior (Blair *et al.*, 2006), and that each most likely responds to very different interventions. Proactive, instrumental, or planned (PIP) is often termed "cold" aggression, and corresponds to what most investigators see as an early form of psychopathic violence. The individual often lacks empathy for the victim of his aggression and may be far more concerned with the outcome or benefit that he derives from the act (Steiner, 2005; Steiner *et al.*, 2005; Blair *et al.*, 2006). At the present time, there is no convincing evidence supporting the use of medications in the treatment of this type of aggression, although several compounds, such as dopamine blockers are of theoretical interest. The inefficacy of psychopharmacological agents against this form of aggression is most likely due to the fact that PIP aggression does not run on a specific neuroarchitecture. In this sense it runs on multiple networks, with many supporting neurotransmitters as do other instrumental behaviors (Blair *et al.*, 2006; Steiner *et al.*, 2006). Conversely, reactive, affective, defensive, or impulsive (RADI) or "hot" aggression is an emotionally charged form that often is poorly thought out and highly reactive to situational stimuli (Steiner *et al.*, 2003b); it runs on readily identifiable neuroarchitecture that has a more limited and better known neurotransmitter profile. For example, it probably involves some dynamic balance of glutamate, norepinephrine, dopamine, serotonin, and gamma-aminobutyric acid (GABA), but there are likely others as well (Blair *et al.*, 2006); the ones listed show direct links to psychopharmacological agents to be considered in treating RADI aggression. As much as the situation permits, attempts to differentiate these forms of aggression should be undertaken, as this will guide treatment strategies and outcome expectations for juvenile delinquents.

When trying to control chronic aggression it is useful to distinguish PIP and RADI subtypes. Compared to age appropriate cohorts, both forms of aggression are elevated in delinquent populations, and co-occur in about five percent of those youths who have clinically significant problems with aggression (Steiner *et al.*, 2005). Clinically significant PIP aggression alone is quite rare in the community, but is often concentrated in juvenile justice settings, and most often correlated with substance abuse, instead of other forms of psychopathology (Wilson *et al.*, in press). Recent research shows that juveniles with the RADI form of aggression respond well to mood stabilizers like lithium carbonate, although side effects make its use problematic. The side effects with other mood stabilizers, especially when delivered as extended release formulations or racemic mixtures are much more benign and less difficult to manage in a population that cannot be easily relied on for compliance and adherence to recommendations (Steiner *et al.*, 2003a; Steiner *et al.*, 2003; Rana *et al.*, 2005; Saxena *et al.*, 2005). The findings in this area of research are preliminary, and further studies are underway to understand the nature of aggression and its responsiveness to pharmacological interventions. A recent consensus panel agreed that RADI aggression is especially common across many different diagnoses, which may suggest that treating the diagnosis may improve the aggression (Jensen *et al.*, in press). As yet, PIP aggression has not been well studied in how it may respond to various treatments but the emerging data suggest that this form of aggression may benefit from limited pharmacological intervention in combination with psychotherapy and structured environments (Vitiello *et al.*, 1990; Vitiello & Stoff, 1997; McDougle *et al.*, 2003).

Evaluation and assessment for psychopharmacology

The cornerstone of sound psychopharmacology is an accurate and detailed psychiatric assessment. The DSM syndromic (American Psychiatric Association, 2000) approach to mental illnesses creates a host of problems when assessing juvenile offenders among whom co-morbidities are the norm. The resulting group of diagnoses often makes it difficult to pursue a sound and rational pharmacological approach, due to the overlapping symptoms and proliferation of diagnoses. With juvenile delinquents it would not be unusual to see three or more concurrent diagnoses in the DSM system. The tragic result of this approach is that children are often placed on multiple medications without a clear understanding of their interactions or of the functional result in helping the juvenile.

Our group prefers an approach more consistent with the *International Classification of Diseases, 10th edition* (*ICD-10*) (World Health Organization, 1992), wherein a principal diagnosis is identified by careful examination of the unfolding behavioral pattern over time. As we know from several recent findings, maladaptive aggression is found to complicate a wide array of diagnoses including mental retardation, pervasive developmental disorders, posttraumatic stress disorder (PTSD), depression, bipolar affective disorder, and attention-deficit/hyperactivity disorder (ADHD). It is especially important to delineate aggression occurring in the context of mental retardation, psychosis, and pervasive developmental disorders, as the profound nature of these disorders affects multiple high level neuroarchitectures in addition to the basic circuitry involved in aggressive behavior. The aggression in the context of these disorders requires a much more comprehensive approach, including techniques to socialize, to help the child comprehend social rules and norms, and to assist in reality testing. Often environmental manipulation (sociotherapy) is a mainstay in the treatment of these diagnoses, and the types of behavioral interventions shown to be effective in this context differ qualitatively from those used in youths where intelligence, reality testing, and knowledge of rules of conviviality is not an issue. Having said this, there is an extensive literature documenting the efficacy and effectiveness of multiple compounds against aggression in profound disorders of executive functioning, which we refer the reader to (Connor, 2002). It will not be discussed here. We will summarize only those trials where the primary recruitment target was a disorder of aggression – conduct disorder (CD), oppositional-defiant disorder (ODD), and intermittent explosive disorder (IED).

The most conservative assumption then would be to treat the principal diagnosis as potently, specifically, and comprehensively as possible. As the principal diagnosis responds, the expectation is that the maladaptive aggression will recede, as has been most clearly demonstrated in the case of ADHD (Connor *et al.*, 2002). Should this prove ineffective and residual symptoms remain, or should there be an inability to establish an initial principal diagnosis, then it is wise to switch to a target symptom approach and to choose pharmacological interventions based on the best estimate of risks and benefits for the individual. As prominent aggression usually poses a danger to the patient and others, it may be necessary to stabilize the situation first while trying to minimize risk to the individual. This may require a secure setting and the use of short-acting agents before consideration is given to long-term strategies and management. It is expected that after the crisis has been resolved, the focus should return to establishing a primary diagnosis and targeting the treatment as specifically as possible.

Every assessment must have a thorough history and physical examination as a starting point. Assessment for neurological findings is of primary importance, as is documentation of any visible evidence of abuse or neglect. It is not unusual to find healed physical scars or wounds that occurred due to recent or remote abuse. Baseline laboratory studies have utility as well. Endocrine dysfunction, neoplastic syndromes, and many other medical problems often present with psychiatric manifestations and can often be easily remedied. Modern psychopharmacology requires that practitioners monitor height, weight, body mass index, nutritional status, intoxicants, vital signs, thyroid panels, kidney functioning, liver functioning, diabetes measures, and other parameters depending on the medication selected. Electrocardiograms (EKGs) could also be needed if certain atypical antipsychotics are used because of their propensity to cause QTc prolongation (Blair *et al.*, 2004).

Practitioners working with problems of aggression need to utilize standardized psychometric instruments as part of an initial assessment. As a first-line screening tool, many juvenile facilities make use of the Massachusetts Youth Screening Instrument, Second Version (MAYSI-2) (Grisso *et al.*, 2001). It is a relatively short instrument that can serve as an indicator for significant dysfunction, and can be done by most front-line personnel. More specialized psychometric or neuropsychological testing may be performed as needed and depending on the circumstance, but in all cases, such instruments should be used to track progress or lack thereof. A recent summary of a range of instruments is available (Connor, 2002).

Another complicating factor is that children are dynamic beings and their behaviors exist along a developmental trajectory (Steiner, 2004; Frick, 2006). What is appropriate at one age may be inappropriate at another. Attention to the juvenile's psychological development is important and must be included in any diagnostic work-up. After a diagnosis is made, or in an acute situation after target symptoms are identified, and are judged to be maladaptive, psychopathological, and not solely induced by the psychosocial milieu in which the youngster currently resides, it is appropriate to move to consideration of the potential use of a pharmacological agent.

Pharmacotherapy for conduct disorder

Juvenile offenders have high rates of meeting diagnostic criteria for conduct disorder. The original framing of the criteria are designed, in part, to help identify these juveniles and channel them towards mental health services. The progenitors in diagnostic nomenclature were termed as either sociopathy or psychopathy. Hervey Cleckley collapsed these concepts in his monograph *The Masks of Sanity* (Cleckley, 1964), which is widely seen as the progenitor for the current understanding of antisocial personality disorder. These concepts have developed over time, and with them has come a great deal of conceptual problems and a significant discrepancy with our emerging understanding of the neurobiology of aggression and violence (Blair *et al.*, 2006). In addition, there are commentators who reasonably argue that the movement to expand concepts of psychopathy into the juvenile period leads to unwarranted labeling, and that such a movement fails to acknowledge that the developmental processes also allow for the possibility of change and rehabilitation (Steiner & Cauffman, 1998; Edens *et al.*, 2001). Thus, it is sometimes wise to separate the processes of diagnostic labeling from

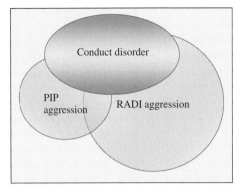

Figure 15.1   Relationship of PIP/RADI aggression to conduct disorder

treatment goals, and to instead view aggression as the target for intervention instead of placing primacy on the overly broad category of conduct disorder.

Both PIP and RADI aggression partially overlap with conduct disorder. Many of the symptoms of CD, IED, and ODD qualify for aggressive acts. They are diagnosed as a disorder because they are presumed to be maladaptive, chronic, persistent, and unresponsive to simple environmental change. At the same time, it is also clear, that much aggressive behavior occurs outside of a psychiatric syndrome, serves a distinct evolutionary purpose, and can be vital for survival. Figure 15.1 clarifies these relationships by showing the functional overlaps of major classes of psychiatric illness and aggression.

Studies of the treatment of conduct disorder have varied and been done with a variety of agents using different research protocols. Table 15.1 reviews all of the major studies that have examined the effects of major classes of medications on conduct disorder, and its related symptomotology, which crudely overlaps with the aggressive patterns described above. As might be expected from the descriptions of aggression above, evidence exists for the use of both atypical antipsychotics and mood stabilizers in the treatment of conduct disorder. Typical and atypical antipsychotics, at low doses, are generally recommended as the first line of intervention, because they have the most data accumulated backing their use (Findling *et al.*, 2005). Their mechanism of action is presumably through the reduction of excitability through dopaminergic blockage, and often non-specific sedation, which occurs within minutes of administration, can be helpful in acute situations at high doses. The more specific effect of dopaminergic blockage usually does not have its onset until days to weeks later, and is maintained for years afterwards. By far the most well studied of the atypical antipsychotics in the treatment of childhood aggression has been the compound risperidone (Findling *et al.*, 2000; Snyder *et al.*, 2002; Findling *et al.*, 2004; Aman *et al.*, 2005;

Table 15.1. Studies of psychopharmacology and conduct disorder by drug class

Study	Medication	Study design/duration	Subjects	Scales used	Results
Antipsychotics, typical					
Campbell *et al.*, 1984	Haloperidol and Lithium	DB RCT/6 wks	N = 61, hospitalized, 5–13 yrs; dx of CD	CPRS (b), CGI, CTQ, CPTQ, TORSA	H & L better than placebo in reducing aggression & conduct problems; more "untoward effects" with H than L.
Aman *et al.*, 1991	Thioridizine and Methylphenidate (MPH)	DB RCT with crossover/9 wks	N = 30, 4–16 yrs, subaverage IQ; dx of CD or ADHD	CTQ, CTRS, DCB, GRTE, RBPC, RLRS	T modestly effective on teacher ratings of conduct problems & hyperactivity; MPH very effective on all teacher ratings.
Greenhill *et al.*, 1985	Thioridizine and Molindone	DB RCT/8 wks	N = 31, hospitalized, 6–11 yrs; dx of CD	CGI, CPRS, CRS, CTQ, DOTES	T & M better than placebo in reducing aggression & conduct problems.
Broche, 1980	Pimozide	DB RCT with crossover/2 mo	N = 10		Social integration was improved.
Joshi *et al.*, 1998	Droperidol	Case series/emergency use	N = 26, hospitalized, mean 9.1 yrs; varied dx, DBD (N = 17)	Subjective rating	Acute aggressive or violent behavior episode resolved such that all subjects returned to milieu in 2 hours after D.
Hameer *et al.*, 2001	Droperidol	Case series/emergency use over 20 wks	N = 6, hospitalized, mean 12 yrs; varied dx	Subjective rating	Hyperactive, violent, and/or combative subjects experienced "profound calming effect" with D.

Antipsychotics, atypical

	Drug	Design/duration	Sample	Measures	Findings
Findling et al., 2000	Risperidone	DB RCT/10 wks	N = 20, 5–15 yrs; dx of CD	RAAPP; CGI, CBCL, CPRS (b)	Aggression on RAAPP significantly improved; no difference in parent rating.
Snyder et al., 2002	Risperidone	DB RCT/7 wks	N = 110, 5–12 yrs, low IQ; dx of DBD, 80% dx of ADHD	ABC, BPI, CGI, CPT, CSI, CVLT, NCBRF	Aggression, hyperactivity, and self-injury significantly improved; no difference between ADHD and non-ADHD subjects.
Findling et al., 2004	Risperidone	Prospective open extension/48 wks	N = 107, 5–12 yo, low IQ; dx of DBD	Safety indicators, CGI, NCBRF	Safe and effective in reducing conduct problems.
Aman et al., 2005	Risperidone	Pooled analysis of 2 DB RCT/6 wks	N = 223 (pooled), 5–12 yrs, low IQ; dx of DBD	NCBRF	Improved social interaction, feelings of self-worth, and reintegration.
Croonenberghs et al., 2005	Risperidone	Open/1 yr	N = 504 kids (32 sites), 5–14 yrs, low IQ; dx of DBD	Safety indicators, CGI, NCBRF	Safe and effective in reducing conduct problems.
LeBlanc et al., 2005	Risperidone	2 RCTs/6 wks	N-163 boys, 5–12 yrs with ODD or CD and co-morbid ADHD or not	NCBRF (selected items)	Aggression was reduced when compared to placebo for boys with below average IQs and comorbid disruptive behaviors
Soderstrom et al., 2002	Olanzapine	Case series	N = 6, 14–19 yrs, male; "extremely aggressive"	Subjective rating	Suggests reduction in aggression.
Stephens et al., 2004	Olanzapine	Single-blind RCT/10 wks	N = 10, 7–13 yrs; dx of Tourette's Syndrome	CBCL	Aggression was significantly reduced.
Masi et al., 2006	Olanzapine	Retrospective case series	N = 23, 16 boys and 7 girls, 11–17 years with CD	KSADS, CGI, MOAS, CGAS	60% were responders to combined medication and non-pharmacological treatments
Findling et al., 2006	Quetiapine	Open/8 wks	N = 17, 6–12 yrs, 16 boys and 1 girl	RAAPPS, NCBRF, CPRS	Significant findings across scales in aggression reduction

Anticonvulsants

	Drug	Design/duration	Sample	Measures	Findings
Kafantaris et al., 1992	Carbamazepine	Open/4 wks	N = 10, hospitalized, 5–10 yrs; dx of CD	CGI, CPRS, CPTQ, GCC	Aggression & explosiveness were significantly reduced.

Table 15.1. (cont.)

Study	Medication	Study design/duration	Subjects	Scales used	Results
Mattes, 1990	Carbamazepine and propanolol	RCT/Varied duration	N = 61, hospitalized, 16 yrs and older; dx of IED	Subjective evaluation	Temper outbursts modestly reduced; suggests C as more effective for IED and P for ADHD.
Cueva et al., 1996	Carbamazepine	DB RCT/9 wks	N = 22, hospitalized, 5–12 yrs; dx of CD	CGI, CPRS, OAS	Not better than placebo in reducing aggression.
Donovan et al., 2000	Valproic Acid	DB RCT with crossover/12 wks	N = 20, 10–18 yrs; dx of DBD	DISC, M-OAS, SCID-V	Improved explosive temper & mood lability
Saxena et al., 2005; Steiner et al., 2003	Valproic Acid	DB RCT/7 wks	N = 71, mean 15 yrs, males; dx of CD, in detention	CGI, WAI, YSR	Self-reported improvement in restraint and impulse control.
Mood stabilizers					
Malone et al., 1994	Lithium	Open/4 wks	N = 8, hospitalized, 9–16 yrs; dx of CD	GCCR, OAS	Aggression was significantly reduced.
Campbell et al., 1984	Haloperidol and Lithium	DB RCT/6 wks	N = 61, hospitalized, 5–13 yrs; dx of CD	CPRS (b), CGI, CTQ, CPTQ, TORSA	H & L better than placebo in reducing aggression & conduct problems; more "untoward effects" with H than L.
Campbell et al., 1995	Lithium	DB RCT/8 wks	N = 50, hospitalized, 5–12 yrs	CGI, CPRS (b), CTQ, GCJCS, POMS, PTQ	L modestly better than placebo in reducing conduct problems, though difference not evident on POMS.
Malone et al., 2000	Lithium	DB RCT/6 wks	N = 40, hospitalized, 10–17 yrs; dx of CD, severe and chronic aggression	CGI, GCJCS, OAS	Aggression was significantly reduced; more than 50% subjects experienced nausea, vomiting and urinary frequency.
Rifkin et al., 1997	Lithium	DB RCT/3 wks	N = 33, hospitalized, 12–17 yrs; dx of CD	BRS, CTRS, HRS-D, OAS	Lithium was not better than placebo in reducing overt aggression.

Antidepressants

Study	Medication	Design/Duration	Sample	Measures	Results
Coccaro et al., 1997	Fluoxetine	DB RCT/12 wks	N = 15, hospitalized, mean 39.4 yrs; IED, personality disorder	OAS	Aggression & irritability were significantly reduced.
Constantino et al., 1997	Fluoxetine, paroxetine, and sertraline	Open/10 + wks	N = 19, hospitalized	MOAS	Aggression was not reduced by any of the SSRI's tested.
Cherek et al., 2002	Paroxetine	RCT/3 wks	N = 12 adults, males; on felony parole	PSAP	Impulsivity was significantly reduced; mixed reduction in aggression.
Armenteros & Lewis, 2002	Citalopram	Open/7 wks	N = 12, 7–15 yrs; 6 + mo of aggression & impulsivity	CBCL, CGI, M-OAS	Impulsivity & aggression were both significantly reduced.
Zubieta & Alessi, 1992	Trazadone	Case series/Varied duration	N = 22, hospitalized, 5–12 yrs; impulsive & aggressive	CPTQ	Aggression, impulsivity, and hyperactivity all subjectively improved.

Stimulants

Study	Medication	Design/Duration	Sample	Measures	Results
Klein et al., 1997	Methylphenidate	DB RCT/5 wks	N = 84, 6–16 yrs; dx of CD, 2/3 also ADHD	CTRS, IAS, QRBPC	Antisocial behavior was significantly reduced; no difference between ADHD and non-ADHD.
Kaplan et al., 1990	Methylphenidate	Mixed Open & DB RCT/7 wks	N = 9, 6 were hospitalized, 13–16 yrs; dx of CD (N = 8) or ODD (N = 1), and ADHD (N = 7)	AABC, CTRS, DICA	Aggression on the AABC was significantly reduced; overall pattern of reduced aggression & hyperactivity.
Hazell & Stuart, 2003	Methylphenidate and Clonidine	DB RCT/6 wks	N = 67, 6–14 yrs, white; dx of ADHD and CD or ODD	CBCL, CPRS, CTRS	Adding C to MPH significantly improved conduct symptoms and had no effect on ADHD symptoms.

Alpha-agonists

Study	Medication	Design/Duration	Sample	Measures	Results
Kemph et al., 1993	Clonidine	Open/1–18 mo	N = 17, 5–17 yrs; dx of CD or ODD	CBCL, RAAP	Aggression was significantly reduced.

Table 15.1. (cont.)

Study	Medication	Study design/duration	Subjects	Scales used	Results
Schvehla et al., 1994	Clonidine	Retrospective/Average of 21 d	N = 18, hospitalized, 6–12 yrs, male; dx of ADHD and CD or ODD	GAF, CGI	Anger, aggression, hyperactivity, & impulsivity all were significantly reduced.
Beta-blockers					
Silver et al., 1999	Propranolol	Mixed Open & DB RCT/Varied duration	N = 20, 18 + yrs; chronic aggression; serious psychiatric dx or MR	CGI, OAS	Aggression was significantly reduced in 7 subjects.
Kuperman & Stewart, 1987	Propranolol	Open/3 + mo	N = 16, 4–24 yrs; physically aggressive	Subjective rating	Frequency and intensity of aggressive outbursts were reduced in 10 subjects.
Mattes, 1990	Carbamazepine and propanolol	RCT/Vaired duration	N = 61, hospitalized, 16 yrs and older; dx of IED	Subjective rating	Temper outbursts modestly reduced; suggests C as more effective for IED and P for ADHD.
Connor et al., 1997	Nadolol	Open/5 mo	N = 12, 9–24 yr, male; developmentally delayed	CGI, Iowa CTRS, OAS	Aggression was significantly reduced.
Buitelaar et al., 1996	Pindolol	DB RCT/4 wks	N = 52, 7–13 yrs; dx of ADHD	ACRS	P and MPH reduced conduct problems and hyperactivity at home equally, but P was less effective than MPH at school and according to psychological testing; significant side effects.

Other

Study	Drug	Design/duration	Sample	Other	Results
Pfeffer et al., 1997	Buspirone	Open/9 wks	N = 25, hospitalized; anxiety & aggression	CGAS, MAVRIC	Aggression was not significantly reduced.
Stanislav et al., 1994	Buspirone	Retrospective/Varied duration	N = 20, hospitalized, 15–55 yrs; varied dx	Subjective rating	Overt aggression was significantly improved for 9/10 subjects given 3 + mo of B.
Vitiello et al., 1991	Diphenhydramine	DB RCT/Emergency use	N = 21, hospitalized, 5–13 yrs; varied dx	CGI, CTRS	D and placebo equally improved aggression.
King et al., 2001	Amantadine	Open/5–14 d	N = 8, hospitalized, 4–12 yrs, males; neurodevelopmental disorder (N = 7)	Subjective rating	Impulse control was improved in all subjects (4 with marked response, 4 with moderate response).

AABC – Adolescent Antisocial Behavior Checklist
ABC – Aberrant Behavior Checklist
ACRS – Abbreviated Conners Rating Scale
BPI – Behavior Problems Inventory
BRS – Behavior Rating Scale
CBC(L) – Child Behavior Checklist
CGAS – Clinical Global Assessment Score
CGI – Clinical Global Impression Scale
CPRS – Conners Parent Rating Scale
CPRS (b) – Children's Psychiatric Rating Scate
CPT – Continuous Performance Task
CSI – Childhood Symptom Inventory
C(P)TQ – Conners (Parent) Teacher Questionnaire
CTRS – Conners Teacher Rating Scale
CVLT – California Verbal Learning Test for Children
DCB – Devereux Child Behavior Rating Scale
DICA – Diagnostic Instrument for Children and Adolescents

Notes to Table 15.1. (cont.)

DOTES – Dosage Order Treatment Emergent Symptoms Scale
GAF – Global Assessment of Functioning
GCC(R) – Global Clinical Consensus Ratings
GCJCS – Global Clinical Judgments Consensus Scale
GRTE – Global Rating of Treatment Effectiveness
HRS-D – Hamilton Rating Scale for Depression
IAS – Iowa Aggression Scale
KSADS – Kiddie Schedule of Affective Disorders and Schizophrenia
MAVRIC – Measure of Aggression, Violence, and Rage in Children
NCBRF – Nisonger Child Behavior Rating Form
(M)OAS – (Modified) Overt Aggression Scale
POMS – Profile of Mood States
PSAP – Point Subtraction Aggression Paradigm
QRBPC – Quay Revised Behavior Problem Checklist
RAAPP – Rating of Aggression Against People and/or Property
RBPC – Revised Behavior Problem Checklist
RLRS – Ritvo-Freeman Real Life Rating Scale for Autism
SCID-V – Structured Clinical Interview for DSM-V
TORSA – Timed Objective Rating Scale for Aggression

Croonenberghs *et al.*, 2005; LeBlanc *et al.*, 2005). Six studies have documented its effectiveness, and four of those studies were randomized clinical trials (RCTs). Findling and colleagues also conducted a 48-week prospective open-label extension study and found that it was safe and effective in the treatment of disruptive behaviors among children with subaverage intelligence at a mean dose of 1.5 mg per day (Findling *et al.*, 2004). More recently, olanzapine (Soderstrom *et al.*, 2002; Stephens *et al.*, 2004; Masi *et al.*, 2006) and quetiapine (Findling *et al.*, 2006) have shown preliminary evidence of efficacy in conduct disordered and aggressive youth.

Among the mood stabilizers, valproate (Donovan *et al.*, 2000; Steiner *et al.*, 2003; Saxena *et al.*, 2005) and lithium (Campbell *et al.*, 1984; Malone *et al.*, 1994; Campbell *et al.*, 1995; Rifkin *et al.*, 1997; Malone *et al.*, 2000), have had randomized controlled trails that have demonstrated efficacy. Carbamazepine (Mattes, 1990; Cueva *et al.*, 1996) has not demonstrated robust effects in the two RCTs conducted in children. Most notably, the Cueva *et al.* (1996) study failed to separate from placebo using validated measures. Presumably, the mechanisms of efficacy with these compounds relates to their ability to activate inhibitory neurotransmitters, such as GABA (Rana *et al.*, 2005), and to perhaps reduce the activating neurotransmitter glutamate, as our group has recently shown in a sample of aggressive bipolar offspring (Chang *et al.*, 2003). Thus, there is an attractive potential complementarity between these two classes of medication: decreasing activation while increasing inhibition across neuroarchitectures relevant to aggression. We have some preliminary evidence that such combinations are potentially more effective in bipolar children (Findling *et al.*, 2003).

The choice of medication will depend on the particular patient, weighing of risks and benefits, and the particular pharmacological properties of each agent. If the clinician judges that activation is the predominant problem, he/she will select the dopaminergic blockers first. If he/she judges aggression is predominantly a lack of self-control, he/she might choose a mood stabilizer first. If there are disturbances in both domains, combination treatment might be the best option (Fig. 15.2).

It should be noted that all of these uses are off-label uses of these medications, and have not been approved for use in this manner by the US Food and Drug Administration (FDA).

Both atypical antipsychotics and mood stabilizers require that the provider assess certain baseline factors, and consistently monitor particular laboratory and physical studies. For all of these medications, baseline weight and vital signs should be done. In addition, hemoglobin A1c and lipid panels should be drawn, prior to initiating treatment with atypical antipsychotics, due to the potential for the development of diabetes and related consequences. For mood stabilizers, basic

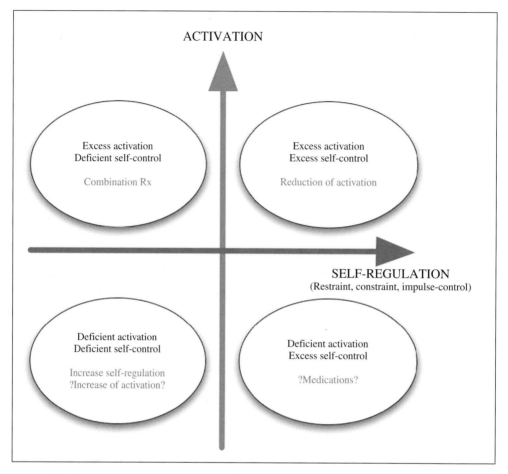

Figure 15.2 Psychopharmacology of maladaptive aggression

chemistries and regular blood levels need to be drawn. Lithium can cause neph-rotoxicity; valproate and carbamazepine can be hepatotoxic. In addition, several of these agents have particular rare side effects that can be lethal, and patients need to be monitored closely for adverse events. Conducting thorough physical examina-tions is especially important among juvenile offenders who, as wards of the state, often lack the authority to make decisions about their care themselves. This state authority and the need to provide mental health care should be taken as a judicious responsibility, and risks and benefits should be documented prior to initiating pharmacotherapy. For a more in-depth review of each medication, the reader is referred to an excellent recent text by Martin and colleagues (Martin, 2003).

Co-morbidity among delinquent populations should be considered the norm (Abram *et al.*, 2003). Several studies suggest that the majority of juveniles in detention not only suffer from illnesses such conduct disorder as described above, but also depression, ADHD, substance use disorders, and anxiety (Feinstein *et al.*, 1998; Abram *et al.*, 2003). It is clearly evident that when addressing the needs of delinquents, conduct disorder and aggression cannot be exclusive targets. Where comorbid conditions exist, they must be addressed, as these may be the driving etiology behind the aggressive behavior or conduct disorder.

Specific classes of medication

Antidepressants

Selective serotonin reuptake inhibitors (SSRIs) are commonly used in pediatric populations in the treatment of depression, obsessive compulsive disorder (OCD), and anxiety, in addition to other disorders. Among the SSRIs, fluoxetine, fluvoxamine, and sertraline have FDA approval in pediatrics for OCD. Fluoxetine alone is also labeled for use in pediatric depression, and has been the subject of a small clinical investigation in juvenile delinquents. This study suggested that fluoxetine was useful in treating eight adolescent substance-dependent males with CD who suffered from major depression that persisted or emerged after four weeks of abstinence (Riggs *et al.*, 1997). Another commonly used SSRI, paroxetine, has demonstrated efficacy in treating social anxiety disorder (Wagner *et al.*, 2004a), OCD (Geller *et al.*, 2004), and depression (Keller *et al.*, 2001). Citalopram likewise has been effective in treating childhood depression (Wagner *et al.*, 2004b). A recent review of the efficacy of all classes of antidepressants in children concludes that only citalopram, fluoxetine, and sertraline have adequately demonstrated superiority to placebo (Wagner, 2005).

Clomipramine, a tricyclic antidepressant, has FDA approval for treating pediatric OCD. Buproprion, which inhibits norepinephrine and dopamine reuptake, has also been used to treat depression, ADHD, and tobacco addiction in children, though no randomized controlled trials have been conducted to confirm its efficacy in juveniles (Wagner, 2005).

Common adverse effects of SSRIs in both adults and children include sexual dysfunction, nausea, drowsiness, constipation, nervousness, and fatigue (Emslie *et al.*, 1997; March *et al.*, 1998; Keller *et al.*, 2001). Following a review of 24 trials, including 4400 depressed children that evidenced an increased risk of suicidality from two percent among the placebo group to four percent among children on antidepressants, the FDA issued a public health advisory in October of 2004 (FDA, 2004). The issue of increased suicide risk remains controversial, as other authors suggest that antidepressants decrease overall suicide rates (Gibbons *et al.*, 2005).

Antipsychotics

Antipsychotics have been used in childhood psychosis, bipolar disorder, conduct disorder, and aggression among other disorders. Typical antipsychotics, with FDA approval for pediatric schizophrenia, include fluphenazine, haloperidol, loxapin, molindone, thiothixene, thioridazine, and trifluoperazine. Chlorpromazine and haloperidol have FDA approval for short-term treatment of hyperactivity and severe behavior problems. Pimozide has FDA approval only for pediatric Tourette's Syndrome. Adverse effects associated with typical antipsychotics are significant, and include extra-pyramidal side effects (EPS) (i.e., akathisia, acute dystonia, and drug-induced Parkinsonism), seizure, weight gain, liver dysfunction, sedation, cardiovascular, and hematological effects. Younger individuals may be at an increased risk of developing EPS (Keepers *et al.*, 1983).

Atypical antipsychotics not only have less risk of EPS, but have the potential to combat schizophrenia resistant to treatment with typical antipsychotics, which is a concern particularly among adolescents with early-onset of the disease (Meltzer *et al.*, 1997). Likely for these reasons and because of the milder side effect profile in general, atypicals are used more commonly than the older class of antipsychotics in pediatric patients, even though the research literature is wanting. None of the atypicals have FDA approval in pediatrics, though off-label usage of olanzapine, quetiapine, ziprasidone, and particularly risperidone is fairly common. One recent review of atypical antipsychotic use in children suggests that they are efficacious in treating psychosis, bipolar disorder, pervasive developmental disorder, and Tourette's, and are likely efficacious in severe ADHD, CD, and mental retardation; however, the authors state that more rigorous clinical investigation is warranted (Cheng-Shannon *et al.*, 2004).

The most common side effects of atypical antipsychotics (which varied by drug) uncovered by this review were cardiovascular effects, weight gain, sedation, sialorrhea, EPS, and hyperprolactinemia. Clozapine requires hematological monitoring due to its risk of leukopenia and agranulocytosis, and is thus seen as a second-line agent. Specific treatment recommendations and guidelines exist for the use of atypical antipsychotics to treat aggressive behavior, and these should be consulted prior to initiating the use of these compounds (Pappadopulos *et al.*, 2003; Schur *et al.*, 2003).

Benzodiazepines

Chlordiazepoxide, diazepam, and lorazepam are among the commonly used benzodiazepines that are FDA approved in children for anxiety. Alprazolam and clonazepam are not labeled for pediatric usage, but both have a long history of off-label use in pediatric populations. Sedation is a common side effect of benzodiazepines, though the class of medications is generally well-tolerated for short-term therapy (Bernstein & Shaw, 1997). Careful consideration must be given to the intended use of these medications, since they can be extremely habituating, which is especially significant in populations like juvenile delinquents who have high rates of co-morbid substance use disorders (Wilson *et al.*, in press).

Second generation hypnotics

Zolpidem is a non-benzodiazepine sedative hypnotic with side effects that include dizziness, lightheadedness, somnolence, headache, and GI upset. Zaleplon and eszopiclone are non-benzodiazepine hypnotics similar to zolpidem that have been more recently developed. None of these have been studied extensively in children, nor do they have pediatric FDA indications.

Mood stabilizers

The anticonvulsant agents carbamazepine and divalproex sodium are used as mood stabilizers in pediatric illnesses such as bipolar disorder, ADHD, and conduct disorder. However, while both drugs have FDA approval for pediatric epilepsy, neither is approved to treat pediatric psychiatric disorders. Nevertheless, increasing evidence has become available on the use of divalproex sodium for the treatment of disruptive behavior disorders (Steiner *et al.*, 2003a; Saxena *et al.*, 2005), and an array of other pediatric psychiatric illnesses (Rana *et al.*, 2005).

Lithium has traditionally been a favored treatment for bipolar disorder in adults and adolescents. While much has been learned about the drug in the last 50 years, the precise mechanisms by which lithium treats acute mania and diminishes recurrence remain largely unknown (Lenox & Hahn, 2000). Lithium is approved by the FDA to treat bipolar disorder in children older than 12 years, but has been used in younger patients. It also has mixed efficacy in treating aggression and irritability, as described in Table 15.1. Side effects of lithium may be significant and include tremor, varied gastrointestinal symptoms, polyuria, hypothyroidism, reversible T-wave depression on electrocardiogram, and neutrophilia (Martin, 2003). Careful monitoring is necessary in children, due to the narrow therapeutic window for lithium, and the ease with which children can become dehydrated in athletic or summer activities, and thus functionally increase the concentration of this ion to toxic levels. Routine blood levels, as well as good psychoeducation are necessary components when dosing lithium.

Stimulants and atomoxetine

ADHD is among the most common psychiatric diagnoses in the United States, and stimulants are the most common medication used to treat the disorder. Stimulants have a long history, and have generated an extremely large treatment literature (Martin, 2003). Methylphenidate is the most commonly studied and prescribed of the stimulants. Dextroamphetamine is a longer acting stimulant than MPH, though longer duration and once daily formulations of MPH have been created (i.e., MPH-SR and concerta). Pemoline is considered second-line stimulant therapy for ADHD due to its associated risk of hepatic failure. Common side effects of stimulants in general include insomnia, decreased appetite, headache, and jitteriness. As with benzodiazepines, consideration must be given to the possible abuse potential of stimulants in youth offenders.

Given the growing black market trade and illegal uses of simulants among children and adolescents (Teter *et al.*, 2003; McCabe *et al.*, 2004; McCabe *et al.*, 2005), it may be preferable to use non-stimulant medications for the treatment of ADHD. Atomoxetine selectively inhibits the reuptake of norepinephrine, but to this point has not been successfully used in depression. Instead, it now has FDA labeling for ADHD in children. Unlike the stimulants, atomoxetine is not a federally controlled substance and has no abuse or diversion potential, therefore making it an extremely promising compound in this population, where we find extremely high rates of SUD (Wilson *et al.*, in press). Atomoxetine was successful in treating ADHD in two studies of children with oppositional-defiant disorder (ODD) (Kaplan *et al.*, 2004; Newcorn, Spencer *et al.*, 2005), but only improved ODD symptoms in one (Newcorn *et al.*, 2005) at high doses up to 2.0 mg/d/kg. In addition, Biederman and colleagues have recently reported that the presence of ODD does not prevent treatment of ADHD when using atomoxetine (Biederman *et al.*, 2005). It is generally well tolerated with no growth, appetite, sleep, or mood interference, and otherwise similar side effect profile to stimulants (Michelson *et al.*, 2001), but transient liver injury has been reported (FDA, 2005). Recent studies by our group have shown atomoxetine to be beneficial in the treatment of RADI aggression (Rana & Steiner, 2005). It appears that in rare cases atomoxetine paradoxically leads to some agitation, and therefore caution should be used when using this medication.

Suicidality

Juvenile offenders are at especially high risk for self-harm during detention or incarceration (Kempton & Forehand, 1992; Battle *et al.*, 1993; Thomas & Penn,

2002; Ruchkin *et al.*, 2003; Farand *et al.*, 2004). There is likely a multifactorial etiology to suicidality that may not be immediately evident, but prompt assessment is always necessary. Studies of inpatient populations have identified several risk factors for suicide attempts including prior suicide attempts, evidence of psychosis, and acuity of suicidal ideation. Fawcett and colleagues suggest that adding severity of anxiety and agitation to current criteria may be beneficial (Busch *et al.*, 2003). Pharmacological interventions can assist with acute anxiety and agitation, including judicious and closely monitored use of benzodiazepines and second generation hypnotics (Fawcett, 2001). In addition to these methods, close observation either with a one-on-one sitter or via regular checks may be needed. If these capabilities are beyond the detention facility, then transfer to an acute inpatient ward may be needed to stabilize a youth offender who is at immediate risk to him or herself. After acute stabilization, consideration can be given to other pharmacological strategies that may offer longer-term benefits if there is an identifiable psychiatric illness present.

In addition, recent FDA warnings have been added to all SSRIs currently on the market due to evidence that suicidal ideation, without increases in completed suicides, occurred in clinical trials for these agents in pediatric studies for depression. The etiology of this process is unclear, but may be linked to the underlying mood disorder combined with the side effects of these medications. Akathesia, agitation, and anxiety are known effects, and juveniles should be monitored closely when being initiated on these medications. Consensus guidelines on the initiation of SSRIs have been published by the American Academy of Child and Adolescent Psychiatry (AACAP, 2001). Among incarcerated juveniles, close monitoring is even more important, given the high rates of suicidal ideation and attempts that occur while in custody.

Integrated treatment planning

Rational psychopharmacology requires integrated treatment. Using the range of tools available to psychiatry is especially important for juveniles who are incarcerated and need intensive rehabilitation. Recent evidence suggests that using psychotherapy in combination with pharmacology has the best outcomes (Steiner, 2004). Nemeroff and colleagues have found in a long-term study of depressed adults, that those with significant histories of childhood trauma are more likely to respond to structured cognitive–behavioral therapy with or without medications, than to medications alone (Nemeroff *et al.*, 2003). The high rates of trauma and PTSD in the delinquent population (Cauffman *et al.*, 1998; Carrion & Steiner, 2000; Plattner *et al.*, 2003), indicate the need for integrated treatment using multiple modalities. In a parallel vein, the MTA study found that medications alone, or medications and behavioral therapy, yielded better outcomes than behavioral therapy alone, or standard community care in the treatment of ADHD and oppositional-defiant disorder (Arnold *et al.*, 2004). Despite the fact that medication and therapy in the MTA study did not separate from medication alone, combination treatment holds the best promise for juvenile offenders given the nature of delinquency.

Williams and colleagues reported that over half of their sample of incarcerated female adolescents were doubtful about the benefits of psychiatric medications, and that those who had positive prior experiences in treatment were more likely to view pharmacotherapy in a positive light (Williams *et al.*, 1998).

While juveniles lack the full authority to refuse treatment and this authority traditionally resides with their parents or guardians, incarcerated delinquents are in a unique situation whereby court officials usually have the authority to determine medical treatment. In some states, parental consent may be required to enable psychiatric treatment (Arroyo, 2001). Unless the situation is emergent, thought should be given to involving the youth and his or her family in treatment decisions as there is evidence from outpatient studies that family therapy can help in reducing aggression (Nickel *et al.*, 2005). In addition, even though compelling treatment while the youth is incarcerated or detained may be legally and even pragmatically possible, the benefits of long-term treatment are likely to be lost when the youth is released from custody unless a good therapeutic alliance is established. In this model, the juvenile needs to be part of the treatment planning, and will hopefully come to see medications as being helpful for maintaining a better quality of life. The period of time in detention or incarceration might then be seen as a starting point for care, with an aim to reduce psychiatric morbidity in order to reduce recidivism. Psychopharmacology can play an important role in this process, and most especially when the youth offender and his or her family is part of the process and engaged with care in a meaningful way.

Consideration should also be given to developing an outpatient plan as the juvenile approaches a period where they may be paroled or released. The overall decision tree would then culminate with a goal of trying to get the juvenile toward appropriate long-term care. This model then focuses less on the acute management of psychiatric issues, which can easily become the focus within institutional environments, and instead tries to view this system within a broader perspective and more of a rehabilitative model. Figure 15.3 outlines the decision tree and goals for care at each level of an integrated treatment plan.

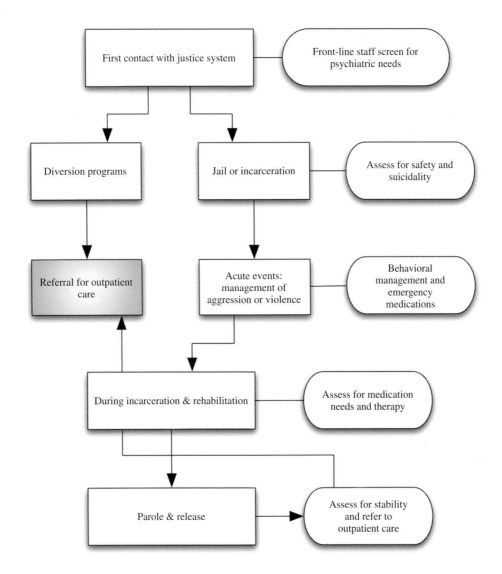

Figure 15.3   Decision tree for integrated treatment planning

Conclusion

Juvenile offenders face an array of psychiatric problems of a multifactorial etiology. Some of these factors can be precipitants of delinquency, while others can be
consequent to incarceration. Prompt assessment and evaluation by trained professionals is an essential component to providing care for juvenile offenders
(Arroyo *et al.*, 2001). The emerging understanding of aggression as one aspect of

delinquency has highlighted two major patterns of aggressive or violent behavior. Differentiating these types of maladaptive aggression is important and can allow better treatment.

As one component of an overall treatment plan, psychopharmacological interventions hold a great deal of promise to improve the lives of youth offenders, and also have the potential to help reduce recidivism by enabling young people to gain better control of their lives. Nevertheless, all medications have risks, and these need to be weighed against the potential benefits in each individual case. Differentiating the reasons for using medications, and the specific targets for treatment can help to allow more prudent and better use of pharmacological interventions. Integrating treatment with psychotherapy and family therapy is also a vital component, especially if these interventions are intended to be lasting parts of the treatment plan for the youth offender.

In all cases, clinicians should strive to use evidenced-based principles for treatment. While many unanswered questions remain in the psychopharmacology of aggression for future randomized controlled studies, multiple consensus papers are available for some guidance (AACAP, 2001; Pappadopulos *et al.*, 2003; Schur *et al.*, 2003; Emslie *et al.*, 2004; Connor *et al.*, 2006; Jensen *et al.*, in press; Steiner *et al.*, 2006). The incarcerated setting offers the opportunity to treat offenders in an optimized quality controlled manner, without externalizing symptoms in juveniles interfering with compliance. The past decade was useful in establishing the nature and extent of disturbances in this population. Now we may proceed to establish evidence-based, or at least practice parameter driven, care in this most difficult population. While there are many political and historical factors contributing to making this a difficult enterprise, we must not cease from bringing modern medicine to those that seem to be most deprived of its benefits.

Notes

An earlier version of this paper was published as Soller *et al.* (2006) Psychopharmacologic treatment in juvenile offenders. The text and tables that appear in this chapter have been revised and updated to reflect the most recent data available at time of publication.

References

AACAP (2001). Practice parameter for the assessment and treatment of children and adolescents with suicidal behavior. *Journal of the American Acadedy of Child and Adolescent Psychiatry*, **40**(7 Suppl), 24S–51S.

Abram, K. M., Teplin, L. A. *et al.* (2003). Comorbid psychiatric disorders in youth in juvenile detention. *Archives of General Psychiatry*, **60**(11), 1097–1108.

Aman, M. G. *et al.* (1991). Clinical effects of methylphenidate and thioridazine in intellectually subaverage children. *Journal of the American Academy of Child and Adolescent Psychiatry*, **30**(2), 246–256.

Aman, M., Buitelaar, J. *et al.* (2005). Pharmacotherapy of disruptive behavior and item changes on a standardized rating scale: pooled analysis of risperidone effects in children with sub-average IQ. *Journal of Child and Adolescent Psychopharmacology*, **15**(2), 220–232.

American Psychiatric Association (2000). *Diagnostic and Statistical Manual of Mental Disorders: DSM-IV-TR*. Washington, DC: American Psychiatric Association.

Armenteros, J. L. & Lewis, J. E. (2002). Citalopram treatment for impulsive aggression in children and adolescents: an open pilot study. *Journal of the American Academy of Child and Adolescent Psychiatry*, **41**(5), 522–529.

Arnold, L. E., Chuang, S. *et al.* (2004). Nine months of multicomponent behavioral treatment for ADHD and effectiveness of MTA fading procedures. *Journal of Abnormal Child Psychology*, **32**(1), 39–51.

Arroyo, W. (2001). Children, adolescents, and families. *Ethics Primer of the American Psychiatric Association*. Washington, DC: American Psychiatric Publishing, Inc., pp. 11–22.

Arroyo, W., Buzogany, W. *et al.* (2001). *Recommendations for Juvenile Justice Reform*. Washington, DC: American Academy of Child and Adolescent Psychiatry.

Battle, A. O., Battle, M. V. *et al.* (1993). Potential for suicide and aggression in delinquents at Juvenile Court in a southern city. *Suicide and Life-Threatening Behavior*, **23**(3), 230–244.

Bernstein, G. A. & Shaw, K. (1997). Practice parameters for the assessment and treatment of children and adolescents with anxiety disorders. American Academy of Child and Adolescent Psychiatry. *Journal of the American Academy of Child and Adolescent Psychiatry*, **36**(10 Suppl), 69S–84S.

Biederman, J., Spencer, T. *et al.* (2005). *Does the Presence of Comorbid ODD Affect Responses to Atomoxetine?* Annual Meeting of the American Psychiatric Association, Atlanta, Georgia.

Blair, J., Taggart, B. *et al.* (2004). Electrocardiographic safety profile and monitoring guidelines in pediatric psychopharmacology. *Journal of Neural Transmission*, **111**(7), 791–815.

Blair, R. J., Coccaro, E. F. *et al.* (2006). Working paper of the AACAP/Stanford/Howard Workgroup on Impulsivity and Aggression. American Academy of Child & Adolescent Psychiatry.

Broche, J. P. (1980). [Use of pimozide (ORAP) in child psychiatry (author's transl)]. *Acta Psychiatrica Belgica*, **80**(3), 341–346.

Buitelaar, J. K., van der Gaag, R. J.*et al.* (1996). Pindolol and methylphenidate in children with attention-deficit hyperactivity disorder. Clinical efficacy and side-effects. *Journal of Child Psychology and Psychiatry*, **37**(5), 587–595.

Busch, K. A., Fawcett, J. *et al.* (2003). Clinical correlates of inpatient suicide. *Journal of Clinical Psychiatry*, **64**(1), 14–19.

Campbell, M., Small, A. M. *et al.* (1984). Behavioral efficacy of haloperidol and lithium carbonate. A comparison in hospitalized aggressive children with conduct disorder. *Archives of General Psychiatry*, **41**(7), 650–656.

Campbell, M., Adams, P. B. *et al.* (1995). Lithium in hospitalized aggressive children with conduct disorder: a double-blind and placebo-controlled study. *Journal of the American Academy of Child and Adolescent Psychiaty*, **34**(4), 445–453.

Carrion, V. G. & H. Steiner (2000). Trauma and dissociation in delinquent adolescents. *Journal of the American Academy of Child and Adolescent Psychiatry*, **39**(3), 353–359.

Cauffman, E., Feldman, S. S. *et al.* (1998). Posttraumatic stress disorder among female juvenile offenders. *Journal of the American Academy of Child and Adolescent Psychiatry*, **37**(11), 1209–1216.

Chang, K., Steiner, H. *et al.* (2003). Studies of offspring of parents with bipolar disorder. *America Journal of Medical Genetics. Part C, Seminars in Medical Genetics*, **123**(1), 26–35.

Cheng-Shannon, J., McGough, J. J. *et al.* (2004). Second-generation antipsychotic medications in children and adolescents. *Journal of Child and Adolescent Psychopharmacology*, **14**(3), 372–394.

Cherek, D. R. *et al.* (2002). Effects of chronic paroxetine administration on measures of aggressive and impulsive responses of adult males with a history of conduct disorder. *Psychopharmacology (Berl)*, **159**(3), 266–274.

Cleckley, H. (1964). *The Mask of Sanity: An Attempt to Clarify Some Issues about the So-Called Psychopathic Personality*. St Louis, MO: Mosby.

Coccaro, E. F., Kavoussi, R. J. & Hauger, R. L. (1997). Serotonin function and antiaggressive response to fluoxetine: a pilot study. *Biological Psychiatry*, **42**(7), 546–552.

Connor, D. F. (2002). *Aggression and Antisocial Behavior in Children and Adolescents: Research and Treatment*. New York, NY: Guilford Press.

Connor, D. F., Ozbayrak, K. R. *et al.* (1997). A pilot study of nadolol for overt aggression in developmentally delayed individuals. *Journal of the American Academy of Child and Adolescent Psychiatry*, **36**(6), 826–834.

Connor, D. F., Glatt, S. J. *et al.* (2002). Psychopharmacology and aggression. I: A meta-analysis of stimulant effects on overt/covert aggression-related behaviors in ADHD. *Journal of the American Academy of Child and Adolescent Psychiatry*, **41**(3), 253–261.

Connor, D. F., Carlson, G. A. *et al.* (2006). Juvenile maladaptive aggression: a review of prevention, treatment, and service configuration and a proposed research agenda. *Journal of Clinical Psychiatry*, **67**(5), 808–820.

Constantino, J. N., Liberman, M. & Kincaid, M. (1997). Effects of serotonin reuptake inhibitors on aggressive behavior in psychiatrically hospitalized adolescents: results of an open trial. *Journal of Child and Adolescent Psychopharmacology*, **7**(1), 31–44.

Croonenberghs, J., Fegert, J. M. *et al.* (2005). Risperidone in children with disruptive behavior disorders and subaverage intelligence: a 1-year, open-label study of 504 patients. *Journal of the American Academy of Child Adolescent Psychiatry*, **44**(1), 64–72.

Cueva, J. E., Overall, J. E. *et al.* (1996). Carbamazepine in aggressive children with conduct disorder: a double-blind and placebo-controlled study. *Journal of the American Academy of Child and Adolescent Psychiatry*, **35**(4), 480–490.

Donovan, S. J., Stewart, J. W. *et al.* (2000). Divalproex treatment for youth with explosive temper and mood lability: a double-blind, placebo-controlled crossover design. *American Journal of Psychiatry*, **157**(5), 818–820.

Edens, J. F., Skeem, J. L. *et al.* (2001). Assessment of "juvenile psychopathy" and its association with violence: a critical review. *Behavioral Sciences and the Law*, **19**(1), 53–80.

Emslie, G. J., Hughes, C. W. *et al.* (2004). A feasibility study of the childhood depression medication algorithm: the Texas Children's Medication Algorithm Project (CMAP). *Journal of the American Academy for Child and Adolescent Psychiatry*, **43**(5), 519–527.

Emslie, G. J., Rush, A. J. *et al.* (1997). A double-blind, randomized, placebo-controlled trial of fluoxetine in children and adolescents with depression. *Archives of General Psychiatry*, **54**(11), 1031–1037.

Farand, L., Chagnon, F. *et al.* (2004). Completed suicides among Quebec adolescents involved with juvenile justice and child welfare services. *Suicide and Life-Threatening Behavior*, **34**(1), 24–35.

Fawcett, J. (2001). Treating impulsivity and anxiety in the suicidal patient. *Annals of the New York Academy of Sciences*, **932**, 94–102; discussion 102–105.

FDA (2004). *FDA Public Health Advisory: Suicidality in Children and Adolescents Being Treated with Antidepressant Medications*. FDA Administration, FDA.

FDA (2005). New warning about ADHD drug. *FDA Consumer*, **39**(2), 3.

Feinstein, R. A., Lampkin, A. *et al.* (1998). Medical status of adolescents at time of admission to a juvenile detention center. *Journal of Adolescent Health*, **22**(3), 190–196.

Findling, R. L., McNamara, N. K. *et al.* (2000). A double-blind pilot study of risperidone in the treatment of conduct disorder. *Journal of the American Academy of Child Adolescent Psychiatry*, **39**(4), 509–516.

Findling, R. L., McNamara, N. K. *et al.* (2003). Combination lithium and divalproex sodium in pediatric bipolarity. *Journal of the American Academy of Child and Adolescent Psychiatry*, **42**(8), 895–901.

Findling, R. L., Aman, M. G. *et al.* (2004). Long-term, open-label study of risperidone in children with severe disruptive behaviors and below-average IQ. *American Journal of Psychiatry*, **161**(4), 677–684.

Findling, R. L., Steiner, H. *et al.* (2005). Use of antipsychotics in children and adolescents. *Journal of Clinical Psychiatry*, **66** (Suppl 7), 29–40.

Findling, R. L., Reed, M. D. *et al.* (2006). Effectiveness, safety, and pharmacokinetics of quetiapine in aggressive children with conduct disorder. *Journal of the American Academy of Child and Adolescent Psychiatry*, **45**(7), 792–800.

Frick, P. J. (2006). Developmental pathways to conduct disorder. *Child and Adolescent Psychiatric Clinics of North America*, **15**(2), 311–331, vii.

Geller, D. A., Wagner, K. D. *et al.* (2004). Paroxetine treatment in children and adolescents with obsessive-compulsive disorder: a randomized, multicenter, double-blind, placebo-controlled trial. *Journal of the American Academy of Child and Adolescent Psychiatry*, **43**(11), 1387–1396.

Gibbons, R. D., Hur, K. *et al.* (2005). The relationship between antidepressant medication use and rate of suicide. *Archives of General Psychiatry*, **62**(2), 165–172.

Greenhill, L. L. *et al.* (1985). Molindone hydrochloride treatment of hospitalized children with conduct disorder. *Journal of Clinical Psychiatry*, **46**(8 Pt 2), 20–25.

Grisso, T., Barnum R. *et al.* (2001). Massachusetts Youth Screening Instrument for mental health needs of juvenile justice youths. *Journal of the American Academy of Child and Adolescent Psychiatry*, **40**(5), 541–548.

Hameer, O. *et al.*(2001). Evaluation of droperidol in the acutely agitated child or adolescent. *Canadian Journal of Psychiatry*, **46**(9), 864–865.

Hazell, P. L. & Stuart, J. E. (2003). A randomized controlled trial of clonidine added to psychostimulant medication for hyperactive and aggressive children. *Journal of the American Academy of Child and Adolescent Psychiatry*, **42**(8), 886–894.

Jensen, P. S., Youngstrom, E. *et al.* (in press). Concensus Report: Impulsive Aggression as a Symptom Across Diagnostic Categories in Child Psychiatry – Implications for Medication Development.'

Joshi, P. T. *et al.* (1998). Use of droperidol in hospitalized children. *Journal of the American Academy of Child and Adolescent Psychiatry*, **37**(2), 228–230.

Kafantaris, V. *et al.* (1992). Carbamazepine in hospitalized aggressive conduct disorder children: an open pilot study. *Psychopharmacol Bull*, **28**(2), 193–199.

Kaplan, S. L. *et al.* (1990). Effects of methylphenidate on adolescents with aggressive conduct disorder and ADDH: a preliminary report. *Journal of the American Academy of Child and Adolescent Psychiatry*, **29**(5), 719–723.

Kaplan, S. L., Heiligenstein, J. *et al.* (2004). Efficacy and safety of atomoxetine in childhood attention-deficit/hyperactivity disorder with comorbid oppositional defiant disorder. *Journal of Attention Disorders*, **8**(2), 45–52.

Karnik, N. S., McMullin, M. A. *et al.* (2006). Disruptive behaviors: conduct and oppositional disorders in adolescents. *Adolescent Medicine Clinics*, **17**(1), 97–114.

Keepers, G. A., Clappison, V. J. *et al.* (1983). Initial anticholinergic prophylaxis for neuroleptic-induced extrapyramidal syndromes. *Archives of General Psychiatry*, **40**(10), 1113–1117.

Keller, M. B., Ryan, N. D. *et al.* (2001). Efficacy of paroxetine in the treatment of adolescent major depression: a randomized, controlled trial. *Journal of the American Academy of Child and Adolescent Psychiatry*, **40**(7), 762–772.

Kemph, J. P. *et al.* (1993). Treatment of aggressive children with clonidine: results of an open pilot study. *Journal of the American Academy of Child and Adolescent Psychiatry*, **32**(3), 577–581.

Kempton, T. & Forehand, R. (1992). Suicide attempts among juvenile delinquents; the contribution of mental health factors. *Behavior Research and Therapy*, **30**(5), 537–541.

King, B. H., Wright, D. M. *et al.* (2001). Case series: amantadine open label treatment of impulsive and aggressive behavior in hospitalized children with developmental disabilities. *Journal of the American Academy of Child and Adolescent Psychiatry*, **40**(6), 654–657.

Klein, R. G. *et al.* (1997). Clinical efficacy of methylphenidate in conduct disorder with and without attention deficit hyperactivity disorder. *Archives of General Psychiatry*, **54**(12), 1073–1080.

Kuperman, S. & Stewart, M. A.(1987). Use of propranolol to decrease aggressive outbursts in younger patients. Open study reveals potentially favorable outcome. *Psychosomatics*, **28**(6), 315–319.

LeBlanc, J. C., Binder, C. E. *et al.* (2005). Risperidone reduces aggression in boys with a disruptive behaviour disorder and below average intelligence quotient: analysis of two placebo-controlled randomized trials. *International Clinical Psychopharmacology*, **20**(5), 275–283.

Lenox, R. H. & Hahn, C. G. (2000). Overview of the mechanism of action of lithium in the brain: fifty-year update. *Journal of Clinical Psychiatry*, **61**(Suppl 9), 5–15.

Malone, R. P., Luebbert, J. *et al.* (1994). The Overt Aggression Scale in a study of lithium in aggressive conduct disorder. *Psychopharmacological Bulletin*, **30**(2), 215–218.

Malone, R. P., Delaney, M. A. *et al.* (2000). A double-blind placebo-controlled study of lithium in hospitalized aggressive children and adolescents with conduct disorder. *Archives of General Psychiatry*, **57**(7), 649–654.

March, J. S., Biederman, J. *et al.* (1998). Sertraline in children and adolescents with obsessive-compulsive disorder: a multicenter randomized controlled trial. *Journal of the American Medical Association*, **280**(20), 1752–1756.

Martin, A. (2003). *Pediatric Psychopharmacology: Principles and Practice*. Oxford, New York: Oxford University Press.

Masi, G., Milone, A. *et al.* (2006). Olanzapine treatment in adolescents with severe conduct disorder. *European Psychiatry*, **21**(1), 51–57.

Mattes, J. A. (1990). Comparative effectiveness of carbamazepine and propranolol for rage outbursts. *Journal of Neuropsychiatry and Clinical Neuroscience*, **2**(2), 159–164.

McCabe, S. E., Teter, C. J. *et al.* (2004). Prevalence and correlates of illicit methylphenidate use among 8th, 10th, and 12th grade students in the United States, 2001. *Journal of Adolescent Health*, **35**(6), 501–504.

McCabe, S. E., Knight, J. R. *et al.* (2005). Non-medical use of prescription stimulants among US college students: prevalence and correlates from a national survey. *Addiction*, **100**(1), 96–106.

McDougle, C. J., Stigler, K. A. *et al.* (2003). Treatment of aggression in children and adolescents with autism and conduct disorder. *Journal of Clinical Psychiatry*, **64** (Suppl 4), 16–25.

Meltzer, H. Y., Rabinowitz, J. *et al.* (1997). Age at onset and gender of schizophrenic patients in relation to neuroleptic resistance. *American Journal of Psychiatry*, **154**(4), 475–482.

Michelson, D., Faries, D. *et al.* (2001). Atomoxetine in the treatment of children and adolescents with attention-deficit/hyperactivity disorder: a randomized, placebo-controlled, dose-response study. *Pediatrics*, **108**(5), E83.

Nemeroff, C. B., Heim, C. M. *et al.* (2003). Differential responses to psychotherapy versus pharmacotherapy in patients with chronic forms of major depression and childhood trauma. *Proceedings of the National Academy of Science USA*, **100**(24), 14293–14296.

Newcorn, J. H., Spencer, T. J. *et al.* (2005). Atomoxetine treatment in children and adolescents with attention-deficit/hyperactivity disorder and comorbid oppositional defiant disorder. *Journal of the American Academy of Child and Adolescent Psychiatry*, **44**(3), 240–248.

Nickel, M. K., Nickel, C. *et al.* (2005). Aggressive female youth benefit from outpatient family therapy: a randomized, prospective, controlled trial. *Pediatrics International*, **47**(2), 167–171.

Pappadopulos, E., Macintyre II, J. C. *et al.* (2003). Treatment recommendations for the use of antipsychotics for aggressive youth (TRAAY). Part II. *Journal of the American Academy of Child and Adolescent Psychiatry*, **42**(2), 145–161.

Pfeffer, C. R., Jiang, H. *et al.* (1997). Buspirone treatment of psychiatrically hospitalized pre-pubertal children with symptoms of anxiety and moderately severe aggression. *Journal of Child and Adolescent Psychopharmacology*, **7**(3), 145–155.

Plattner, B., Silvermann, M. A. *et al.* (2003). Pathways to dissociation: intrafamilial versus extra-familial trauma in juvenile delinquents. *Journal of Nervous and Mental Disease*, **191**(12), 781–788.

Rana, M. & Steiner, H. (2005). *Atomoxetine Decreases RADI (Reactive/Affective/Defensive/Impulsive) Aggression in ADHD*. Annual Meeting of the American Psychiatric Association. Atlanta, Georgia: APA.

Rana, M., Khanzode, L. *et al.* (2005). Divalproex sodium in the treatment of pediatric psychiatric disorders. *Expert Review of Neurotherapeutics*, **5**(2), 165–176.

Rifkin, A., Karajgi, B. *et al.* (1997). Lithium treatment of conduct disorders in adolescents. *American Journal of Psychiatry*, **154**(4), 554–555.

Riggs, P. D., Mikulich, S. K. *et al.* (1997). Fluoxetine in drug-dependent delinquents with major depression: an open trial. *Journal of Child and Adolescent Psychopharmacology*, **7**(2), 87–95.

Ruchkin, V. V., Schwab-Stone, M. *et al.* (2003). Suicidal ideations and attempts in juvenile delinquents. *Journal of Child Psychology and Psychiatry*, **44**(7), 1058–1066.

Saxena, K., Delizonna, L. *et al.* (2005). *Divalproex Sodium in Outpatients with Disruptive Behavior Disorders*. Annual Meeting of the American Psychiatric Association. Atlanta, Georgia: APA.

Saxena, K., Silverman, M. A. *et al.* (2005). Baseline predictors of response to divalproex in conduct disorder. *Journal of Clinical Psychiatry*, **66**(12), 1541–1548.

Schur, S. B., Sikich, L. *et al.* (2003). Treatment recommendations for the use of antipsychotics for aggressive youth (TRAAY). Part I: a review. *Journal of the American Academy of Child and Adolescent Psychiatry*, **42**(2), 132–144.

Schvehla, T. J., Mandoki, M. W.*et al.* (1994). Clonidine therapy for comorbid attention deficit hyperactivity disorder and conduct disorder: preliminary findings in a children's inpatient unit. *Southern Medical Journal*, **87**(7), 692–695

Silver, J. M., Yudofsky S. C. *et al.* (1999). Propranolol treatment of chronically hospitalized aggressive patients. *Journal of Neuropsychiatry and Clinical Neuroscience*, **11**(3), 328–335.

Snyder, R., Turgay, A. *et al.* (2002). Effects of risperidone on conduct and disruptive behavior disorders in children with subaverage IQs. *Journal of the American Academy of Child and Adolescent Psychiatry*, **41**(9), 1026–1036.

Soderstrom, H., Rastam, M. & Gillberg, C. (2002). A clinical case series of six extremely aggressive youths treated with olanzapine. *European Child and Adolescent Psychiatry*, **11**(3), 138–141.

Soller, M. V., Karnik, N. S. *et al.* (2006). Psychopharmacologic treatment in juvenile offenders. *Child and Adolescent Psychiatric Clinics of North America*, **15**(2), 477–499.

Stanislav, S. W., Fabre, T. *et al.* (1994). Buspirone's efficacy in organic-induced aggression. *Journal of Clinical Psychopharmacology*, **14**(2), 126–130.

Steiner, H. (2004). *Handbook of Mental Health Interventions in Children and Adolescents: an Integrated Developmental Approach*. San Francisco, CA: Jossey-Bass Publishers.

Steiner, H. (2005). *Primary and Secondary Disorders of Aggression in Youth: Mood Stabilizers, Atypicals, and Stimulants*. Annual Meeting of the American Psychiatric Association. Atlanta, Georgia: APA.

Steiner, H. & Cauffman, E. (1998). Juvenile justice, delinquency, and psychiatry. *Child and Adolescent Psychiatric Clinics of North America*, **7**(3), 653–672.

Steiner, H., Petersen, M. L. *et al.* (2003a). Divalproex sodium for the treatment of conduct disorder: a randomized controlled clinical trial. *Journal of Clinical Psychiatry*, **64**(10), 1183–1191.

Steiner, H., Saxena, K. *et al.* (2003b). Psychopharmacologic strategies for the treatment of aggression in juveniles. *CNS Spectrums*, **8**(4), 298–308.

Steiner, H., Delizonna, L. *et al.* (2005). *Does the Two-Factor Model of Aggression Hold Incarcerated Delinquents?* Annual Meeting of the American Psychiatric Association. Atlanta, Georgia: APA.

Steiner, H., Blair, R. J. *et al.* (2006). Working Paper of the AACAP/Stanford/Howard Workgroup on Impulsivity and Aggression. American Academy of Child and Adolescent Psychiatry.

Stephens, R. J., Bassel, C. & Sandor, P. (2004). Olanzapine in the treatment of aggression and tics in children with Tourette's syndrome – a pilot study. *Journal of Child and Adolescent Psychopharmacology*, **14**(2), 255–266.

Teplin, L. A., Abram, K. M. *et al.* (2002). Psychiatric disorders in youth in juvenile detention. *Archives of General Psychiatry*, **59**(12), 1133–1143.

Teter, C. J., McCabe, S. E. *et al.* (2003). Illicit methylphenidate use in an undergraduate student sample: prevalence and risk factors. *Pharmacotherapy*, **23**(5), 609–617.

Thomas, C. R. & Penn, J. V. (2002). Juvenile justice mental health services. *Child and Adolescent Psychiatric Clinics of North America*, **11**(4), 731–748.

Vermeiren, R. (2003). Psychopathology and delinquency in adolescents: a descriptive and developmental perspective. *Clinical Psychology Reviews*, **23**(2), 277–318.

Vermeiren, R., Jespers, I. *et al.* (2006). Mental health problems in juvenile justice populations. *Child and Adolescent Psychiatric Clinics of North America*, **15**(2), 333–351, vii–viii.

Vitiello, B. & Stoff, D. M. (1997). Subtypes of aggression and their relevance to child psychiatry. Journal of the American Academy of Child and Adolescent Psychiatry, **36**(3), 307–315.

Vitiello, B., Behar, D. *et al.* (1990). Subtyping aggression in children and adolescents. *Journal of Neuropsychiatry and Clinical Neuroscience*, **2**(2), 189–192.

Vitiello, B., Hill, J. L. *et al.* (1991). P.r.n. medications in child psychiatric patients: a pilot placebo-controlled study. *Journal of Clinical Psychiatry*, **52**(12), 499–501.

Wagner, K. D. (2005). Pharmacotherapy for major depression in children and adolescents. *Progress in Neuropsychopharmacology and Biological Psychiatry*, **29**(5), 819–826.

Wagner, K. D., Berard, R. *et al.* (2004a). A multicenter, randomized, double-blind, placebo-controlled trial of paroxetine in children and adolescents with social anxiety disorder. *Archives of General Psychiatry*, **61**(11), 1153–1162.

Wagner, K. D., Robb, A. S. *et al.* (2004b). A randomized, placebo-controlled trial of citalopram for the treatment of major depression in children and adolescents. *American Journal of Psychiatry*, **161**(6), 1079–1083.

Wasserman, G. A., McReynolds, L. S. *et al.* (2003). Psychiatric disorders in incarcerated youths. *Journal of the American Academy of Child and Adolescent Psychiatry*, **42**(9), 1011.

Williams, R. A., Hollis, H. M. *et al.* (1998). Attitudes toward psychiatric medications among incarcerated female adolescents. *Journal of the American Academy of Child and Adolescent Psychiatry*, **37**(12), 1301–1307.

Wilson, J. J., Karnik, N. S. *et al.* (in press). Substance Dependence and Psychopathology among Incarcerated Adolescents.

World Health Organization (1992). *The ICD-10 Classification of Mental and Behavioural Disorders: Clinical Descriptions and Diagnostic Guidelines.* Geneva: World Health Organization.

Zubieta, J. K. & Alessi, N. E. (1992). Acute and chronic administration of trazodone in the treatment of disruptive behavior disorders in children. *Journal of Clinical Psychopharmacology*, **54**(12), 346–351.

16

Evidence-based treatment for justice-involved youth

Eric Trupin

The past ten years have seen a rapid increase in the development of evidence-based interventions for youth; however, many challenges remain. These factors include the challenges associated with service delivery, the importance of initial engagement, and the complex nature of the problem (Wasserman *et al.*, 2000). On the other hand, treatment research in this area (and the more global child and adolescent treatment research) has moved considerably toward recognizing the need for "empirically supported" treatment. In 1995, the American Psychological Association Division 12 Task Force on Promotion and Dissemination of Psychological Procedures was charged with the task of identifying treatment approaches with demonstrated "efficacy." Efficacy refers to the ability to bring about the desired change under ideal conditions, and an efficacious program is one with scientific evidence demonstrating positive changes among those who receive the treatment. This term is contrasted with the word "effective," which refers to the likelihood that a person will comply with a given treatment. An effective program has the ability to produce positive change in the general population. In a comprehensive review of the literature, the APA's Task Force (Levant, 1995) established the validity of numerous treatment approaches. They applied the terms "empirically validated" or "empirically supported" and "probably efficacious" to represent therapeutic approaches with varying degrees of scientific evidence.

The list of therapies deemed valid or "well-established" and probably efficacious was updated in 1998 (Chambless *et al.*, 1998) and again in 2001 (Chambless & Ollendick, 2001). O'Donohue, Buchanan and Fisher (2000) provided a synthesis of the characteristics associated with empirically supported treatment. They agreed empirically supported treatments should have:

(a) a skill development focus;
(b) a problem-focus;
(c) continuous assessment of progress;
(d) some type of homework/out-of-session work; and
(e) a recognition of the importance of the therapeutic relationship.

The Mental Health Needs of Young Offenders: Forging Paths toward Reintegration and Rehabilitation, eds. Carol L. Kessler and Louis J. Kraus. Published by Cambridge University Press. © Cambridge University Press 2007.

Most empirically-supported treatments focus on specific risk factors for delinquency, as well as systemic and behavioral targets of the youth and family. The identification of risk factors for youth involved in the juvenile justice system requires both a life-span and an ecological perspective. In a comprehensive review of risk factors for youth violence, Hawkins *et al.* (2000) identified risk factors from a developmental perspective, as well as from an ecological or systems point of view. Risk factor identification begins with the recognition that prenatal exposure to teratogens (e.g., tobacco, alcohol, and illicit drugs) is a risk factor for poor fetal growth and neurodevelopmental impairment. Complications during pregnancy have been found to be associated with violent offenders (Kandel & Mednick, 1991). Significant stressors in the home and in particular the synergistic effects of multiple stressors (e.g., unemployment, housing conditions, and family/marital discord) are associated with poor parenting practices. Parents' ability to monitor and provide structure for their children presents as a significant risk factor beginning in early childhood. These stressors are also associated with poor maternal life outcomes with the end result of multiple successive births to families with limited financial and social supports.

A meta-analysis of treatment outcome studies for children and adolescents provided additional support for behaviorally- and parent-focused intervention for children and adolescents (Weisz *et al.*, 1995).

Research on empirically supported treatments (ESTs) has resulted in positive changes in the psychotherapy field, including the integration of curricula on ESTs in training programs (Chambless & Ollendick, 2001). However, this research has also been instrumental in suggesting a framework for evaluating programs. For example, a well-established program must have at least two randomized controlled trials (RCTs) demonstrating that it will result in the desired outcomes compared with a control condition (placebo or wait-list control). In some cases, a large series of rigorous single-case studies are accepted as meeting the minimum criteria. To receive this classification, a program must use a treatment manual or well-specified protocol, specify the characteristics of the sample, and result in the desired outcomes by at least two different research teams (Chambless & Ollendick, 2001). Treatments placed in a validated, but less well-established category ("probably efficacious") must have at least one RCT demonstrating superiority of the treatment over a control condition or a small series of single-case studies. Programs deemed "promising" have some evidence (e.g., a case series) indicating improvements attributable to the treatment approach. Although this framework has been criticized on a number of dimensions (e.g., heavy emphasis on quantitative data; Chambless & Ollendick, 2001), few can argue against the value of contrasting treatment approaches to distill the components necessary for desired change.

Treatment can and should occur at different stages. In this chapter we will pinpoint the conceptual foundations and treatment strategies for early intervention, and community-based treatment programs, and will provide case examples illustrating the unique features of each approach. In addition, we will present two promising transition programs with implications for treatment of youth in secure programs prior to their participation in community-based aftercare treatments.

Early intervention and community-based treatment programs are intended to provide alternatives to secure facilities for juveniles involved in criminal activity. These approaches are analogous to strategies used in public health to prevent, control, and reduce the impact of illness on quality of life, morbidity, and mortality.

Program classifications

Early intervention

Early intervention programs primarily seek to identify and counter negative influences in youths' lives that are likely to lead to escalated antisocial behavior and are typically applied to youth prior to incarceration in secure facilities. Two examples of early intervention programs include diversion programs and mentoring programs.

Diversion programs

Diversion programs are designed to minimize the negative impacts of incarceration, such as stigmatization and negative peer relationships, by diverting youth involved in first-time or misdemeanor crimes from entering secure facilities (Shelden, 1999). The tenets of this early intervention approach are based on labeling research (Schur, 1971). This research suggests that labeling behaviors as deviant creates a class of individuals who are deemed "outsiders" as a result of engaging in behaviors that are outside the norm of appropriate behavior (Schur, 1971). "Outsiders" are more likely to continue engaging in antisocial behaviors as a result of how others react or label their behaviors. Research also shows that association with a negative peer group, as is the case in incarceration settings, plays a key role in the escalation of an existing delinquency problem (Elliot, Huizinga, & Ageton, 1985).

Key intervention strategies and targets for change

Diversion programs target youth with minor offenses (e.g., truancy, shoplifting) and aim to stop future recidivism by targeting specific risk factors for recidivism such as parent–child relations, youth self-esteem, and youth decision-making.

Parents, teachers, and correctional staff refer youth to diversion programs if the youth appears to be at risk for continued criminal behavior. Referrals can occur either before or during the adjudication process. Once referred, the youth and family become involved in a number of different activities. Common elements in diversion programs include a diagnostic assessment, counseling, tutoring, job training, community service restitution, and substance abuse treatment. Youth participate in psychoeducational treatment groups to learn anger management, conflict resolution, decision-making, substance abuse, peer pressure, and self-esteem. Parents can also receive training in parenting styles and decision-making. The family receives training as a relational unit in communication. The length of treatment can vary from four weeks to six months (Davidson *et al.*, 1985). Many programs are associated with the 4-H organization (Cummings & Clark, 1993). If the youth successfully completes the diversion program, his/her criminal charges are suspended.

Evaluation

There is conflicting evidence on the efficacy of diversion programs. Early diversion programs were found to actually increase recidivism and perceived labeling (Polk, 1995). However, later programs have shown more success. The Washington State Institute for Public Policy (WSIPP) found a Washington-based diversion program to have significant effects in reducing recidivism. This program features community members, family members, a youth counselor, and the youth developing the youth's treatment plan, which can include community service, restitution, and/or counseling. Research by WSIPP for this program suggested a significant (5.1 percent) drop in recidivism at six months post-program completion for participants compared to their recidivism rates established prior to completing the program, as well as substantial cost-savings to taxpayers in the amount of $2,775 per participant (Barnoski, 1997).

In a study examining the effectiveness of Back-on-Track, an after-school diversion program that uses a multimodal approach for the treatment of early-career juvenile offenders, Myers *et al.* (2000) found program completers were significantly less likely than matched controls to have committed subsequent criminal offenses at 12 months. In addition, they have significantly fewer subsequent criminal charges at 9- and 12-month follow-up intervals than the control group. However, generalizability remains an issue as dropout rates continue to be high (27 percent) after enrollment.

Predictors and correlates of success

Diversion programs continue to be popular alternatives to incarceration for many reasons, including active involvement from community members and families in solving problems of delinquency and the emphasis on restorative justice. However, there are a number of limitations to diversion programs. Before entering a diversion program, youth must admit guilt to the crime and agree to the terms of the diversion program. Youth who are unwilling or unable to complete the requirements of the diversion programs or who reoffend must return to court for sentencing and detention. Little formal emphasis is placed upon motivation or commitment strategies to encourage youth and families to remain in the programs when difficulties arise. In addition, family involvement is essential and often mandatory in most diversion programs, so when parents or family members refuse to engage or are unable to support their child in the program, the youth is often unable to complete the program as well.

Mentoring programs

Mentoring programs endeavor to provide youth with adult role models to serve both a supportive and an advocacy function. This approach is based loosely on the modeling component of social cognitive theory (Bandura, 1985), although it originated in the late 19th century as an extension of the "friendly visitor" model (Grossman & Garry, 1997). Adult role models establish relationships with youth to model and reinforce positive development in all domains of life (school, sports, career, art, and family). The Big Brothers Big Sisters of America (BBBS) programs are among the most widely known examples of mentoring programs, and include perhaps the clearest understanding of program parameters which include:

- complete orientation for all volunteers
- volunteer screening including written applications, background checks, extensive interviewing, and a home assessment
- youth assessment, including written applications, child and parent interviews, and a home assessment
- matching protocols that consider the need of the youth, abilities of volunteers, preferences of the parent, and capacity of program staff
- supervision of the volunteers via contacts with parents, volunteers, and youth at regular intervals during the program.

Key intervention strategies and targets for change

Younger adolescents (c.12 years) are referred to mentoring programs when they have begun to exhibit delinquent behavior and are deemed at risk for continued delinquency. In a large evaluation of the JUMP initiative, Novotney and colleagues (2000) reported that the most prominent risk factors across 7399 youth included school problems (69 percent; e.g., poor grades, school behavior), social/family problems (54 percent), and delinquency (13 percent; fighting). Alcohol, nicotine, and drug use were not prevalent in this population (2.35 percent, 2.1 percent and

3 percent respectively). Teen pregnancy was also very low (1.5 percent among females); the latter factors reflecting the early intervention nature of mentoring programs.

Services are delivered by volunteers who interact regularly and build relationships with a single youth. Typically, the mentoring relationship lasts approximately one year.

Evaluation

The BBBS program has assessed the outcomes of youth who have participated in their programs compared to their non-participating peers. After 18 months, participating youth showed significant decreases in drug use and assaultive behavior and increases in successful academic behavior, attitudes, and relationships with parents and peers (McGill, Mihalic & Grotpeter, 1998). In addition, preliminary reports indicate other mentoring programs can reduce recidivism (Barnoski, 2002a). Future reports may indicate significant cost-savings for these types of programs.

Predictors and correlates of success

Limitations of mentoring programs include the unavailability of adult mentors for the vast numbers of youth seeking this type of supportive relationship (Novotney et al., 2000). This is particularly true for male mentors. To counter this limitation, programs are beginning to partner with businesses and encourage employers to grant leave time to their employees to participate in mentoring programs (Davidson et al., 1990). Another limitation is the lack of specificity of treatment targets. Mentoring programs recruit and train mentors yet most programs do not specify how treatment should be delivered or the content of the mentoring sessions. Programs may vary widely and process evaluation measures, besides matching and satisfaction, are left unspecified.

The success of mentoring programs is contingent on the strength of the mentor–mentee relationship. This requires matching youth and adults on characteristics that are deemed important for effective mentoring. Among the characteristics found most important are matching by gender and ethnicity, and the length of commitment on the part of the mentor (Novotney et al., 2000). In their evaluation of several mentoring programs associated with the JUMP initiative, Novotney and colleagues found equivalent satisfaction levels without gender matching, but same-sex matching resulted in improvements in gang and drug avoidance.

The success of these programs at this time seems heavily dependent on demonstrated quality recruitment methods from churches and other pro-social environments, as well as the early intervention to low-risk clients to affect behavior change prior to the development of long-term or entrenched behavior patterns.

Community-based treatment programs

Community-based treatment programs provide rehabilitative services to youth and families in the home and community, primarily as an alternative to incarceration in secure settings. This type of service delivery represents a shift from previous responses to juvenile crime including punitive approaches or individualized treatment in an office or institutional setting. This shift is accompanied by a change in attitude toward families, from that of a dysfunctional cause of the child's psychopathology to an effective partner with professionals (Duchnowski *et al.*, 2000). Two types of community-based programs include multisystemic therapy (MST) and functional family therapy (FFT).

Multisystemic therapy

Multisystemic therapy is based on systems theory and the theory of social ecology. Multisystemic therapy services are individualized to the characteristics and behaviors of each individual and his/her particular social ecology with assessment and intervention occurring in the natural ecology. Services are delivered in the home, school, and community (Schoenwald & Rowland, 2002).

Key intervention strategies and targets for change

MST targets youth engaged in serious antisocial behavior and their families. Ongoing research is examining the effects of MST on youth with a variety of serious emotional disorders and emotional problems (Schoenwald & Rowland, 2002). Multisystemic therapy employs several different types of interventions integrated from structural and strategic family therapies, parent management techniques, cognitive behavior therapy, and problem-focused interventions at the system level. It targets and incorporates multiple systems including the family, school, community, church, and peer groups, relying heavily on initial and continued commitment strategies to engage and motivate stakeholders in the youth's treatment.

Multisystemic therapy services are provided for three–five months per family depending on the seriousness of the problems and the success of the interventions. Therapists, typically master's-level or highly skilled bachelor's-level individuals, are available to their clients 24 hours a day, 7 days a week, and each therapist works with only four–five families at a time. Frequency, duration, and intensity of the treatment varies in accordance with the needs of each family (Schoenwald & Rowland, 2002). Individual therapy for adolescent substance use or mental illness are provided if ecological change does not result in a reduction of substance use and psychiatric symptoms, or if improvements in the ecology are impeded by the youth's substance use or psychiatric symptoms.

Treatment goals are developed in collaboration with the family, and family strengths are built upon and used as primary change agents. The overarching goals of MST are to reduce the rates of antisocial behavior in the youth, reduce out-of-home placements, and empower families to resolve future difficulties.

Evaluation

Since the completion of early studies indicating favorable effects of MST (Henggeler *et al.*, 1986, Brunk *et al.*, 1987), there have been larger, more recent randomized clinical trials documenting the clinical effectiveness and cost-effectiveness of MST with youth who engage in serious antisocial behavior. In a randomized study comparing MST with individual therapy, Borduin *et al.* (1995) found that youth who received MST were significantly less likely to be rearrested than those who received individual counseling. For those who did recidivate, MST youths were less likely to be arrested for violent crimes and drug offenses. Results from a randomized study by Henggeler *et al.* (1992) showed that MST was effective at reducing rates of criminal activity and institutionalization. In addition, families that received MST reported increased family cohesion and decreased adolescent aggression with peers in comparison with the comparison group. Results from various studies also indicate that MST may be more cost-effective than traditional services (Schoenwald *et al.*, 1996; Washington Institute for Public Policy, 1998).

Predictors and correlates of success

A large factor in MST's success is the emphasis on quality assurance and account-ability of therapists for outcomes. Significant resources are devoted to ongoing therapist training and clinical consultation to maintain treatment integrity and fidelity. Multisystemic therapy therapists are clinically supervised on a routine basis, and are held responsible for achieving outcomes within families by contin-uous engagement and the removal of barriers to success. A major goal of clinical supervision is to continually assess the effects of therapist interventions on the family in order to make adjustments in the treatment plan to fit the needs of the family (Henggler & Borduin, 1995).

Functional family therapy

Although commonly used as an intervention program, Functional family therapy (FFT) is considered by some as a prevention approach to reduce the likelihood of violent and serious offending (Wasserman *et al.*, 2000). Functional family therapy is a family behavioral intervention that employs well-established techniques from applied behavior analysis (Sulzer-Azaroff & Mayer, 1977) to increase family communication and improve problem-solving abilities. Functional family therapy has been implemented in a variety of treatment settings with demonstrated efficacy.

Key intervention strategies and targets for change

Target populations range from at-risk pre-adolescents to youth with very serious problems such as conduct disorder, violent acting-out, and substance abuse. While FFT targets youth aged 11–18, younger siblings of referred adolescents often become part of the intervention process.

A major goal of FFT is to use specific skills such as reframing to improve family communication while decreasing negativity and blaming between family members. The family is treated as a whole, so that both strengths and problems within the family are attributed as relational issues, instead of sole issues of particular individuals. Specific techniques used in FFT include contingency management and contracting, token economy, and social reinforcement. Parents are taught how to establish and communicate clear rules and consequences for their child's behavior by creating contracts that link prosocial child behavior with specific rewards. A token economy (a point system used to monitor prosocial behavior in exchange for additional privileges) is often used to provide a link between behaviors and consequences.

The FFT intervention is typically spread over a three-month period and the intensity of services varies depending on the needs of the family. On average, eight–twelve sessions are provided for mild cases and up to 30 hours of direct service (e.g., clinical sessions, telephone calls, and meetings) are provided for more difficult cases (Sexton & Alexander, 2000). Functional family therapy therapists pay particular interest in building "balanced alliances" with all family members to avoid the appearance of siding with one family member or another. Goals for treatment are based upon the goals of the family, and the therapist assists the family in achieving "small obtainable changes" in order to introduce successes into the family (Alexander & Parsons, 1982). The FFT program is divided into four distinct phases:

(1) Introduction or impression
(2) Motivation
(3) Behavior change
(4) Generalization.

Treatment goals are developed for each family and must be "matched" to the family culturally and contextually, taking into consideration the values and norms of the family, as well as the phase of treatment in which the family is participating (Alexander & Parsons, 1982).

Evaluation

Results from both randomized trials and non-randomized comparison group studies indicate that FFT significantly reduces recidivism for various juvenile offense patterns (Alexander *et al.*, 2000). In a summary of outcome findings from FFT studies conducted over the last 30 years, Sexton and Alexander (2000) report that FFT can reduce adolescent rearrest rates by 20–60 percent when compared with no treatment, other family therapy interventions, and traditional juvenile court services.

Predictors and correlates of success

As with MST, FFT places a high priority on quality assurance measures and outcome evaluation. A significant factor in FFT's success is the emphasis on adherence, fidelity, and clinical consultation for therapists. This includes adherence measures for in-session characteristics as well as family interaction processes, leading the FFT program to produce therapists who can demonstrate sensitivity as well as the ability to focus and structure family contacts in order to produce the best outcomes.

Multidimensional treatment foster care

Multidimensional treatment foster care (MTFC) is a model that has demonstrated effectiveness with severely emotionally disturbed, antisocial children and adolescents who would otherwise be treated in group care (Chamberlain & Reid, 1998). The philosophy behind MTFC is that the most effective treatment for youth who exhibit antisocial behavior is likely to take place in a family environment in which systematic control is exercised over the contingencies governing the youth's behavior. Multidimensional treatment foster care parents are the primary treatment agents for youth in the program, and the youth's own biological/ step/adoptive/relative families participate in the treatment in preparation for reunification with their child at the program's end (Fisher & Chamberlain, 2000).

Key intervention strategies and targets for change

The objectives of the MTFC program are to provide youth with close supervision, fair and consistent limits, predictable consequences for rule breaking, a supportive relationship with at least one mentoring adult, and limited exposure and access to delinquent peers (Fisher & Chamberlain, 2000). There are three primary mechanisms within the model that contribute to positive outcomes:
(1) proactive approach to reducing problem behaviors;
(2) implementation of an individualized behavior management system within the foster home; and
(3) separation and stratification of members of the treatment team including behavior support specialists, youth therapists, consulting psychiatrists, case managers, and clinical supervisors (Fisher & Chamberlain, 2000).

In addition, the unification plan to ultimately unite the youth with the biological family occurs through the provision of family therapy to the biological family and by teaching the interventions used in MTFC to the biological parents. Closely supervised home visits are conducted throughout the youth's MFTC placement, and the biological parents are encouraged to have frequent contact with the program regarding their child's progress (Chamberlain & Mihalic, 1998).

Evaluation

Evaluations of MTFC youth compared with non-participating control youth indicate a reduction in incarceration days, arrest rates, runaway behaviors, hard drug use, and quicker community placement rates from secure settings (Chamberlain & Mihalic, 1998). Other evaluations on therapeutic foster care (TFC) programs indicate TFCs to be cost-effective as a result of the above-mentioned outcomes. Research also shows some TFC programs to increase the treatment program completion rates (Chamberlain, 1998).

Promising programs

In addition to the empirically supported program examples mentioned (diversion, mentoring, multisystemic therapy, functional family therapy, and multidimensional treatment foster care), we would like to introduce two promising programs for juveniles that have some evidence indicating improvements attributable to the treatment approach: family integrated therapy (FIT) and dialectical behavior therapy (DBT).

Family integrated therapy

This treatment project is currently being piloted in Washington State, and is designed to transition high-risk, high-need juvenile offenders with co-occurring disorders of mental illness and chemical dependency from secure facilities back into their home communities. The program is based upon multisystemic therapy (MST), providing ecological interventions to the youth and family, but incorporates components from motivational enhancement therapy (MET) and dialectical behavior therapy (DBT). Youth receive intensive family- and community-based treatment targeted at the multiple determinants of serious antisocial behavior by individual providers who are available 24 hours per day, 7 days per week. The program strives to promote behavior change in the youth's home environment, emphasizing the systemic strengths of family, peers, school, and neighborhoods to facilitate change. This intervention stresses the transition process and begins during the youth's final two months in the secure residential setting, and continues for four–six months while the youth is under parole supervision.

Predictors and correlates of success

Like MST and FFT programs, family integrated therapy also places a high emphasis on therapist and program adherence and fidelity, and is currently piloting a
therapist-adherence measure. This tool objectively measures therapist effectiveness from the perspective of the family. The first results show the therapists
assessed are adhering to MST principles at a level consistent with achieving
positive outcomes. Families report FIT therapists are conducting productive
sessions, are engaging families in problem-solving, and are improving the ways
families interact with each other.

Perhaps one of the finest aspects of this program is the emphasis placed on
motivation and engagement of families. This program specifically targets juveniles
who represent the most high risk for recidivism and the most complex treatment
needs: co-occurring mental illness and chemical dependency. For many reasons,
the families of these youth are very difficult to engage in treatment and community
intervention. This has prompted FIT therapists to become very persistent, persua-
sive, and creative in creating hope and motivating families to engage in the treatment process. A continual assessment method is used to first assess what factors
motivate the family in order for therapists to get a "foot in the door," and then
joint assessment with the family and in clinical consultation is used to determine
treatment planning.

Preliminary reports regarding engagement indicate the FIT program is demonstrating success in engaging families to at least participate in the program, which is
very promising for this population. Future studies will indicate whether or not
decreases in criminal behavior, substance use, mental health symptomotology;
increases in school and work participation; relationship improvements; and general quality of life improvements; will be present.

Dialectical behavior therapy

Dialectical behavior therapy (DBT) is empirically supported for treatment of
borderline personality disorder in the adult female population (Koons *et al.*,
2001; Evans *et al.*, 1999; Linehan *et al.*, 1999; Linehan *et al.*, 1991); however, for
many reasons, DBT is being tested and implemented in an "off-the-shelf" fashion
for a variety of different populations. One population for which the use of DBT has
produced promising data is in the treatment of mentally ill juvenile offenders in
secure settings.

The symptoms for borderline personality disorder which DBT is highly effective
in treating include parasuicidal and suicidal behavior, and emotional dysregulation, or "high emotional vulnerability plus an inability to regulate emotions"
(Linehan, 1993). Individuals suffering from emotional dysregulation have the
following traits:

- quick emotional reactions
- easily provoked into emotional reactions
- extreme and intense emotional reactions to cues
- slow return to emotional baseline.

Mentally ill youth in secure settings demonstrate many of the same characteristics and symptoms as adults with borderline personality disorder. These youth demonstrate a continued inability to stabilize or regulate their own behavior, and do not respond to traditional behavioral interventions. These youth often engage in impulsive and reckless behaviors including suicide attempts, parasuicidal behaviors, assault, and excessive property damage. It should be noted that many of these youth demonstrate behaviors that would warrant inpatient psychiatric care were they to remain in the community.

Because the numbers of assaults and parasuicidal behaviors had significantly increased in one Washington State secure juvenile facility, the program received resources to implement dialectical behavior therapy to train staff to respond effectively and therapeutically to these specific behaviors. Dialectical behavior therapy incorporates a broad array of cognitive behavioral strategies and has been shown to be highly effective in the reduction of suicidal and self-mutilating behaviors, as well as other typical problems of borderline personality disorders and other mental illness. Though DBT is a validated outpatient model, the Washington juvenile program effectively modified aspects of the treatment for a secure residential setting. The use of behavioral analysis to identify drivers of specific behaviors, individual counseling, contingency management, and skills groups in emotion regulation, interpersonal effectiveness, distress tolerance, and mindfulness are integrated components of this program. Bachelor's-level staff were able to implement the program because of the user-friendly assessment method (behavioral analysis) and a manualized skill set; however, regular training and consultation from DBT experts to refine clinical concepts of contingency management, targeting behaviors, and treatment planning was essential to successful implementation.

Predictors and correlates of success

Results indicate significant decreases in the number of parasuicidal behaviors, assaults, and general behavior problems in the mentally ill population in this program, as well as a decrease in the use of punitive responses by staff (Trupin *et al.*, 2002). In addition, preliminary reports indicate this DBT program reduces recidivism in mentally ill juveniles (Barnoski, 2002b). This research will be continued to determine if significant cost-savings are also associated with the DBT program.

A major strength and probable predictor of the success of this program is the ongoing consultation and training for direct-care staff from DBT experts. While

Table 16.1. Treatment approaches and their respective frameworks, goals, targets, and intervention strategies

Treatment	Theoretical framework	Goals for treatment	Intervention strategies	Evidence of outcomes
Diversion programs	• Labeling research	• Identify and counter negative influences leading to antisocial behavior • Reduce recidivism • Reduce number of offenses • Reduce cost to justice system • Minimize stigma	• Community-involved treatment planning • Psychoeducational treatment groups (anger management, decision-making, communication skills) • Parent groups • Individual specialized treatment (mental health, chemical dependency) • Youth job placement, restitution, and community service	• Fixed evaluations of efficacy • Lowered recidivism rates in most recent studies • Substantial cost savings • Dropout rates a concern
Mentoring programs	• Role modeling (a component of social cognitive theory)	• Reduce delinquency and gang involvement • Reduce school dropout • Improve academic performance	• One-to-one mentoring with a supportive adult, preferably matched to youth based on gender and ethnicity • Reinforcement of positive development in all life domains (school, sports, family, etc.)	• Few outcome studies performed • One study shows decreases in drug use and assault • Preliminary reports indicate cost-effectiveness
Functional family therapy	• Applied behavior analysis	• Refocus problem definition • Reduce negativity and blaming within family • Increase hope • Understand family contexts • Obtain small obtainable changes • Motivation of family to participate in treatment	• Parent–child contracting • Teaching problem-solving skills • Family-centered goal development • Match interventions to family • Constant assessment • Reframing • Introducing therapeutic themes • Teaching family communication skills	• Reduced rearrest rates • Reduced recidivism • Increased family cohesion

Table 16.1. (cont.)

Treatment	Theoretical framework	Goals for treatment	Intervention strategies	Evidence of outcomes
Multisystemic therapy	• Family systems theory • Social ecology theory	• Reduce out-of-home placements • Reduce serious antisocial behavior • Decrease emotional disorders and problems • Empower families to resolve difficulties	• Involvement of multiple systems for change (school, family, work, peers, church) • 5:1 family/therapist ratios • Family-driven goal development • Problem-focused interventions • Parent management skills • Cognitive–behavioral techniques • Consistent assessment • Commitment and motivation strategies • Individual therapy for specialized treatment areas (mental health, substance abuse)	• Decreased arrest rates • Reduced rates of criminal activity and institutional placements • Increased family cohesion • Decreased youth aggression • Demonstrated cost-effectiveness
Multidisciplinary treatment foster care	• Family systems theory	• Decrease youth aggression • Decrease recidivism • Reducing problem behaviors • Family reunification	• Contingency management • Family therapy • Limited access to delinquent peers • Individualized behavior management programs	• Reduction in incarceration days, arrest rates and runaway behaviors • Decrease in drug use

Model	Theory	Goals	Treatment components	Outcomes
			• Educational groups (anger management, decision-making, alcohol/drug education, self-esteem) • Involvement of tertiary providers in treatment planning and implementation	• Quicker community placement rates from secure settings • Cost-effectiveness • Increase in treatment completion rates
Family integrated therapy	• Family systems theory • Social ecology theory	• Reduce out-of-home placements • Reduce serious antisocial behavior • Decrease emotional disorders and problems • Decrease substance abuse • Empower families to resolve difficulties	• Constant systems and individual analysis • Involvement of multiple systems for change (school, family, work, peers, church) • Parent management skills • Motivation and engagement strategies • Building of community connections to family • Contingency management • Skills training • Individual treatment for specialized needs	• Promising results: decreased chemical use, mental health symptomotology, parole revocations, increased school and work performance, improved social functioning, decreased recidivism
Dialectical behavior therapy	• Cognitive–behavioral theory	• Reduction in suicidal and parasuicidal behaviors • Increase in emotion regulation • Increase in skill acquisition and use	• Skills groups • Contingency management • Individual therapy • Consultation to the client	• Promising results: decreased suicidal behavior, assault • Increased ability to participate in treatment programs

an adherence tool does not exist for DBT yet, the consistent use of trained DBT consultants is essential to achieve successful outcomes for clients. In addition, the understanding and support for the DBT model from high- and mid-level administrators and managers in this program represents their use of effective strategies to overcome barriers to successful implementation of DBT (Swenson, Torrey & Koerner, 2002). DBT has been modified for other juvenile populations, with promising results (Miller *et. al.*, 1997; Miller & Rathus, 2000). We anticipate many juvenile programs in both community and residential settings to present compelling data regarding this application of DBT in the future.

Key elements of effective treatment service provision

Several themes are present in most of the programs described above and are essential components to achieve successful outcomes for clients.

Qualities of effective providers

The first characteristics of effective service provision focus on the qualities of individual providers. In many of the evidence-based programs, therapists having qualities of warmth, cultural sensitivity, as well as the skills to motivate clients and focus interventions without alienating clients is essential. We see these therapist traits highlighted in programs such as FFT, MST, and the FIT program. Although experience is an important component for effective service provision in any treatment approach, experienced youth caseworkers have been found to be especially important in diversion programs (Dryfoos, 1990).

Training and protocol adherence

All of the noted programs, with the exceptions of mentoring and perhaps MTFC, cited manualized treatments and intensive training as essential to achieving significant positive outcomes for clients. As noted by Chambless and Ollendick (2001), treatments deemed efficacious should include either a treatment manual or well-specified protocol. Equally important is the need for high staff-to-family ratios to facilitate more frequent contact between the provider and the client (Wasserman *et al.*, 2000), which is particularly evident in the low ratios demonstrated in MST, FFT, FIT, and MTFC.

Clinical supervision

Despite differences in key intervention strategies and goals for treatment across treatment approaches, consistent and on-going supervision is required to achieve successful outcomes. The professional credentials of the supervisor may vary; however, consistent clinical supervision with stated goals for supervision is key to the success of the programs discussed. The length of supervision per client/family is far less variable. In most cases, therapists receive approximately one hour of supervision per week.

Collaboration with stakeholders in the system

Most of the strategies discussed in this chapter include a collaborative component to the model. Early intervention and community-based treatment programs, place the youth and family together at the center of the treatment process, but also reach out to all members of the family's community to elicit support. This may include extended family members, members of the church, school personnel including teachers and coaches, community center staff, probation and parole officers, court staff, and case managers. These efforts of collaboration, demonstrated in every program discussed, have proven especially effective in changing high-risk behaviors and increasing positive, prosocial behaviors in at-risk youth.

Conclusions

Alternative approaches to the punitive model of crime control have gained increasing prominence with evidence that juvenile incarceration solely focused on custody does not solve the problem.

The treatment strategies described in this chapter primarily focus on systemic or ecological changes rather than youth-focused changes. Although there are excellent examples of empirically validated youth-focused interventions (Weisz *et al.*, 1995), it is our belief that effective approaches for this population of youth need to target the ecology and address interpersonal factors that may not be ameliorated without system-level change. Antisocial behavior results from a complex set of risk factors that evolve within multiple contexts. As such, interventions for children and adolescents in the juvenile justice system require change across these systems.

While the implementation of evidence-based services is logical given the research and demonstrated proof of positive outcomes in the field, we must also emphasize the complexity and difficulty of translating and replicating programs from setting to setting. All of the common characteristics of evidence-based programs highlighted in this chapter must be attended to and fulfilled, including:

- qualities of effective providers
- training and protocol adherence
- clinical supervision
- collaboration with stakeholders in the system.

A strength of all of the programs is the ability of bachelor's-level therapists to apply the treatment, under the clinical supervision of a treatment expert. This makes implementing evidence-based programs in routine settings very attractive to state and local agencies. However, without an emphasis placed upon adherence and fidelity, one cannot guarantee the duplication of positive outcomes. Therefore, state and local agencies who wish to implement evidence-based programs should have a clear plan for training and implementation that will address all these issues. Treatment providers and agencies should also have a clear understanding and adhere to the research for the applicability of the treatment to the population for which the agency intends to implement.

Policy recommendations and future direction

With the influx of new research, we now have at our disposal a battery of manualized, discreet interventions, which have demonstrated significant positive outcomes for juvenile justice populations, from youth who are low-risk to high-risk for recidivism as well as for youth with complex treatment needs such as mental illness and chemical dependency. These programs, when implemented according to adherence and fidelity standards, have been shown to reduce specific risk factors related to recidivism and increase positive protective factors, thereby improving public safety as well as individual family outcomes. In addition, because of their effective uses as alternatives to long-term incarceration and commitments to other secure settings, such as inpatient psychiatric hospitals and short-term detention settings, significant cost-savings to taxpayers can be realized through the implementation of such programs.

Policy-makers at the federal and state level, as well as clinical program administrators, are recognizing the social and fiscal benefits of implementing evidence-based programs to address the serious problem of juvenile delinquency in our country. The need to implement programs that produce significant outcomes within the context of cost-effectiveness is essential, particularly during times of fiscal uncertainty. Already, the public, legislators, and advocacy groups are beginning to hold direct-service providers, programs, and agencies accountable for the failure to implement programs that generate fiscal and clinical outcomes. At the same time, some legislative bodies are rewarding and allocating funding to agencies who choose to implement evidence-based programs. (Washington State RCW 13.40.510)

It is our recommendation that this trend of fiscal reinforcement expand to assist state and local agencies in implementing known evidence-based interventions and in having the ability to incorporate the latest innovative models for difficult populations and settings as research becomes available. This is indeed an exciting time in the area of juvenile justice treatment and more significant advances in adolescent behavioral sciences are certain to follow.

Case example 1

Edward is a 15-year-old youth who has been arrested for shoplifting compact discs from a local music store. The county prosecutor has reviewed Edward's case and has recognized him as a first-time offender with strong family support. After consulting with the manager of the music store, the prosecutor referred Edward to the local diversion program. There, the store manager, Edward, his parents, and two other community members (a volunteer parent and volunteer high school student) sit together to discuss Edward's crime and his applicability for the diversion program. Edward is allowed to admit to his crime and tell the group the events that he experienced before and after he committed the crime.

The group discusses an appropriate plan for community service and restitution, and decides together that Edward will perform 100 hours of community service and will pay $75 in restitution to the store manager. In addition, Edward is placed on six months' probation, in which he agrees to attend school regularly, find part-time employment, and meet regularly with his probation counselor. Upon assessment, the youth does not show signs of mental illness or chemical dependency, so he will not undergo specialized treatment; however, based upon the events leading to the crime, he will be required to attend job skills classes and communication skills classes. Edward agrees to fulfill his treatment plan, and his parents agree to support Edward in meeting the requirements of the plan. Edward is assigned a probation counselor.

Edward decided to volunteer at a nursing home as part of his community service. With help from his probation officer, he was able to find a part-time job at a fast-food restaurant and has paid his restitution. Edward and his parents met with his probation counselor twice per month, and the probation counselor often checked on Edward spontaneously at school.

A year has now passed since the initial offense. Edward attends high school, has maintained his part-time employment, and has not reoffended. The conviction has been removed from his legal file.

Case example 2

Tina is a 13-year-old youth who lives in an inner-city neighborhood with her single mother and an eight-year-old brother. Tina's mother, Jane, works two jobs to support her children, and is worried that Tina does not receive enough supervision. While her younger son, Bobby, attends after-school programs, Tina is often left on her own. Tina has started to hit her younger brother more often, is not doing well in school, and shares an overall negative attitude. Jane cannot afford to pay for many of the sports leagues and other hobbies in which Tina is interested and this has been a subject of many arguments within the home. Jane made a call to a local mentoring program in her area and arranged for Tina to participate in the program.

Tina is assigned a mentor named Noelle. Noelle is 28 years old, and works as a nurse in a doctor's office. Noelle was matched to Tina as they are both African-American and have stated interests in music and sports. Noelle is proficient in the guitar, and Tina is in the choir at her school.

Case example 2 (cont.)

Noelle and Tina's first meeting was a little awkward, so they decided to attend a movie to get accustomed to being in each other's company without having to make extended conversation. Over the next few months, however, Noelle and Tina met once per week and built upon their initial meeting. Tina was able to have someone to talk to and share concerns with, and together they learned how to rollerblade and play soccer at the public park. Noelle was able to give Tina beginning lessons for the guitar.

Jane immediately noticed a change in her daughter's attitude at home, although it took several months for her grades to improve. Noelle talked to Jane on the telephone after each visit with Tina, to keep the family abreast of the content of the visits. Tina's jealousy of her brother's activities decreased, as now she had her own special activities with Noelle, and the assaultive behaviors toward her brother decreased.

At the end of the year, Tina had improved grades, had joined the school jazz band, and started to associate with other girls her age in the choir. Though Jane still has to work many hours to support her family, she is not as worried about her daughter, Tina, who has made many positive changes in the last year through the mentoring program.

Case example 3

Tiffany is a 16-year-old youth who has had prior convictions for shoplifting and misdemeanor assault. Currently, she has been arrested for stealing her mother's car, and has been referred to a multisystemic therapy (MST) community-based treatment program, in lieu of time in a secure facility, based upon court assessment and the presence of family support.

An MST therapist, Jim, is assigned to the family, and meets initially with the entire family to gauge the family's level of engagement and commitment to the treatment program. Each family member is encouraged to state his or her goals for the treatment process, and together, the family makes a list of goals. Tiffany would like to get a part-time job and earn her GED, while her mother would like to see Tiffany remain drug-free. Tiffany's father would like to see the relationship with Tiffany and her mother improve to provide more harmony within the family, especially during mealtimes. Tiffany's nine-year-old brother, Sean, just wants "everyone to get along."

Over the next four months, Jim is able to work within the family to help improve the communication skills between Tiffany and her mother. Tiffany's parents learn concepts of contingency management and reinforcement, and are able to provide incentives to Tiffany as she maintains a part-time job, while consistently monitoring her school attendance and homework completion. With coaching from the MST therapist, logical consequences are applied by Tiffany's parents when she hits her younger brother, and, gradually, this behavior dissipates. The MST therapist is able to work individually with Tiffany regarding her substance abuse, and Tiffany is rewarded by her parents for providing clean urinalysis tests. After three months of working individually with the MST therapist on substance abuse issues, Tiffany is connected with an AA group in her community.

During the fifth month of the MST service, Tiffany and her mother get into a heated argument about attending a concert, and Tiffany runs away from home, staying away for the entire night. When Tiffany returns the next day, the MST therapist is able to work with the family to discuss what happened to incite the argument, and teaches replacement interventions to conflict as an alternative to automatically calling the police, as has happened every time in the past. The family invents a "contract" for future problems, and each family member has roles and obligations to fulfill in the contract the next time a problem arises. Tiffany makes the commitment not to run away during family conflict.

At the end of the fifth month, the family demonstrates many new skills and decides they are ready to end the formal treatment program. Tiffany has remained drug-free and has not committed any new crimes. While her relationship with her mother is not ideal, both have acquired new communication skills and seem willing to practice them.

Case example 4

Terrance is a 12-year-old who has had significant problems with truancy from school. His parents, the school system, and the juvenile court jointly referred the family into a functional family therapy (FFT) program operated by the juvenile court. Terrance's family was assigned an FFT therapist, who waited for Terrance to be released from juvenile detention to meet with the entire family at once in order to assess and engage the family as a whole.

When the FFT therapist, Susan, met with the family, she became aware of a significant amount of hostility within the family, particularly between Terrance's parents, Dione and Robert. Susan assessed her first priority as a therapist was to decrease the negativity between family members in order to improve communication and increase warmth. Susan used the FFT techniques of restatement and reframing to help Terrance's parents understand the frustration all members of the family were feeling. Once Terrance and his parents recognized the underlying hurt and loss all were experiencing during arguments, tempers began to diminish and communication began to improve.

The family agreed to meet with the FFT therapist once per week for 12 weeks, and by the end of the first session, all members seemed relatively hopeful about investing in the treatment program. Terrance stated that this was the first time in a long time that he could talk with his parents without an argument ensuing.

Over the next few weeks, the family decided to work on having family dinners without arguments and sarcasm present. The family's goal started at one dinner without conflict per week, and slowly moved up from there, once they started experiencing success with the goal. The family would discuss their progress and learn new ways of communicating each time they met with the FFT therapist, Susan. Susan was also available to the family for consultation on at least two occasions by phone, when Terrance and his mother found themselves unable to disengage from a verbal argument at home.

Robert and Dione were able to invent a set of rewards for Terrance when he attended school and punishments for when he chose not to attend school. Terrance was able to

Case example 4 (cont.)

give input to the contract. Although Terrance's school attendance was not perfect, his truancy did decrease, and, more importantly, Robert and Dione were able to administer consequences to Terrance consistently without arguing and blaming each other or Terrance.

At the end of the 12 weeks, the level of anxiety and overall anger within the family had decreased. Dione realized that her husband, Robert, would not become more available at this time to assist her in supervising and parenting Terrance due to his line of work, and she was able to recognize other kinds of support he is able to provide to her regarding parenting. Terrance's truancy did diminish, and he became more interested and able to share school projects and events with his parents as he received positive attention. Robert came to understand how to begin to control his own judgments and anger and stated he was willing to continue practicing new skills. The FFT therapist, Susan, connected the family with school officials and a family therapist in their community, for possible future reference and consultation.

Case example 5

Julio is a 16-year-old youth who served a two-year sentence in a secure juvenile facility for felony assault. Julio has been assessed as chemically dependent on alcohol and meth-amphetamines, and was able to attend an inpatient treatment program while incarcerated. He is also diagnosed with major depression and anxiety, for which he is prescribed psychotropic medication. Julio and his family were referred to the family integrated therapy (FIT) program approximately four months prior to his scheduled release date from the juvenile facility. Upon release, Julio was placed under six months of community parole supervision and simultaneously participated in the FIT program.

The FIT therapist assigned to Julio's case traveled to the juvenile facility where Julio was housed two months prior to Julio's release date to meet with the youth. They discussed the program parameters and, more importantly, Julio was able to tell the FIT therapist his goals for his upcoming release. Julio stated he was very concerned about his placement with his mother, as she had difficulty finding work and lived in a small one-bedroom apartment with little or no furniture. Julio was concerned his mother would not be able to keep the apartment and would leave Julio to his own devices in the community. Julio was also concerned about having his medications available, and was very anxious about seeing his old gang friends again.

Prior to Julio's release, the FIT therapist was also able to meet with Julio's mother, Rosa, after several attempts to set up a meeting. Rosa did not seem very receptive to participating in the program and viewed the FIT therapist as someone to "fix" her son. The FIT therapist ended up taking Rosa to breakfast and engaged her in her son's treatment using MET strategies. Rosa expressed some of the same concerns as her son, and also added that she was very concerned about Julio's potential drug use when he returned to her home. The FIT therapist arranged to take Rosa to see Julio before he was released in order to talk about these issues and jointly plan to deal with all of these concerns, in addition to the parole requirements that Julio would be expected to meet.

Julio was released, and over the next six months the FIT therapist worked with the family to integrate Julio into the community. The FIT therapist coached Rosa to be effective in working with school officials to allow Julio back into regular school, instead of the alternative school he had attended before. Rosa thought this transition to be a high priority in order to distance Julio from the gang friends with which he had associated at the school when he committed his offense. The FIT therapist also assisted Julio and Rosa to obtain medical coupons to pay for Julio's psychotropic medications, and the FIT therapist was able to work individually with Julio on his drug and alcohol issues until a suitable NA meeting near the home was found.

Julio attended job interviews without much success. The FIT therapist used DBT's behavioral analysis with Julio to determine specifically what was getting in the way of Julio's success, and together they determined Julio's anxiety was causing problems during the interviews. The family consulted with Julio's doctor, who adjusted Julio's medication in addition to teaching Julio behavioral techniques to manage his anxiety.

During the third month, Julio went through a period of leaving home and staying out all night, which was a violation of his parole conditions. The FIT therapist, the parole counselor, Rosa and Julio met and determined that Julio was extremely frustrated as he did not have any privacy at his mother's apartment, and had been sleeping on the floor. The FIT therapist arranged for a used hide-away couch to be donated to the family, which allowed Julio to have a bed to sleep in. Julio agreed to stay at home at night and avoided a parole revocation.

The FIT therapist met with the family two–three times per week for the entire eight months in the program, and was able to accommodate Rosa's work schedule. Julio did not reoffend, but did have many trials in dealing with his own mental health issues and with the temptation of hanging out with his old criminal friends. He and his mother were able to learn communication skills and improved their understanding of one another's goals. They discovered that most of their goals overlapped. Both were able to maintain employment, and, when the program ended, the family was arranging to move into a two-bedroom apartment. The FIT therapist was able to help the family take advantage of community-based mental health counseling and public assistance for health insurance.

Case example 6

Amy is a 17-year-old youth incarcerated for selling heroine and felony assault. She has a long history of inpatient psychiatric hospitalizations and self-harming behaviors. While incarcerated, Amy was referred to an inpatient program to treat her chemical dependency; however, her assaultive behavior toward her peers and staff, as well as her willingness to self-mutilate made her unable to continue in the treatment program. Amy was transferred to the mental health unit within the secure facility.

Case example 6 (cont.)

Amy's behaviors did not improve initially. In fact, the night she transitioned into the program, Amy cut her stomach several times with a plastic hair barrette she obtained from another girl. After taking precautionary measures to keep Amy safe that night, her counselor sat with her after a 24-hour period and walked Amy through a behavioral analysis for her self-harming behavior. The analysis showed Amy to be suffering from anxiety and a lack of sleep, but the analysis also showed Amy was angry and humiliated from an argument with several of the other girls in the program. Amy and her counselor discussed these drivers of her behavior and alternative ways of handling extreme emotions, such as anger and shame. Her counselor introduced Amy to a set of skills in DBT known as emotion regulation skills and gave her a workbook that outlined all of the skills.

In a staff consultation meeting, the staff team also reviewed Amy's behavioral analysis and discovered that Amy had received much attention from staff and her peers for the self-harming behavior in addition to the relief of painful emotion she received from the act of cutting herself. The staff team devised a plan to remove the positive attention she received from them after maladaptive behavior, although they recognized they would not be able to remove the other reinforcers to her behavior.

As part of the program, Amy attended treatment groups, learning and practicing all of the DBT skills. During individual sessions with her counselor, Amy reviewed specific behaviors and feelings she had been having, and discussed her specific practice and use of emotion regulation skills. Staff made a point to reward Amy for any use of adaptive skills, regardless of her proficiency, and did not reinforce her for self-harming behaviors or ideation.

Though Amy's self-harm ideation initially increased, the staff recognized this as an "extinction burst" and maintained their program plan. Eventually, Amy's use of self-harm to cope with intensely painful feelings decreased; however, her use of assault seemed to increase. Again, Amy performed behavioral analysis with her counselor to determine drivers of her behavior, and with the staff team, invented behavioral contracts for how others in the unit would react to her maladaptive behavior.

After a year in the mental health unit, Amy's self-harm and assaultive behavior had stabilized to a point where she could transition to the chemical dependency treatment program. Amy immediately experienced intense anxiety and frustration, but her counselors from the mental health unit were able to provide consultation to her in using her acquired DBT skills to stabilize herself. Amy was eventually able to complete the drug and alcohol treatment program. The staff coached Amy to share the DBT skills she found to be effective with her mother, who was then also able to assist Amy to generalize the skills as she returned home. She was released into the community upon completion of her sentence and, with help from the institutional mental health staff, was able to connect with a mental health/chemical dependency outpatient treatment provider in her community who was familiar with the DBT protocols and skills set.

References

Alexander, J. F. & Parsons, B. V. (1982). *Functional Family Therapy: Principles and Procedures.* Carmel, CA: Brooks/Cole.

Alexander, J. F., Pugh, C., Parsons, B. V., & Sexton, T. L. (2000). Functional family therapy. In D. S. Elliott, ed., *Blueprints for Violence Prevention* (Book 3), 2nd edn. Boulder, CO: Center for the Study and Prevention of Violence. Institute of Behavioral Science, University of Colorado.

Bandura, A. (1985). *Social Foundations of Thought and Action: A Social Cognitive Theory.* New York, NY: Plenum.

Barnoski, R. (1997). *Fast Tracking Youth to Diversion in Thurston County: A Preliminary Analysis.* Washington State Institute of Public Policy.

Barnoski, R. (2002a). *Preliminary Findings for the Juvenile Rehabilitation Administration's Mentoring Program.* Washington State Institute for Public Policy.

Barnoski, R. (2002b). *Preliminary Findings for the Juvenile Rehabilitation Administration's Dialectical Behavior Therapy Program.*

Borduin, C. M., Mann, B. J., Cone, L. T. *et al.* (1995). Multisystemic treatment of serious juvenile offenders: long-term prevention of criminality and violence. *Journal of Consulting and Clinical Psychology*, **63**, 569–578.

Brunk, M., Henggeler, S. W. & Whelan J. P. (1987). A comparison of multisystemic therapy and parent training in the brief treatment of child abuse and neglect. *Journal of Consulting and Clinical Psychology*, **55**, 311–318.

Chamberlain, P. (1998). *Treatment Foster Care: Family Strengthening Series.* Washington, DC: US Department of Justice (*OJJDP Bulletin*, NCJ 1734211).

Chamberlain, P. & Mihalic, S. F. (1998). *Blueprints for Violence Prevention, Book Eight: Multidimensional Treatment Foster Care.* Boulder, CO: Center for the Study and Prevention of Violence.

Chamberlain, P. & Reid, J. (1998). Comparison of two community alternatives to incarceration for chronic juvenile offenders. *Journal of Consulting and Clinical Psychology*, **6**(4), 624–633.

Chambless, D. L. & Ollendick, T. H. (2001). Empirically supported psychological interventions: controversies and evidence. *Annual Reviews of Psychology*, **52**, 685–716.

Chambless, D. L., Baker, M. J., Baucom, D. H. *et al.* (1998). Update on empirically validated therapies, II. *The Clinical Psychologist*, **51**, 3–16.

Cummings, S. & Clark, R. W. (1993). Juvenile diversion programs. *Journal of Extension*, **31**(1).

Davidson, W. S. II, Redner, R., Admur, R., & Mitchell, C. (1990). *Alternative treatments for troubled youth: The case of diversion from the justice system.* New York, NY: Plenum.

Dryfoos, J. (1990). *Adolescents at Risk: Prevalence and Prevention.* New York, NY: Oxford University Press.

Duchnowski, A. J., Kutash, K. & Friedman, R. M. (2002). Community-based interventions in a system of care and outcomes research. In B. Burns and K. Hoagwood, eds., *Community Treatment for Youth: Evidence-Based Interventions for Severe Emotional and Behavioral Disorders.* New York: NY: Oxford University Press, pp. 91–116.

Elliott, D. S., Huizinga, D. & Ageton, S. S. (1985). *Explaining Delinquency and Drug Use*. Beverly Hills, CA: Sage Publications.

Evans, K., Tyrer, P., Catalan, J. *et al.* (1999). Manual assisted cognitive-behaviour therapy (MACT): a randomized controlled trial of a brief intervention with bibliotherapy in the treatment of recurrent deliberate self-harm. *Psychological Medicine*, **29**, 19–25.

Fisher, P. A. & Chamberlain, P. (2000). Multidimensional treatment foster care: a program for intensive parenting, family support, and skill building. *Journal of Emotional and Behavioral Disorders*, **8**(3), 155–164.

Grossman, J. B. & Garry, E. M. (1997, April). Mentoring – a proven delinquency prevention strategy. *OJJDP Bulletin*, NCJ.

Hawkins, J. D., Herrenkohl, T. I., Farrington, D. P. *et al.* (2000). Predictors of youth violence. *OJJDP Bulletin*, NCJ.

Henggeler, W. W., Rodick, J. D., Borduin, C. M. *et al.* (1986). Multisystemic treatment of juvenile offenders: effects on adolescent behavior and family interactions. *Developmental Psychology*, **22**, 132–141.

Henggeler, S. W., Melton, G. B. & Smith, L. A. (1992). Family preservation using multisystemic therapy: an effective alternative to incarcerating serious juvenile offenders. *Journal of Counseling and Clinical Psychology*, **60**(6), 953–961.

Henggler, S. W. & Borduin, C. M. (1995). Multisystemic treatment of serious juvenile offenders and their families. In I. M. Schwartz, ed., *Family- and Home-Based Services*. Lincoln: University of Nebraska Press.

Kandel, E. & Mednick, S. A. (1991). Perinatal complications predict violent offending. *Criminology*, **29**, 519–529.

Koons, C. R., Robins, C. J., Tweed, J. L. *et al.* (2001). Efficacy of dialectical behavior therapy in women veterans with borderline personality disorder. *Behavior Therapy*, **32**, 371–390.

Levant, R. F. (2005). Evidenced-based practice in psychology. *Monitor in Psychology*, **36**(2), 5.

Linehan, M. M. (1993). *Cognitive Behavior Therapy for the Treatment of Borderline Personality Disorder*. New York, NY: Guilford Press.

Linehan, M. M., Armstrong, H., Suarez, A., Almon, D. & Heard, H. (1991). Cognitive-behavioral treatment of chronically parasuicidal borderline patients. *Archives of General Psychiatry*, **48**, 1060–1064.

Linehan, M. M., Schmidt, H. & Dimeff, L. A. (1999) Dialectical behavior therapy for patients with borderline personality disorder and drug dependence. *American Journal of Addictions*, **8**, 279–292.

McGill, D. E., Mihalic, S. F. & Grotpeter, J. K. (1998). *Blueprints for Violence Prevention, Book Two: Big Brothers Big Sisters of America*. Boulder, CO: Center for the Study and Prevention of Violence.

Miller, A. L. & Rathus, J. H. (2000). Dialectical behavior therapy: adaptations and new applications. *Cognitive and Behavioral Practice*, **7**, 420–425.

Miller, A. L., Rathus, J. H., Linehan, M. M., Wetzler, S. & Leigh, E. (1997). Dialectical behavior therapy adapted for suicidal adolescents. *Journal of Practical Psychiatry and Behavioral Health*, **3**, 78–86.

Myers, W. C., Burton, P. R. S., Sanders, P. D. *et al.* (2000). Project Back-on-Track at 1 year: A delinquency treatment program for early-career juvenile offenders. *Journal of the American Academy of Child and Adolescent Psychiatry*, **39**, 1127–1134.

Novotney, L. C., Mertinko, E., Lange, J. & Baker, T. K. (2000, September). Juvenile mentoring programs: a progress review. *ODDJP Bulletin*, NCJ 182209.

O'Donohue, W., Buchanan, J. A. & Fisher, J. E. (2000). Characteristics of empirically supported treatments. *Journal of Psychotherapy Practice and Research*, **9**(2), 69–74.

Polk, K. (1995). Juvenile diversion: a look at the record. In P. M. Sharp and B. W. Hancock, eds., *Juvenile Delinquency*. Englewood Cliffs, NJ: Prentice Hall.

Schoenwald, S. K. & Rowland, M. D. (2002). Multisystemic therapy. In B. Burns and K. Hoagwood, eds., *Community Treatment for Youth: Evidence-Based Interventions for Severe Emotional and Behavioral Disorders*. New York: NY: Oxford University Press, pp. 91–116.

Schoenwald, S. K., Ward, D. M., Henggeler, S. W., Pickrel, S. G. & Patel, H. (1996). MST treatment of substance abusing or dependent adolescent offenders: costs of reducing incarceration, inpatient, and residential placement. *Journal of Child and Family Studies*, **5**, 431–444.

Schur, E. (1971). *Labeling Deviant Behavior: Its Sociological Implications*. New York, NY: Harper and Row.

Sexton, T. L. & Alexander, J. F. (2000). *Functional Family Therapy* (Bulletin). Washington, DC: Department of Justice, Office of Justice Programs, Office of Juvenile Delinquency Prevention.

Shelden, R. G. (1999, September). Detention diversion advocacy: an evaluation. *OJJDP Bulletin*, NCJ 171155.

Sulzer-Azaroff, B. & Mayer, G. R. (1977). *Applying Behavior-analysis Procedures with Children and Youth*. New York: Holt, Rinehart and Winston.

Swenson, C. R., Torrey, W. C. & Koerner, K. (2002). Implementing dialectical behavior therapy. *Psychiatric Services*, **53**(2), 171–177.

Trupin, E. W., Stewart, D. G., Beach, B. & Boesky, L. (2002). Effectiveness of a dialectical behaviour therapy program for incarcerated female juvenile offenders. *Child and Adolescent Mental Health*, **7**(3), 121–127.

Washington Institute for Public Policy (1998). *Watching the Bottom Line: Cost-Effective Interventions for Reducing Crime in Washington*. Olympia, WA: Evergreen State College.

Wasserman, G. A., Miller, L. S. & Cothern, L. (2000, April). Prevention of serious and violent juvenile offending. *OJJDP Bulletin*, NCJ 178898.

Weisz, J. R., Weiss, B., Han, S. S., Granger, D. A., & Morton, T. (1995). Effects of psychotherapy with children and adolescents revisited: a meta-analysis of treatment outcome studies. *Psychological Bulletin*, **117**, 450–468.

Weisz, J. R., Doss, J. R., Jensen, A. & Hawley, K. M. (2005). Youth psychotherapy outcome research: a review and critique of the evidence base. *Annual Review of Psychology*, **56**, 337–363.

17

Community alternatives to incarceration

Christopher R. Thomas

Introduction

The central reason behind the creation of the juvenile justice system at the beginning of the twentieth century was the belief, that in contrast to adult offenders, delinquents were amenable to change in their antisocial behaviors. Therefore, the juvenile courts sought to capitalize on this opportunity and provide rehabilitation, not solely punishment. The rate of recidivism among young offenders certainly supports the notion of developing programs aimed at reforming delinquents (Snyder, 1988). The reduction in youth crime and its personal and economic costs to the individual and communities easily justify the expense of intervention (Schoenwald *et al.*, 1996). In addition, it has been estimated that each delinquent that continues onto an adult criminal career costs society $1.3–1.5 million (Cohen, 1998).

The founding principle of the opportunity for rehabilitation has been questioned from the start as to whether effective interventions truly exist with juvenile delinquents. Early intervention efforts were based on an individualized approach to meeting the needs of the particular youth before the court. While some intervention models were based on theoretical speculations regarding the causes of delinquency, few were derived from direct research on the causes and correlates of antisocial behavior in youth. Most reflected an application of general models of psychopathology and treatment to the special case of delinquency, such as Aichhorn's psychoanalytic approach (Aichhorn, 1935). A series of research reviews in the late 1970s supported the popular belief that "nothing works" with delinquents (Lipton *et al.*, 1975; Greenberg, 1977; Romig, 1978; Sechrest *et al.*, 1979). The increase in youth violence in the late 1980s further intensified the debate as to whether juvenile justice was truly able to deal with youth crime, especially violent offenses (Woolard *et al.*, 2001). In response, many states altered their handling of young offenders, by lowering the age of adult culpability or facilitating the use of transfer to adult criminal courts, especially for more serious delinquents (Jenson & Howard, 1998).

The Mental Health Needs of Young Offenders: Forging Paths toward Reintegration and Rehabilitation, eds. Carol L. Kessler and Louis J. Kraus. Published by Cambridge University Press. © Cambridge University Press 2007.

While discouraging in tone, the earlier negative reviews of delinquency intervention programs pointed out that most intervention studies suffered from deficits in methodological rigor and research design. Further analysis revealed promising approaches and factors related to efficacy (Gendreau & Ross, 1979; Palmer, 1983; Lipsey, 1992). Beginning in the 1990s, reports of improved programs with better evaluation began to appear, demonstrating effective methods in dealing with adjudicated youth (Palmer, 1994; Davidson et al., 1990; Schoenwald et al, 1996; Greenwood, 1996; Lipsey & Wilson, 1998; Woolfenden et al., 2001).

Effective community based interventions offer several advantages over residential programs. The most obvious is the cost savings, with funds devoted to treatment services rather than the additional burden of facilities. More important is the ability to treat the youth within the context of home and community. The treatment team can directly assess the family and neighborhood factors that contribute to continued delinquency and determine what resources are available for change. Changes are measured within the environment that the youth must return to and improve in for the program to be successful. If the safety and containment of adjudicated youth permit, community based interventions are preferable.

Meta-analytic studies on the efficacy of delinquency interventions

While there have been a number of thorough reviews of community based delinquency programs, they are limited as are all literature reviews. The central problem is finding a standard metric on which to combine and compare the information presented in disparate studies. Merely counting whether outcomes were positive or negative is inadequate to accumulate results across reports, since studies will vary in significance by sample size or difference from control. In addition, single studies are often unable to produce definitive conclusions about any treatment approach that can be generalized to other settings or populations, because of sampling and measurement limitations. Meta-analysis addresses the issues of statistically compiling and comparing results across various studies (Cook et al., 1992). Comparisons are usually made by determining the effect size for each treatment. Effect size is the ratio of the change associated with a particular intervention to the standard deviation.

In one of the first applications of meta-analytic techniques on community based interventions with adjudicated youth, Gottschalk and colleagues analyzed 90 studies reported between 1967–1983 (Gottschalk et al., 1987). Programs were selected on the basis of focus on adjudicated youth and treatment occurring within the youth's community. The studies comprised over 11 000 subjects and most were published after 1975. The average treatment duration was 22 weeks with a median of 15 weeks, and the average total service was 42 hours with a median of 15 hours.

The authors of this meta-analysis noted a number of problems in the research design of the surveyed studies, including the lack of treatment implementation measures, infrequent use of random assignment to treatment, and that 50 percent of the studies had no control group or only utilized a "treatment as usual" comparison. The authors were unable to reject the null hypothesis of no treatment effect for the 90 studies in considering the outcome measures of overall effectiveness, recidivism, and behavior. This observation would appear to support the conclusion of the previous less systematic reviews that nothing is effective in reducing delinquency. The effect sizes in studies using a pre/post design were larger than those with experimental control design, but this probably reflected the influence of other factors in pre/post comparisons such as selection or historical artifact. The authors noted that the type of intervention was related to effectiveness, with behavioral, educational/vocational, and group therapy programs showing the greatest trend toward improvement. In addition, they found that the number of treatment hours was positively correlated to effect size. The authors cautioned that most of the interventions may not have been powerful enough to demonstrate effect because of short duration or poor quality of implementation. They concluded that while there were possible conditions for effective community interventions with delinquents, that more rigorous design was required to demonstrate this. Other early meta-analyses of delinquency interventions published at about the same time considered both institutional and community programs together (Garrett, 1985) or evaluated only studies with control groups (Whitehead & Lab, 1989; Andrews *et al.*, 1990). Lipsey (1992) in his review of these studies pointed out that while the authors drew differing conclusions about the mean efficacy of the various delinquency programs, they all found similar results with about 0.25–0.30 standard deviation superiority for the treatment over control comparison.

Lipsey's (1992) report on the variability of treatment effects was a major advance in meta-analysis of delinquency programs. A massive effort, it included 443 studies that were coded for 154 items and analyzed across a number of variables. While a wide variety of outcomes were considered, the most common measures of treatment impact were related to reduction in recidivism. Considering the direction of differences in outcome between treatment and control, Lipsey found a significant difference for treatment, with 285 programs favoring treatment, 131 favoring control, and 27 favoring neither. To measure the overall magnitude, he calculated the n-adjusted effect size. Only 397 of the studies were included in this part of the analysis as they supplied sufficient information to determine the effect size. The unweighted mean effect size was 0.172 and the inverse-variance weighted mean was 0.103 that was statistically significant. This result did not appear due to other factors that may have influenced the studies, such as non-randomization of subjects. He concluded that, in general, treatment to reduce delinquency produces a positive but relatively modest effect, with treated juveniles having on average a 0.10 standard deviation reduction in delinquency. This is more meaningful, he points out, when you consider this is equivalent to a reduction in recidivism from a hypothetical baseline of 50 percent to 45 percent. It is also important to recognize that this is just the average effect size, and that specific programs may demonstrate more robust results. Regression analysis found a modest but positive correlation between treatment effect size and the duration, frequency, and amount of treatment. In other words, more intensive treatments tended to have greater impact. This observation was complicated by the inclusion of programs for institutionalized youth. The strongest correlation with effect size was for variables related to type of treatment. Overall, the more structured and focused treatments were generally found to be more effective. Treatment programs employing skills training, behavioral techniques, or multimodal approaches tended to have a greater positive impact than other types of intervention, with effect sizes ranging from 0.20–0.32. Of equal importance, some treatments appeared to produce negative results, including shock incarceration or "scared straight" programs. In other words, delinquents were more likely to reoffend after receiving these treatments.

In an important follow-up analysis, Lipsey and Wilson (1998) evaluated 200 studies on interventions with serious delinquents, both institutionalized and non-institutionalized. Selection criteria for studies in this analysis included programs that focused on adjudicated delinquents with records of prior property or person offenses, or the focus of treatment was physically aggressive behavior. Most of the programs used random assignment or matched controlled design. The interventions were usually mandated and most participants were under court authority during treatment. Of the programs analyzed, 117 were for non-institutionalized delinquents. Lipsey and Wilson reported that the largest proportion of the effect size variance among these interventions was related to characteristics of the delinquents receiving treatment. Treatment effects were greater for delinquents with mixed prior offenses than for those with mostly property prior offenses. Programs that reported all of the delinquents having prior offense records also showed a greater treatment effect than those programs where only most of the delinquents had prior offense records. The influences of these two variables on treatment effectiveness were independent and indicate that the greatest treatment effect sizes are with more serious offenders. This supports the so-called "risk principle" (Andrews *et al.*, 1990), that treatment of delinquents is most effective with those youth at the greatest risk for recidivism. It is directly opposite the more prevalent opinion that interventions are ineffective with serious delinquents. In comparing treatment types, marked differences were again found in effect sizes.

Those programs based on interpersonal skills training, individual counseling, or behavioral techniques demonstrated the greatest positive effect sizes. Following behind this group in treatment effect size were programs that utilized multiple services (or multimodal approaches) and restitution. As in the earlier meta-analysis, several treatment approaches were found to be consistently non-effective, including wilderness challenge, early release, deterrence, and vocational training programs. The amount of treatment was also found to be a strong contributing factor to program outcome. Duration of treatment was positively correlated with outcome, although the number of treatment hours per week was negatively correlated. Overall, the intervention programs studied in this meta-analysis produced significant results with the more effective programs reducing recidivism by as much as 40 percent.

Meta-analytic studies have provided more detailed overview of community based delinquency programs. Countering the previous view that little could be done to rehabilitate young offenders, they have shown that programs can produce significant results. They also describe the characteristics of the most effective approaches. In addition, there is evidence that programs can make a difference with violent delinquents and those with records of prior offenses.

Individual interventions

Many features of delinquency would appear to favor individual interventions. The heterogeneous nature of antisocial behavior supports an individualized approach to specific risks and deficits. Many of the associated individual features, such as impulsivity, poor social skills, or problem-solving deficits, are obvious treatment targets with established interventions. The juvenile justice system is also in a better position to order and enforce treatment with an individual than it can with parents or an entire family. In practice, the overall results of individual intervention programs for delinquents have been mixed.

Traditional insight or relationship based therapies are among the most frequently employed individual modalities with delinquents (Mulvey *et al.*, 1993), but in general have not produced strong results (Lipsey, 1992; Kazdin, 2000). This may have more to do with the non-directive and unstructured characteristics of this approach rather than the specific modality (Gordon & Arbuthnot, 1987; Lipsey, 1992). One individual treatment study that produced significant results did employ a more organized and defined approach with reality therapy techniques (Bean, 1988). The intervention consisted of twelve weekly one-hour sessions using reality therapy to help young offenders regain control by learning goal setting and self-assessment, coupled to detailed plans of action. This approach includes aspects of skills training discussed in further detail later. While most individual treatments rely on trained professional counselors, one program with significant impact for high risk delinquents on probation used community volunteers (Moore, 1987). Those delinquents randomly assigned to a community volunteer had significantly fewer arrests during probation compared to controls. In addition they exhibited significant improvements on the California Psychological Inventory scales for achievement via conformance, responsibility taking, socialization, self-control, and socialization. The authors of the study note that the volunteers were carefully screened and matched with the delinquents, which may present difficulty in replicating this program in other communities.

Skills training therapies encompass a variety of treatments that share a basic goal of educating participants in new modes of thinking or behavior. These include problem-solving skills training and social skills training for delinquency interventions. Both employ cognitive–behavioral techniques in addressing identified deficits exhibited by antisocial youth (Kennedy, 1984; Fonagy & Kurtz, 2002). Youth with antisocial behaviors have difficulty thinking of alternatives for interpersonal problems and conflict, misperceive the feelings and motivations of others, and cannot appreciate the consequences of their actions (Spivak & Shure, 1974). A particular difficulty in their misperception of others' intent is assuming that others are hostile or aggressive when cues are vague (Crick & Dodge, 1994).

Extensive treatment studies have demonstrated the efficacy of social skills training or problem-solving skills training with disruptive behavior in youth (Fonagy & Kurtz, 2002), but there are fewer reports on community based treatments with young offenders (Cunliffe, 1992) and some have questioned its impact with adolescents (Taylor *et al.*, 1999). In one study, male delinquents were randomly assigned to social skills training, support, or no treatment (Spence & Marzillier, 1981). Improvements in behavior were noted after completion of the twelve one-hour treatment sessions and maintained at three-month follow up. Recidivism was also lower, but not significantly different in comparison to the control groups.

A social skills training approach designed for violent delinquents is aggression replacement training (ART) (Goldstein & Glick, 1994). This program teaches participants impulse and anger control through structured sessions and group discussion over ten weeks. In an 18-month follow-up evaluation, ART overall produced significant reductions in felony recidivism, but not for total recidivism or violent reoffense (Barnoski, 2004). Treatment results in this study depended on the competency of treatment implementation, with competent ART programs averaging 19 percent in felony recidivism as compared to 26 percent for incompetent ART programs and 25 percent for controls. In addition, the highly competent ART programs produced a significant reduction in total recidivism in addition to felony recidivism in comparison to controls.

Problem-solving skills training was compared to mentoring in a non-random trial with non-violent misdemeanor or first felony offense delinquents (Blechman *et al.*, 2000). Only 37 percent of those receiving problem-solving skills training were rearrested after two years as compared to 51 percent of those assigned to mentoring and 46 percent of those sent to juvenile diversion. Although condition assignment in the study was non-random, propensity analysis controlling for differences between the groups for original arrest charge, demographics, and psychological status indicated problem-solving skills training was superior to mentoring in reducing recidivism.

Family interventions

A wide range of family factors have been identified as increasing risk of delinquency, including family cohesion and attachment, harsh or erratic discipline, parental rejection, lack of parental supervision, family disruption, and abuse (Burke *et al.*, 2002). It is understandable then that a great deal of attention has been focused on developing treatments directed at the family in dealing with delinquency. A meta-analysis of eight studies employing family interventions found that youth receiving treatment spent significantly less time in institutions and were at significantly reduced risk for recidivism up to three years after intervention (Woolfenden *et al.*, 2001). There was also a significant reduction in self-reported delinquency although there was some heterogeneity in the results (Woolfenden *et al.*, 2002). Family interventions can even significantly reduce delinquency in siblings (Klein *et al.*, 1977). Three family based interventions that have received extensive evaluation and produced significant improvements with delinquency are functional family therapy (FFT), multisystemic therapy (MST), and multidimensional treatment foster care (MTFC).

Functional family therapy seeks to address problem behavior from the understanding of the functions they serve in the family system (Alexander & Parsons, 1982). Treatment aims at altering family interactions and communication into more adaptive and productive patterns. Treatments range from 10–30 one-hour sessions, depending on the difficulties of the family. Specific therapist skills are employed with three discrete phases of treatment that are outlined in a therapy manual. The first phase is engagement and motivation of the family for change. The next phase focuses on behavior changes with identified problems. The final phase helps the family to generalize their problem-solving skills to other areas. Each of the phases incorporate assessment and intervention components that deal with identified factors influencing family interactions. Delivery of services is flexible, and sessions can be held in the home or at a clinic by one or two therapist teams. Therapists carry caseloads of 10–12 families. Clinical trials have demonstrated it to be an effective intervention with delinquents, including those involved in violence and substance abuse (Alexander *et al.*, 1994). Functional family therapy was shown to be more effective than group home placement in treating previously incarcerated delinquents with multiple prior offenses (Barton *et al.*, 1985). During the 15-month follow-up period, only 60 percent of those receiving FFT were rearrested as compared to 93 percent of those placed in group homes. Functional family therapy has also been shown to be an effective intervention for youth in rural areas (Gordon *et al.*, 1995). An evaluation of FFT in Washington State found that the reduction in recidivism depended on the competency of the therapists (Barnoski, 2004). In this study, the overall recidivism rate was not significantly different for delinquents receiving FFT in comparison to the control group, but there was a significant reduction in recidivism for those youth receiving FFT from competent therapists. Furthermore, the reduction in recidivism continued at 6-, 12-, and 18-month follow-up assessment. The cost–benefit analyses found FFT generated $10.69 in reduced crime costs for every dollar spent in therapy.

Multisystemic therapy is an intensive, brief, in home treatment based on a social systems model (Bronfenbrenner, 1979) in dealing with delinquent behavior. Multisystemic therapy was designed as a community based alternative for delinquents who would otherwise need residential placement. Treatment efforts are directed at the family, peer, school, and neighborhood systems and the relationships between them as they influence behavior (Henggeler *et al.*, 1998). The goal of treatment is to empower the family and youth to deal with issues in a more adaptive and constructive fashion (Henggeler *et al.*, 1992). Using a family preservation approach, the counselor works with the family in their home and community with frequent and sometimes daily contact. The duration of treatment is usually three months. Counselors typically handle no more than five cases at a time because of the frequency and intensity of contact with families. Therapy is guided by a treatment manual in accordance with the nine principles of MST (Henggeler *et al.*, 1994). Randomized trials of MST produced significant improvements with serious, violent, and substance abusing delinquents and their families (Borduin *et al.*, 1995; Henggeler *et al.*, 1993). Trials have found MST to be a culturally competent treatment and to have similar positive results in both urban and rural communities. Multisystemic therapy is also reported to be effective with adolescent sexual offenders (Borduin *et al.*, 1990).

Often with delinquents, the family is unavailable for involvement with home based interventions, or the family situation requires temporary placement out of the home. Multidimensional treatment foster care provides a model for a structured family based approach in these situations. It is a community based alternative to residential placement, utilizing specially trained and supervised foster families to provide intensive treatment for young offenders (Chamberlain & Mihalic, 1998). Foster parents are trained in behavioral management techniques derived from coercion theory (Patterson *et al.*, 1992). It is a multimodal intervention with weekly family and individual therapy sessions as well as supervision by a treatment case manager. The individual sessions use a social skills training approach reinforced by the family sessions. In comparison to residential care services as usual, delinquents receiving MTFC had significant reductions in rearrest and self-reported delinquency at one year after leaving treatment (Chamberlain & Reid, 1998). Further analysis of this study showed that family management skills and deviant peer association functioned as mediators of treatment effect on subsequent delinquency (Eddy & Chamberlain, 2000). In reviewing this and two previous treatment studies (Chamberlain, 1990; Chamberlain & Reid, 1994), the Task Force on Community Preventive Services recommended this intervention for prevention of violence in adolescents with a history of chronic delinquency (Hahn *et al.*, 2005).

Programs with minimal or negative effects

It is also instructive to consider delinquency programs that have failed to produce the desired results. Two examples that have received a great deal of popular attention are "wilderness challenge" and "boot camp." Wilderness challenge programs are based on the concept of experiential learning (Gass, 1993). Delinquents participate in physically challenging activities that will hopefully instill personal confidence and better self-control. Many of the tasks can only be accomplished through group coordination and effort, with the intention of developing better communication and interpersonal skills. Unfortunately, the outcome studies of interventions based on this model have consistently shown relatively weak improvements at best (Lipsey & Wilson, 1998). The program features that appeared to be associated with improved outcome were the intensity of the physical training and the presence of additional therapy (Wilson & Lipsey, 2000). Boot camp began as a concept to shorten adult criminal sentences and decrease crowding and costs, as well as reduce recidivism by providing a more intensive correctional program using a military model of strict discipline and drill. The concept was expanded to juvenile justice in the 1990s as a get-tough approach to rising youth violence. By 1995, state and local agencies operated 30 juvenile boot camps across the nation (Parent, 2003). Concern was raised by reports from initial research that indicated higher rates of recidivism in some cases for those sentenced to boot camps, especially those that emphasized a military rather than a rehabilitative approach (Henggeler & Schoenwald, 1994; McKenzie *et al.*, 1995). Further evaluation found that the rate of recidivism with juvenile boot camps was essentially not reduced and that most improvements were associated with the educational or community follow-up components (Peters, 1997; Parent, 2003). While many factors could potentially affect the impact for wilderness challenge and boot camp, it is interesting to note that in both cases, positive findings were associated with additional ancillary features, not the core intervention. Both programs were also based on concepts of what might help, rather than interventions for known factors contributing to delinquency and antisocial behavior.

Of greatest concern are programs that despite the best intentions actually make problems worse. A common public misconception is that there is no harm in trying new interventions with youth already exhibiting antisocial behavior. Even the most well reasoned efforts may have unforeseen effects and actually exacerbate delinquency. This was true with the Cambridge-Somerville Study of the 1930s, a program based on the sensible idea of pairing a social worker with a delinquent and his family for individualized counseling. Long-term follow-up found that those receiving this service were at greater risk for increased antisocial behavior than the control group (McCord, 1993). A more recent example of a harmful intervention is the popular "scared straight" or shock incarceration programs. The intent is to deter further offending by exposing delinquents to the harsh realities of incarceration through organized visits to prisons and lectures by adult inmates. Originally the program claimed to have significant success (Finckenauer, 1982). Rigorous outcome studies, however, found the intervention produced negative results with participating delinquents having higher rates of recidivism than if nothing was done (Petrosino *et al.*, 2000; Petrosino *et al.*, 2002). Even more surprising is that in spite of the evidence of the intervention increasing rates of delinquency, scared straight remains popular. In one case, when evaluation revealed the negative impact of the California San Quentin Utilization of Inmate Resources, Experiences, and Studies program, the evaluation was discontinued, not the program (Finckenauer *et al.*, 1999).

Special issues and future directions

In order to better address the multifaceted nature of delinquent behavior, more programs are emphasizing a systems approach in treatment. As already described, MST views the focus of intervention to be the multiple social systems involving the delinquent. Another example of a multicomponent, contextual program in community based interventions is Project Back-on-Track (Myers *et al.*, 2000), which offers adjudicated youth and their parents a month-long series of multiple services. Treatment includes group and family therapy, parent groups, educational sessions, community service programs, and empathy training. Participating youth are involved in sessions two hours a day, four days a week for a total of 32 contact hours, while parents attend a total of 15 contact hours. Those completing treatment were at significantly less risk for recidivism at one-year follow-up in comparison to controls. "Wraparound" programs have sought to individualize services by coordinating the efforts of multiple agencies and providers depending on the individual needs of the youth, with the goal of reducing out-of-home placements (Clarke & Clarke, 1996). Wraparound Milwaukee provides each youth with a care coordinator, who identifies and facilitates needed services. Decreased recidivism and problem severity is attributed to the intervention, with the average number of arrests falling 85 percent during one-year follow-up (Mendel, 2000). The proportion of youth with two or more offenses dropped from 45 percent in the year prior to program entry to 11 percent in the year after entering treatment. The Office of Juvenile Justice and Delinquency Prevention has advocated for coordination and cooperation among different agencies and groups in providing services at a program level (Wilson & Howell, 1993). The Galveston Island Youth Programs (Thomas *et al.*, 2002) developed prevention and intervention programs that shared the resources and personnel of law enforcement, city parks and recreation, schools, and community groups, targeting specific identified risk factors within the community. Juvenile arrests dropped 83 percent for violent offenses and 39 percent for non-violent offenses during the five-year project.

A particular problem confronting community based interventions is the high rate of co-morbid mental disorder in delinquents (Thomas & Penn, 2002). One study found among detained youth that almost 60 percent of males and more than 66 percent of females met criteria for a psychiatric disorder other than conduct disorder (Teplin *et al.*, 2002). In a specific program to address this, arrested and detained youth in Illinois were screened for psychotic or mood disorders, linked to community mental health services and monitored (Lyons *et al.*, 2003). Among those screened, 75 percent were successfully referred to ongoing treatment. Functioning improved in home, community, and school and only 42 percent were rearrested in the following year compared to the state-wide average of 72 percent. Wraparound programs are also well suited to addressing co-morbid mental health problems through individualized planning (Kamradt, 2000).

Most delinquency programs are understandably targeted at the largest age-group of adolescent offenders, although child delinquents under the age of 13 are at the greatest risk for going on to become serious and violent juvenile offenders (Loeber *et al.*, 2003). Developmentally appropriate programs addressing the special needs and risks of this population need to be developed (Burns *et al.*, 2003). The 8% Early Intervention Program was developed specifically for juvenile offenders under the age of 15 (Schumacher & Kurz, 1999). It was so named because this group represents eight percent of the total probation caseload, but they account for more than half of all repeat offenses. Young offenders are identified at the time of court referral and a multisystemic approach is utilized to address family and academic problems as well as behaviors in the community.

Conclusion

Research on outcomes of community based interventions has justified the goal of rehabilitation for delinquents, and the creation of the juvenile justice system. Structured interventions with sufficient duration delivered by well trained counselors appear to deliver the greatest benefit, even with serious and chronic delinquents (Lipsey & Wilson, 1998; Barnoski, 2004). The creation of multimodal, multiagency, and systems based interventions address the multiple problems contributing to and associated with antisocial behavior in youth. Several resources disseminate the methods and findings of proven and promising delinquency interventions to assist in community planning, including the Center for the Study and Prevention of Violence, Blueprints for Violence Prevention, (Mihalic *et al.*, 2001) and the Office of Juvenile Justice and Delinquency Prevention, What's Promising/What Works (Montgomery *et al.*, 1994; Sherman *et al.*, 1998). Further study is still needed to improve the efficacy of interventions and clarify the indications for specific techniques to better individualize treatment planning. Clearly, no single community based intervention program has proven to be effective in all cases of delinquency, and it is unlikely that one will ever be developed given the heterogeneous nature of antisocial behavior (Catalano *et al.*, 1999). In addition, individual community risk factors and resources vary greatly so that the optimal intervention plan will also differ from setting to setting. The National Council on Crime and Delinquency and the Office of Juvenile Justice and Delinquency Prevention have reaffirmed the original promise of the juvenile court with the policy of graduated sanctions, matching young offenders to appropriate punishment, and treatment on the basis of offense and individual needs (Krisberg *et al.*, 1995). This approach envisions a flexible response in dealing with adjudicated youth, providing a variety of interventions involving multiple services. Current program development and research support this view in response to delinquency and the promise of community alternatives to incarceration.

References

Aichhorn, A. (1935). *The Wayward Youth New York*. New York, NY: Viking Press.

Alexander, J. F. & Parsons, B. V. (1982). *Functional Family Therapy*. Monterey, CA: Brooks/Cole.

Alexander, J. F., Holtzworth-Munroe, A. & Jameson, P. B. (1994). The process and outcome of marital and family therapy research: review and evaluation. In A. E. Bergin and S. L. Garfield, eds., *Handbook of Psychotherapy and Behavior Change*, 4th edn. New York, NY: John Wiley & Sons.

Andrews, D. A., Zinger, I., Hoge, R. D. *et al.* (1990). Does correctional treatment work? A clinically relevant and psychologically informed meta-analysis. *Criminology*, **28**(3), 369–404.

Barnoski, R.. (2004). *Outcome Evaluation of Washington State's Research-Based Programs for Juvenile Offenders*. Olympia, WA: Washington State Institute for Public Policy.

Barton, C., Alexander, J. F., Waldron, H., Turner, C. W. & Warburton, J. (1985). Generalizing treatment effect of functional family therapy: three replications. *American Journal of Family Therapy*, **13**, 16–26.

Bean, J. S. (1988). The effect of individualized reality therapy on the recidivism rates and locust of control orientation of male juvenile offenders. *Dissertation Abstracts International*, **49**(06), 2370B.

Blechman, E. A., Maurice, A., Buecker, B. & Helberg, C. (2000). Can mentoring or skill training reduce recidivism? Observational study with propensity analysis. *Prevention Science*, **1**(3), 139–155.

Borduin, C. M., Henggeler, S. W., Blaske, D. M. & Stein, R. (1990). Multisystemic treatment of adolescent sexual offenders. *International Journal of Offender Therapy and Comparative Criminology*, **34**, 105–113.

Borduin, C. M., Mann, B. J., Cone, L. *et al.* (1995). Multisystemic treatment of serious juvenile offenders: long-term prevention of criminality and violence. *Journal of Consulting and Clinical Psychology*, **63**, 569–578.

Bronfenbrenner, U. (1979). *The Ecology of Human Development: Experiments by Nature and Design*. Cambridge, MA: Harvard University Press.

Burke, J. D., Loeber, R. & Birmaher, B. (2002). Oppositional defiant disorder and conduct disorder: a review of the past 10 years, Part II. *Journal of the American Academy of Child and Adolescent Psychiatry*, **41**(11), 1275–1293.

Burns, B. J., Howell, J. C., Wiig, J. K. *et al.* (2003). Treatment, services and intervention programs for child delinquents. *Child Delinquency Bulletin*. Washington, DC: US Department of Justice, Office of Juvenile Justice and Delinquency Prevention NCJ # 193410.

Catalano, R. F., Loeber, R. & McKinney, K. C. (1999). School and community interventions to prevent serious and violent offending. *Juvenile Justice Bulletin*. Washington, DC: US Department of Justice, Office of Juvenile Justice and Delinquency Prevention NCJ# 177624.

Chamberlain, P. (1990). Comparative evaluation of specialized foster care for seriously delinquent youth: a first step. *Community Alternatives: International Journal of Family Care*, **2**, 21–36.

Chamberlain, P. & Mihalic, S. F. (1998). *Blueprints for Violence Prevention, Book Eight: Multidimensional Treatment Foster Care*. Boulder, CO: Center for the Study and Prevention of Violence.

Chamberlain, P. & Reid, J. B. (1994). Differences in risk factors and adjustment for male and female delinquents in treatment foster care. *Journal of Child and Family Studies*, **3**, 23–39.

Chamberlain, P. & Reid, J. B. (1998). Comparison of two community alternatives to incarceration for chronic juvenile offenders. *Journal of Consulting and Clinical Psychology*, **66**(4), 624–633.

Clark, H. B. & Clarke, R. T. (1996). Research on the wraparound process and individualized services for children with multisystem needs. *Journal of Child and Family Studies*, **5**(1), 1–5.

Cohen, M. A. (1998). The monetary value of saving a high risk youth. *Journal of Quantitative Criminology*, **14**, 5–33.

Cook, T., Cooper, H., Cordray, D. *et al.*, eds. (1992). *Meta-Analysis for Explanation: A Casebook.* New York, NY: Russell Sage.

Crick, N. R. & Dodge, K. A. (1994). A review and reformulation of social information processing mechanisms in children's social adjustment. *Psychological Bulletin*, **115**, 74–101.

Cunliffe, T. (1992). Arresting youth crime: a review of social skills training with young offenders. *Adolescence*, **27**(108), 891–901.

Davidson, W. S., Redner, R., Amdur, R. I. & Mitchell, C. M. (1990). *Alternative Treatments for Troubled Youth: The Case of Diversion from the Justice System.* New York, NY: Plenum.

Eddy, J. M. & Chamberlain, P. (2000). Family management and deviant peer association as mediators of the impact of treatment condition on youth antisocial behavior. *Journal of Consulting and Clinical Psychology*, **68**(5), 857–863.

Finckenauer, J. O. (1982). *Scared Straight and the Panacea Phenomenon.* Englewood Cliffs, NJ: Prentice-Hall.

Finckenauer, J. O., Gavin, P. W., Hovland, A. & Storvoll, E. (1999). *Scared Straight and the Panacea Phenomenon Revisited.* Prospect Heights, Ill: Waveland Press.

Fonagy, P. & Kurtz, A. (2002). Disturbance of conduct. In Fonagy, P., Target, M., Cottrell, D., Phillips, J. & Kurtz, Z., eds., *What Works for Whom: A Critical Review of Treatments for Children and Adolescents.* New York, NY: Guilford Press, pp. 106–192.

Garrett, C. J. (1985). Effects of residential treatment on adjudicated delinquents: a meta-analysis. *Journal of Research in Crime and Delinquency*, **22**, 287–308.

Gass, M. A. (1993). *Adventure Therapy: Therapeutic Applications of Adventure Programming.* Dubuque, IA: Kendall Hunt Publishing Co.

Gendreau, P. & Ross, B. (1979). Effective correctional treatment: bibliotherapy for cynics. *Crime and Delinquency*, **25**, 463–489.

Goldstein, A. P. & Glick, B. (1994). Aggression replacement training: curriculum and evaluation. *Simulation and Gaming*, **25**, 9–26.

Gordon, D. A. & Arbuthnot, J. (1987). Individual, group and family interventions. In Quay, H. C., ed., *Handbook of Juvenile Delinquency.* New York, NY: John Wiley & Sons, pp. 290–324.

Gordon, D. A., Graves, K. & Arbuthnot, J. (1995). The effect of functional family therapy for delinquents on adult criminal behavior. *Criminal Justice and Behavior*, **22**, 60–73.

Gottschalk, R., Davidson, W. S., Gensheimer, L. K. & Mayer, J. P. (1987). Community-Based Interventions. In Quay, H. C., ed., *Handbook of Juvenile Delinquency.* New York, NY: John Wiley & Sons, Inc., pp. 266–289.

Greenberg, D. F. (1977). The correctional effect of corrections: a survey of evaluations. In Greenberg, D. F., ed., *Corrections and Punishment.* Beverly Hills, CA: Sage.

Greenwood, P. W. (1996). Responding to juvenile crime: lessons learned. *The Future of Children, The Juvenile Court*, **6**(3), 75–85.

Hahn, R. A., Bilukha, O., Lowy, J. *et al.* (2005). Task force on community preventive services. The effectiveness of therapeutic foster care for the prevention of violence: a systematic review. *American Journal of Preventive Medicine*, **28**(2 Suppl 1), 72–90.

Henggeler, S. W. & Schoenwald, S. J. (1994). Boot camps for juvenile offenders: just say no. *Journal of Child and Family Studies*, **3**, 243–245.

Henggeler, S. W., Melton, G. B. & Smith, L. A. (1992). Family preservation using multisystemic therapy: an effective alternative to incarcerating serious juvenile offenders. *Journal of Consulting and Clinical Psychology*, **60**(6), 953–961.

Henggeler, S. W., Melton, G. B., Smith, L. A., Schoenwald, S. K. & Hanley, J. (1993). Family preservation using multisystemic therapy: long-term follow-up to a clinical trial with serious juvenile offenders. *Journal of Child and Family Studies*, **2**, 283–293.

Henggeler, S. W., Schoenwald, S. J., Pickrel, S. G., *et al.* (1994). *Treatment Manual for Family Preservation Using Multisystemic Therapy*. Columbia, SC: SC Health and Human Services Finance Commission.

Henggeler, S. W., Schoenwald, S. J., Borduin, C. M., Rowland, M. D. & Cunningham, P. B. (1998). *Multisystemic Treatment of Antisocial Behavior in Children and Adolescents*. New York, NY: Guilford Press.

Jenson, J. M. & Howard, M. O. (1998). Youth crime, public policy, and practice in the juvenile justice system: recent trends and needed reforms. *Social Work*, **43**(4), 324–334.

Kamradt, B. (2000). Wraparound Milwaukee: aiding youth with mental health needs. *Juvenile Justice*, **7**(1), 14–23.

Kazdin, A. E. (2000). *Psychotherapy for Children and Adolescents: Directions for Research and Practice*. New York, NY: Oxford University Press.

Kennedy, R. E. (1984). Cognitive behavioral interventions with delinquents. In Meyers, A. W., Craighead, W. E., eds. *Cognitive Behavior Therapy with Children*. New York, NY: Pergamon Press.

Klein, N. C., Alexander, J. F. & Parsons, B. V. J. (1977). Impact of family systems intervention on recidivism and sibling delinquency: a model of primary prevention and program evaluation. *Journal of Consulting and Clinical Psychology*, **45**, 469–474.

Krisberg, B., Currie, E., Onek, D. & Wiebush, G. (1995). Graduated sanctions for serious, violent and chronic juvenile offenders. In J. C. Howell, B. Krisberg, J. D. Hawkins, & J. J. Wilson, eds., *A Sourcebook: Serious, Violent, and Chronic Juvenile Offenders*. Thousand Oaks, CA: Sage Publications, pp. 142–170.

Lipsey, M. (1992). Juvenile delinquency treatment: a meta-analytic inquiry into the variability of effects. In T. Cook, H. Cooper, D. Cordray, *et al.*, eds., *Meta-analysis for Explanation: A Casebook*. New York, NY: Russell Sage, pp. 83–127.

Lipsey, M. & Wilson, D. (1998). Effective intervention for serious juvenile offenders: a synthesis of research. In R. Loeber & D. Farrington, eds., *Serious and Violent Juvenile Offenders: Risk Factors and Successful Interventions*. Thousand Oaks, CA: Sage, pp. 313–345.

Lipton, D., Martinson, R. & Wilks, J. (1975). *The Effectiveness of Correctional Treatment: A Survey of Treatment Evaluation Studies*. New York, NY: Praeger.

Loeber, R., Farrington, D. P. & Petechuk, D. (2003). Child delinquency: early intervention and prevention. *Child Delinquency Bulletin*. Washington, DC: US Department of Justice, Office of Juvenile Justice and Delinquency Prevention, NCJ# 186162.

Lyons, J. S., Griffin, G., Quintenz, S., Jenuwine, M. & Shasha, M. (2003). Clinical and forensic outcomes from the Illinois mental health juvenile justice initiative. *Psychiatric Services*, **54**(12), 1629–1634.

McCord, J. (1993). The Cambridge-Somerville study: a pioneering longitudinal experimental study of delinquency prevention. In J. McCord & R. E. Trembly, eds., *Preventing Antisocial Behavior.* New York, NY: Guilford Press, pp. 196–206.

McKenzie, D. L., Brame, R., McDowall, D. & Souryal, C. (1995). Boot camp prisons and recidivism in eight states. *Criminology*, **33**(3), 327–357.

Mendel, R. A. (2000). *Less Hype, More Help: Reducing Juvenile Crime, What Works and What Doesn't.* Washington, DC: American Youth Policy Forum.

Mihalic, S., Irvin, K., Elliott, D., Fagan, A. & Hansen, D. (2001). Blueprints for violence prevention. *Juvenile Justice Bulletin.* Washington, DC: US Department of Justice, Office of Juvenile Justice and Delinquency Prevention, NCJ # 187079.

Montgomery, I. M., Torbet, P. M., Malloy, D. A. *et al.* (1994). *What Works: Promising Interventions in Juvenile Justice, Program Report.* Washington, DC: US Department of Justice, Office of Juvenile Justice and Delinquency Prevention, NCJ # 150858.

Moore, R. H. (1987). Effectiveness of citizen volunteers functioning as counselors for high-risk young male offenders. *Psychological Reports*, **61**, 823–830.

Mulvey, E., Arthur, M. & Reppucci, N. (1993). The prevention and treatment of juvenile delinquency. *Clinical Psychology Review*, **13**, 133–167.

Myers, W. C., Burton, P. R., Sanders, P. D. *et al.* (2000). Project Back-on-Track at 1 year: a delinquency treatment program for early-career juvenile offenders. *Journal of the American Academy of Child and Adolescent Psychiatry*, **39**(9), 1127–1134.

Palmer, T. (1983). The effectiveness issue today: an overview. *Federal Probation*, **46**, 3–10.

Palmer, T. (1994). *A Profile of Correctional Effectiveness and New Directions for Research.* Albany, NY: SUNY Press.

Parent, D. G. (2003). *Correctional Boot Camps: Lessons from a Decade of Research.* Washington, DC: U.S. Department of Justice, National Institute of Justice. NCJ# 197018.

Patterson, G. R., Reid, J. B. & Dishion, T. J. (1992). A social learning approach, 4. *Antisocial Boys.* Eugene, OR: Castalia.

Peters, M., Thomas, D. & Zamberlan, C. (1997). *Boot Camps for Juvenile Offenders.* Washington, DC: U.S. Department of Justice, Office of Juvenile Justice and Delinquency Prevention, NCJ # 164258.

Petrosino, A., Turpin-Petrosino, C. & Finckenauer, J. O. (2000). Well-meaning programs can have harmful effects! Lessons from experiments of programs such as scared straight. *Crime and Delinquency*, **46**(3), 354–379.

Petrosino, A., Turpin-Petrosino, C. & Buehler, J. (2002). "Scared Straight" and other juvenile awareness programs for preventing juvenile delinquency. *The Cochrane Database of Systematic Reviews* Issue 2. Art. No.CD002796. DOI:10.1002/14651858.CD002796.

Romig, D. A. (1978). Diversion from the juvenile justice system. In D. A. Romig, ed., *Justice for our Children.* Lexington MA: Lexington Books, pp. 117–123.

Schoenwald, S., Thomas, C. & Henggeler, S. (1996). Treatment of serious antisocial behavior. In T. Scruggs & M. Mastropieri, eds., *Advances in Learning and Behavioral Disabilities*, Vol. 10 (Part B, Intervention Research). Greenwich, CT: JAI Press, Inc., pp. 1–21.

Schumacher, M. & Kurz, G. (1999). *The 8% Solution: Preventing Serious, Repeat Juvenile Crime.* Thousand Oaks, CA: Sage Publications, Inc.

Sechrest, L., White, S. P. & Brown, E. D. (1979). *The Rehabilitation of Criminal Offenders: Problems and Prospects*. Washington, DC: National Academy of Sciences.

Sherman, L. W., Gottfredson, D. C., MacKenzie, D. L. *et al.* (1998). Preventing crime: what works, what doesn't, what's promising. *Research in Brief*. Washington, DC: US Department of Justice, National Institute of Justice, NCJ # 171676.

Snyder, H. (1988). *Court Careers of Juvenile Offenders*. OJJDP.

Spence, S. H. & Marzillier, J. S. (1981). Social skills training with adolescent male offenders: II. Short-term, long-term and generalizing effects. *Behavior Research and Therapy*, **19**, 349–368.

Spivak, G. & Shure, M. B. (1974). *Social Adjustment of Young Children*. San Francisco, CA: Jossey-Bass.

Taylor, T. K., Eddy, J. M. & Biglan, A. (1999). Interpersonal skills training to reduce aggressive and delinquent behavior: limited evidence and the need for an evidence-based system of care. *Clinical Child and Family Psychology Review*, **2**(3), 169–182.

Teplin, L. A., Abrams, K. M., McClelland, G. M., Dulcan, M. K. & Mericle, A. A. (2002). Psychiatric disorders in youth in juvenile detention. *Archives of General Psychiatry*, **59**(12), 1133–1143.

Thomas, C. & Penn, J. (2002). Juvenile justice mental health services. *Child and Adolescent Psychiatric Clinics of North America*, **11**(4), 731–748.

Thomas, C., Holzer, C. & Wall, J. (2002). The island youth programs: community interventions for reducing youth violence and delinquency. *Adolescent Psychiatry*, **26**, 125–143.

Wasserman, G. A., Keenan, K., Tremblay, R. E. *et al.* (2003). *Risk and Protective Factors of Child Delinquency*, Child Delinquency Bulletin Series. Washington, DC: US Department of Justice, Office of Juvenile Justice and Delinquency Prevention, NCJ# 193409.

Whitehead, J. T. & Lab, S. P. (1989). A meta-analysis of juvenile correctional treatment. *Journal of Research in Crime and Delinquency*, **26**(3), 276–295.

Wilson, J. J. & Howell, J. C. (1993). *Comprehensive Strategy for Serious, Violent and Chronic Juvenile Offenders*. Washington, DC: US Department of Justice, Office of Juvenile Justice and Delinquency Prevention, NCJ# 143453.

Wilson, S. J. & Lipsey, M. W. (2000). Wilderness challenge programs for delinquent youth: a meta-analysis of outcome evaluations. *Evaluation and Program Planning*, **23**, 1–12.

Woolard, J. L., Fondacaro, M. R. & Slobogin, C. (2001). Informing juvenile justice policy: directions for behavioral science research. *Law and Human Behavior*, **25**(1), 13–24.

Woolfenden, S. R., Williams, K. & Peat, J. (2001). Family and parenting interventions in children and adolescents with conduct disorder and delinquency aged 10–17. *The Cochrane Database of Systematic Reviews*, Issue 2. Art. No.CD003015.DOI:10.1002/1465185.CD003015.

Woolfenden, S. R., Williams, K. & Peat, J. K. (2002). Family and parenting interventions for conduct disorder and delinquency: a meta-analysis of randomized controlled trials. *Archives of Disease in Childhood*, **86**(4), 251–256.

18

Innovative problem-solving court models for justice-involved youth

Carol L. Kessler

The traditional adjudication process for youth has been wrought with such difficulties as overcrowded detention centers, delay in processing cases, and ineffective case dispositions. The US juvenile justice system, in response to the pressure of an increase in youth crime in the 1980s, resorted to increased detention and transfer to adult court. Punitive models threatened to overtake the heart of the juvenile justice system – a system predicated on the commitment to offer youth rehabilitation and integration into their communities.

Despite a trend toward punishment, committed teams of judges, lawyers, law enforcement officers, probation officers, community leaders, and mental health providers have fashioned creative alternatives to traditional adjudication. They aim to address such root causes of delinquent behavior as mental illness, substance abuse, academic failure, and family disintegration. The process of adjudication is transformed into a therapeutic, rehabilitative approach, wherein young people's needs are assessed and addressed. Youth at risk are seen as youth in need of support – a term that youth advocates coined for themselves at a recent meeting convened by the American Bar Association's Youth at Risk Initiative.

Problem-solving courts search for young people's strengths, and endeavor to support youth with needed educational, vocational, health, and mental health services. They seek to deliver services in a culturally relevant, developmentally appropriate manner, and they strive to link youth to effective aftercare.

These courts embody a model of restorative justice. Reparations are made by the youth to his/her community and by the community to their youth. The court holds the community accountable for providing needed services, and monitors the youth's rehabilitative progress. Youth are spared detention in overcrowded facilities, where threats of violence may exacerbate an underlying mental disorder that is unlikely to be identified or treated due to lack of sufficient mental health professionals in detention facilities (Koppelman, 2005). Detention and isolation with offenders is avoided, and substituted with the possibility of a road toward a prosocial, productive life.

The Mental Health Needs of Young Offenders: Forging Paths toward Reintegration and Rehabilitation, eds. Carol L. Kessler and Louis J. Kraus. Published by Cambridge University Press. © Cambridge University Press 2007.

Youth courts

An alternative to traditional adjudication that has become an integral component of the US Juvenile Justice System is most commonly known as youth court. Other names for this model are peer court, teen court, and peer jury. These courts are a cost-effective, creative manner of addressing predominantly young first offenders. They have grown in number and popularity, since they decrease the backlog in an overtaxed system, ensuring timely consequences to offending behavior. They have become an instrument of prevention and early intervention for youth at risk. Though studies are few in number, most youth courts boast low recidivism rates and high rates of program completion. They enjoy broad community support of offenders, victims, and legal professionals (Godwin, 1996).

The youth court model evolved gradually over the last half century. Its precursor was the bicycle court of the 1940s that addressed teen cyclists' traffic violations (Butts & Buck, 2002). From this model, an obscure crime prevention program emerged with a handful of teen courts emerging in the 1960s. A court in Odessa, Texas developed in 1976 and is identified by many as a national model (Godwin, Steinhart & Fulton, 1998). In the past decade, youth courts have grown exponentially throughout the US. Whereas in 1994, 78 such courts were functioning, by 2005, 1035 courts had developed nationwide, reflecting a 1330 percent increase in a ten-year period (Pearson & Jurich, 2005).

Rapid growth of youth courts has been facilitated by the creation of a National Youth Court Center in Lexington, Kentucky. The Office of Juvenile Justice and Delinquency Prevention established this center in 1999 to offer training and technical assistance to existing and developing youth courts. They maintain a database and a clearinghouse of information regarding courts throughout the US. Communication is facilitated through their website – www.youthcourt.net. The center develops national guidelines for youth courts. The center is supported in its mission by the US Department of Health and Human Services, Substance Abuse and Mental Health Services Administration, the US Department of Education, and the US Department of Transportation's National Highway Safety Administration. The American Bar Association has been instrumental in developing the Youth Court Center's curriculum for youth volunteers. In addition to the National Youth Court Center, a National Youth Court Alliance of federal, state, and local agencies has emerged to promote this now widespread model of juvenile justice (Vickers, 2000).

Youth courts are now woven throughout the US juvenile justice system in a myriad of settings. Some function within juvenile courts, juvenile probation departments, or law enforcement agencies. Schools house other youth courts. Still others are operated by private, non-profit organizations (Pearson, 2003).

Youth courts differ in their settings and their styles of operation, yet they commonly serve those young first offenders who would typically receive minimal or no attention from an overtaxed juvenile justice system. Advocates of the youth court model point out the benefit of immediate, meaningful consequences to law-breaking behaviors. A 2005 review of youth courts found that referred teens ranged from age 11–17, with volunteer court staff ranging from age 13–21 years. Youth are referred by judges, police, probation officers, and schools. Cases typically involve vandalism, theft, disorderly conduct, minor assault, alcohol possession, minor drug offenses, larceny, or truancy. Offenses are primarily misdemeanors or status offenses, though some youth courts handle felonies as well (Pearson & Jurich, 2005).

Youth courts are a specialized diversion program that has become a primary diversion option in the US. Entry is voluntary, and in 90 percent of courts is contingent upon admission of guilt. Courts function to impose meaningful sanctions; if fulfilled, delinquency charges are dismissed. Sentences vary, yet they are constructive, seeking restitution and reparation. They typically include letters of apology to victims; community service; mental health and/or substance abuse treatment; anger management training; and service to the youth court. Youth encounter the concept of making amends for hurtful behaviors (Pearson & Jurich, 2005).

Youth courts are thus staffed by former offenders and/or by community volunteers. Some courts are linked with schools that integrate the service-learning model developed by the National Youth Court Center with their social science curriculum (Pearson, 2003). Youth earn credits for youth court involvement. Training typically lasts 16–20 hours. Educational goals achieved include conflict-resolution; balance of rights with responsibilities; public speaking; and knowledge of courtroom proceedings (Butts & Buck, 2002).

Court proceedings vary somewhat between four basic models. Adults serve as judge in a few instances. More often adults occupy administrative positions – seeking grant funding; coordinating liaisons with community agencies. Most courts are staffed by youth in the roles of judge, jury, defense attorney/youth advocate, prosecutor/community impact evaluator, bailiff, and clerk. Cases tend to be heard in this setting within two–four weeks from time of hearing. Prosecutors speak on behalf of the victim and the community, whereas defending counsel points out mitigating factors. Hearings last for about one hour, and conclude with a determination of sentences. Sentences are typically completed within one–three months (Pearson & Jurich, 2005).

Rather than ignore first offenders or place them with youth whose antisocial behaviors are more entrenched, peer courts hold youth immediately accountable, and place them in a context where peer pressure can produce favorable, prosocial results. Youth are tried by a jury of their peers, who don't condone law-breaking behaviors. They encounter peers who model prosocial attitudes (Butts & Buck, 2000). Sentences may include relationships with adult mentors, employed within the broader agency housing the court.

Youth encounter a court of their peers that seeks to provide restorative justice. By participating in court, the accused youth is educated about the legal system and about the impact of his/her behavior on the community, on the victims, and on himself. Sentences afford youth the opportunity to have a positive impact on their community. The court process provides an arena for teens to practice such life skills as problem-solving and communicating with a diverse group of peers. Youth learn to listen to one another, to negotiate conflict, and to respect authority (Godwin, 1996).

Respect for authority increases as youth are empowered themselves. In teen court, youth are given responsibility to sentence peers, and to make decisions regarding program management. Beyond court walls, youth are sentenced with community service that empowers them to address problems that are at the root of delinquency. Entrusting youth with meaningful roles endows them with confidence and self-esteem.

Links between teen courts and schools, businesses, and faith communities develop as community service placements are generated. Teen courts portray youth as a valuable resource; community agencies are challenged to provide the necessary tools for youth to change themselves and their communities. Teen courts thereby challenge communities' negative stereotypes of their youth, and mobilize communities to form alliances with youth in a collective struggle against crime. Youth are provided with a path toward civic engagement, wherein they take pride in and ownership of the well-being of their neighborhood (Pearson & Jurich, 2005).

In Red Hook, Brooklyn, truant youth were sentenced to provide tutoring to grade school children. Other delinquency charges were repaired through service in a soup kitchen or at the local health clinic (Anderson, 1999). In the South Bronx, New York, Youth Force's Youth Court provides identification cards to facilitate safe interaction with police and to minimize arrests. Peers help youth to formulate educational and vocational goals; they also facilitate referrals to appropriate educational, recreational, vocational, and mental health resources. Community service in the Bronx may involve sentencing a youth involved in vandalism to a tenant-organizing campaign, or a substance offender to service in a hospital unit of crack-addicted newborns (South Bronx Community Justice Center, 1999). Youth Force has also been instrumental in identifying stores that sell liquor to youth (Kessler, 2000). Teen courts' community involvement has led to communities regaining pride in their youth.

Indeed, youth courts have rapidly gained popularity, despite few studies to document their effectiveness. The American Youth Policy Forum has recently conducted a national survey of the teen court model. In November 2004, forms were mailed nationwide requesting feedback from 500 youth court coordinators; 365 coordinators responded. Data compiled from their feedback indicated that an average of 89 percent of youth sentenced completed their sanctions. Between 100 000 and 125 000 youth were served each year by 100 000 youth volunteers. The average annual budget for a youth court was $49 000 per year, or $430 per youth served. Most courts received state and/or local funding (Pearson & Jurich, 2005).

This national review concluded that youth courts are a cost-effective alternative, that boast high completion rates and low recidivism rates. These statistics may partially reflect the low-risk population served – i.e., young first offenders, willing to admit their guilt are perhaps the least likely to reoffend (Pearson & Jurich, 2005).

The American Youth Policy Forum survey notes that youth courts have gained the support of judges, probation officers, law enforcement officers, teachers, and prosecutors. Youth and their families also report satisfaction with the process. Youth served reportedly have improved grades and more positive attitudes toward authority (Pearson & Jurich, 2005).

To address the lack of outcome studies, the Urban Institute conducted the Evaluation of Teen Courts Project. This project involved a quasi-experimental evaluation of four program sites, wherein teen court participants were matched with traditional juvenile justice system quasi-controls. All four sites – Alaska, Arizona, Maryland, Missouri – boasted low six-month recidivism rates, ranging from six–nine percent. Over 90 percent of parents and youth were pleased with the youth court experience. In two of the four sites, teen court graduates were significantly less likely to reoffend than traditional court graduates (Butts, Buck & Coggeshall, 2002).

While further studies are warranted, those available indicate that youth courts are a cost-effective alternative that promise to promote volunteerism, and to transform the relationship between court and community into a partnership for prosocial youth development. Youth courts demonstrate the potential of community-based programs that hold youth accountable to one another, and to the surrounding neighborhood. When provided with alternatives to detention, adolescents who offend can be channeled to educational and clinical resources in the community, while they make reparations for the harm inflicted by their actions. With limited cost, youth enrich themselves, as they contribute in a creative, constructive manner to one another and to the community.

Restorative justice conferences

Young offenders, less than 13 years of age, pose a unique challenge to the justice system that has been studied by the Office of Juvenile Justice and Delinquency

Prevention's Study Group on Very Young Offenders. Since their delinquent acts tend to be mild in nature, they tend to be dismissed by an overwhelmed system that fails to hold young youth accountable. However, these youth are at considerable risk of reoffending, with 60 percent of ten-to twelve-year-olds returning to court, and 80 percent of returning offenders, becoming court-involved once again.

Creative responses to non-violent first offenders are restorative justice conferences. Young people who acknowledge guilt are referred to a facilitator-led meeting with their victim, the victim's supporters, and their own support network. This group discusses the offense, and the resultant harm to the victim, and to the victim's and youth's support groups. The meeting concludes with a signed reparation agreement, that defines amends that the youth is expected to make.

Restorative justice conferences base their effectiveness on "principles of control, deterrence, and reintegrative shaming" (McGarrell, 2001). The latter principle declares that accountability and respect are critical factors in retaining youth as members of their community. Justice conferences, rather than labeling youth, forge a path toward reintegration and right-relation.

Early outcome studies are promising. A restorative justice experiment in Indianapolis boasts an 82.6 percent completion rate, compared to 57.7 percent completion for youth in a control group referred to other diversion programs. Furthermore, the restorative justice program's recidivism rate six months after completion was 13.5 percent less than that of the control group. Anecdotally, both victims and youth were grateful for their level of involvement in the justice-promoting process.

Juvenile mental health courts

Whereas youth courts emerged out of the unique context of young people interfacing with the justice system, other youth specialty courts have been modeled after adult counterparts. Ironically, juvenile courts, which were established in the US at the end of the nineteenth century to create a rehabilitative response to youth offenses, have become increasingly more punitive, with rising rates of detention and transfer to adult courts. Meanwhile, during the past few decades, adult courts, overwhelmed by the needs of deinstitutionalized mentally ill adults who became embroiled with the criminal justice system, have developed mental health specialty courts (Bureau of Justice Assistance, 2000). In these adult specialty courts, a model of therapeutic jurisprudence echoes the original concept of a rehabilitative juvenile court.

With therapeutic jurisprudence, the judge sits at the center of a team that integrates mental health and criminal justice disciplines, with the goal of promoting the well-being of the person subject to the legal proceeding (Kessler, 2005). The judge serves as a continual monitor of the progress of an individual interfacing with the criminal justice system. The judge offers praises and/or sanctions when appropriate, and holds families, schools, and mental health agencies accountable as well (Steadman *et al.*, 2001).

Youth mental health courts are an example of such specialty courts modeled after previously established adult mental health courts. Adult mental health courts originally were established in Florida in 1997, and the first youth mental health court was formed on February 14, 2001 in Santa Clara County, California. Its name was changed from mental health court to Court for the Individualized Treatment of Adolescents, or CITA, when stigma deterred youth from volunteering to agree to its services.

CITA was established to meaningfully address delinquent behavior, not merely as an act to punish, but as a non-specific symptom. CITA recognized that many youth who become embroiled in the criminal justice system have undiagnosed, untreated mental illness. In the traditional justice system, these illnesses often remain unassessed and unaddressed. Rates of mental illness are estimated to range between 50–70 percent of youth who become "mired in a system ill-equipped to rehabilitate them" (Arredondo *et al.*, 2001).

Failure to take mental illness into account leaves such legal concerns as competence and culpability unaddressed. Detention of mentally ill youth may violate that individual's right to be free of cruel and unusual punishment. Absence of treatment impedes the justice system's supposed goals of rehabilitation and community safety. If the root cause of delinquent behavior is mental illness, which is neither diagnosed nor treated, disturbed and dangerous behaviors are likely to recur. Suffering of both the offender and the community are likely to be protracted.

Developers of mental health courts recognized the silo effect of two systems – mental health and juvenile justice – working independently to address the needs of the same severely emotionally and behaviorally disturbed youth who commit delinquent acts. Neither system has been able to meet these youths' needs alone. Yet traditionally, communication and collaboration between systems has been sparse. The goal of courts such as CITA is to build bridges between "silos" by creating an interdisciplinary model, fueled by cross-training and teamwork (Arredondo *et al.*, 2001).

Existing resources are thereby realigned in a cost-effective, efficient manner, with the guidance of a strong judicial leader. One judge oversees a team of mental health worker, probation officer, defense attorney, and prosecutor; treatment thereby becomes a crucial component of the court process. An integrated system is created where mentally ill youth exhibiting delinquent behavior may be identified, held accountable, and linked to humane treatment in the least restrictive, most culturally sensitive manner possible.

Multiple professionals provide follow-up and case management to youth and their families. Family is included in interactions with court and with service providers. Relatives are provided with psycho-education, and are linked to supportive services. The mental health specialty court thereby aims to decrease recidivism; to enhance community safety; to appropriately match services to needs; to decrease the misuse of detention; and to promote the psychosocial well-being of youth and families.

Santa Clara County's CITA has narrowly defined its eligibility criteria to youth diagnosed with a "biologically determined illness," with a genetic component, that contributes to criminal activity. Specific disorders include major depressive disorder, bipolar disorder, schizophrenia, severe anxiety disorder, severe attention-deficit/hyperactivity disorder, mental retardation, autism, pervasive developmental disorder, and such organic disorders as head injury. Youth who solely are diagnosed with conduct disorder, oppositional-defiant disorder, adjustment disorder, or personality disorder are excluded from CITA. Legally, youth are referred after committing misdemeanors, felonies, or parole violations. Youth who were older than 14 at the time of a violent offense are not eligible for CITA (Arredondo et al., 2001).

To determine eligibility for CITA, all youth brought into custody are screened. In addition to administering the MAYSI, screening includes a search of the mental health department data; information from parents, schools, and mental health professionals; and a chart review. Of 1700 youth admitted to detention in Santa Clara County, MAYSI administration found that 37 percent had endured severe trauma, 19 percent were depressed, 9 percent were psychotic, and 8 percent had suicidal ideation. In CITA's experience, most youth referred for their services were diagnosed with affective disorders and with mental retardation, and the most common offense was threatening behavior (Arredondo et al., 2001).

Screening is the first step, and identifies youth to refer to CITA's mental health court coordinator and probation officer. These court workers may consult with a psychiatrist before determining eligibility. If youth and family, in consultation with a defense attorney, approve transfer to CITA, the prosecution screens for risk to the community. If deemed eligible and willing, a comprehensive assessment is conducted by the mental health court coordinator before developing an individualized treatment plan. Assessment minimally includes the DISC, interviews of parents, and a home visit. Treatment plans consider therapy, medication, and wraparound services, and they are formulated through a strength-based, family-focused, culturally sensitive lens.

The judge ultimately determines the youth's disposition, after weighing safety of the community, mental health issues, and the youth's need for accountability. This same judge and an integrated team reviews treatment plans every one–three months at a CITA hearing. At this hearing, treatment adherence and school progress are assessed. Between hearings, a probation officer meets at least twice monthly with the youth, as well as twice monthly with either youth, family, school, or treatment provider. The probation officer attends school meetings where individualized educational plans are reviewed, and assists in the formulation of treatment plans by mental health providers. The probation officer serves to supervise the youth, to connect with community resources, and to provide feedback to the judge. At hearings, the judge may elect to enforce such legal sanctions as electronic monitoring or brief detention; the judge may also remand the youth for inpatient psychiatric treatment or for review of psychopharmacologic interventions.

Youth remain on probation with periodic hearings for at least one year. If they consistently demonstrate progress, they may graduate to intensive aftercare. Prior to their release, the CITA team meets with youth, family, school, and supportive services to identify ongoing issues, and resources that might address them. The youth is then transferred in a timely manner to the least restrictive level of care (Arredondo *et al.*, 2001).

CITA boasts the efficient creation of an integrated system that effectively processes youth with mental illness, clarifying rates of psychiatric diagnoses, and identifying resources for treatment of mentally ill youth with delinquent behavior. This specialized court equips the judge with appropriate dispositional alternatives, and thereby decreases rates of detention. Family, school, and community are more effectively engaged in promoting rehabilitation. Recidivism is also expected to decrease, since meaningful aftercare is fashioned for each youth.

Youth mental health courts are in their infancy. The CITA model has been replicated, with minor variations, in two counties within the US. Hard data and vigorous outcome studies are lacking. The Bazelon Center for Mental Health Law has expressed concern that mental health courts may be creating a system wherein youth are arrested in order to channel them to appropriate services. Their critique states that the true root cause of youth interfacing with the justice system is the lack of early intervention, prevention, and treatment of mental illness. Indeed, schools tend to adopt zero tolerance policies that rely on suspension, expulsion, and police intervention, rather than assessment and therapeutic intervention. Whereas five percent of US school children are estimated to suffer from mental disorder and/or functional impairment, less than one percent receive special education services (Harris & Seltzer, 2004).

The Bazelon Center views specialty courts as "too little, too late," and as potentially stigmatizing to youth who have been denied needed services, and now bear a history of court involvement. This legal advocacy center argues that cases that may have been dismissed or received minimal sanctions are caught in the net of the specialty court system with questionable results. The Bazelon Center raises relevant concerns and points to the need for investment in outcome studies, to ensure that therapeutic jurisprudence is indeed effective.

The judge of Santa Clara's CITA boasts positive results. Recidivism in this specialty court is rated at 7 percent, compared to 25 percent in the general population (Arredondo, 2001). These data are helpful, but clearly inconclusive.

Juvenile drug courts

Juvenile drug courts are a recent addition to the juvenile justice system. They were adapted from an adult specialty drug court model that is based on the notion of therapeutic jurisprudence – a notion that is the foundation of the US's juvenile justice system. Adult drug courts were developed in the 1980s, with the first court established in Dade County, Miami, Florida in 1989 (Drug Court Clearinghouse, 1999). They arose in response to an escalating epidemic of substance abuse met with harsh drug laws that resulted in the flooding of the criminal justice system with non-violent substance abusers.

Punitive measures and incarceration created a revolving door of relapsing, reoffending individuals, who failed to receive meaningful sanctions or services (Roberts, Brophy & Cooper, 1997). In 1997, more than 60 percent of offenders were imprisoned for drug-related crimes, and more than 75 percent of incarcerated individuals had substance abuse problems (Drug Court Clearinghouse, 1999).

Neither treatment services nor court systems operating in isolation were effective. Studies indicated that effective substance abuse treatment is dependent on length of involvement, regardless whether treatment is voluntary or mandated (Drug Court Clearinghouse, 1999). Drug courts were established to integrate justice and treatment systems in a model of therapeutic jurisprudence that upholds both community safety and restorative justice.

A judge holds both service providers and defendants accountable, through regular status hearings, frequent urinalyses, and through the integrated work of a team of attorneys, probation officers, case managers, and treatment providers. Sanctions or praise are offered in rapid response to defendants' misdeeds or success, respectively. Adult drug courts quickly spread throughout the US through federal funding and the technical assistance of the Drug Court Planning Office (Roberts et al., 1997).

Outcome studies are limited in their methodology and scope, yet they boast high rates of retention. An average of 70 percent of drug dependent offenders remained in or graduated from treatment programs; this is more than double the retention rate for traditional treatment (Drug Court Clearinghouse, 1999). Participants decrease their drug use and criminal activity while enrolled in the drug court. More than 25 percent had failed to succeed in a previous program. An average of 47 percent of participants graduate (Belenko, 2001).

Adult drug courts boast cost-effectiveness by decreasing jail bed days; they also free up these beds for more serious offenders. Furthermore, program graduates have benefited from vocational training, and are more likely to become employed (Drug Court Clearinghouse, 1999). In Miami, for every dollar spent on drug courts, seven dollars are saved elsewhere in the criminal justice system (Makkai, 1998). A review of research on drug courts from June 1999 – April 2001, concluded that these courts receive considerable local support, and provide intensive, long-term treatment to offenders with a long history of substance use and criminal justice contacts, as well as high rates of social and health problems (Belenko, 2001).

An average of two or three participants in adult drug courts are parents of minor children, who are at risk for developing problems with substances (Drug Court Clearinghouse, 1999). Some adult drug courts have developed a prevention component, intervening with children of participants. Family drug courts have emerged to address issues of custody, visitation, and charges of abuse or neglect against substance dependent parents, with the goal of court-supervised treatment leading to family reunification (Drug Court Clearinghouse, 1999).

The popular drug court model was later adapted to serve those juvenile offenders who use substances. Since 1995, juvenile drug courts have become a national movement supported at a federal level by the Bureau of Justice Assistance. Given the multigenerational nature of addiction, many of these youth's family members have appeared before adult or family drug courts. Developers of juvenile drug courts soon realized that they address much more complex problems, since they must interface with youth's peer group, family, and school, and must provide developmentally appropriate services in order to be effective (Drug Court Clearinghouse, 1999). Furthermore, the notion of family must extend beyond traditional, biological ties to include stepparents, godparents, or neighbors in the youth's support system.

Youth served most frequently have used alcohol and/or marijuana, with cocaine, crack, methamphetamine, heroin, and toxic inhalants becoming more prevalent (Drug Court Clearinghouse, 1999). The average age at first use is 10–12 years, with some using as early as age 8. Substance-using youth, aged 13–17 years, present with non-violent misdemeanors, felonies, or status offenses; they rarely meet the full criteria for substance dependence (Cooper, 2001).

A 2001 review of juvenile drug courts noted that participants tend to be older, White male alcohol or marijuana users, with serious educational problems, and previous court involvement. This review noted that 57 percent were between 16–17 years of age; 83 percent were male; 49 percent were White; 24 percent were African-American: 23 percent were Hispanic. Thirty percent had not received previous treatment, whereas 83 percent had previous court involvement. There were high rates of mental health problems, and prevalent histories of physical and sexual abuse (Belenko, 2001).

Juvenile drug courts aim to respond swiftly with appropriate sanctions and services, monitored by a judge. They hope to provide skills to youth, and to promote accountability to the community. They seek to strengthen families. Youth are equipped with tools and supports that may empower them to lead substance-free, crime-free, healthy, productive lives.

There are considerable variations in the structure of juvenile drug courts throughout the US. Sixteen strategies have been identified by a workgroup convened by the National Drug Court Institute, as essential for the framework of a juvenile drug court. This group consisted of court officials, prosecutors, defense attorneys, treatment providers, educators, and researchers (Bureau of Justice Assistance, 2003). The strategies they outlined are:

1. collaborative planning – involvement of judge, prosecutor, public defender, probation, school, social services, treatment providers, community organizations
2. teamwork – an interdisciplinary, systemic approach
3. clearly defined target population and eligibility criteria, identifiable through a screening instrument
4. judicial involvement and supervision – judge "in loco parentis"
5. monitoring and evaluation – strengths-based biopsychosocial assessment
6. community partnerships
7. comprehensive treatment planning, with quarterly reviews; plans for vocational training, recreation, education, substance abuse treatment, mental health services in the least restrictive environment
8. developmentally appropriate services
9. gender-appropriate services
10. cultural competence
11. focus on strengths
12. family engagement
13. educational linkages
14. drug testing – frequent, random, observed
15. goal-oriented incentives and sanctions
16. confidentiality.

Courts vary in their approach to pleas and sentences. Most are post-adjudicatory in nature, serving youth whose guilt has been established, via plea or adjudication. Performance in the program determines whether the sentence will be deferred or suspended, and whether the charge will be dismissed. Some courts operate with a diversion model that delays prosecution until treatment is completed. Most prosecutors prefer the post-adjudicatory model, which gives more leverage for sentencing should youth fail to complete the program (Blumenthal Guigui *et al.*, 2004).

Juvenile drug courts share in an effort to screen early for substance-using offenders, and to provide immediate, individually tailored, court-supervised treatment (Peters & Peyton, 1998). Treatment aims to embrace health, mental health, educational, family, and recreational needs in a culturally sensitive, gender-appropriate manner, and is monitored by regular status hearings. Communication with community agencies, treatment providers, and schools is critical. Frequent urine toxicology monitors substance use. A multisystemic, family-based approach is frequently used to promote community-based care. Length of treatment ranges from 9–18 months.

A judge, with commitment to the needs of substance-using youth, provides continuity, and responds with consistent sanctions or praise, as appropriate. Successful youth transition to aftercare is sought, where youth who fail to engage or progress may be mandated to more restrictive interventions, such as residential treatment programs (Cooper, 2001).

Outcome studies have been limited by the variations encountered among juvenile drug courts, and by the lack of data regarding long-term impact. Reviewers of available data, are concerned with the "black box" of juvenile drug courts (Blumenthal Guigui *et al.*, 2004). Youth enter and leave, yet the various interventions they encounter are not explicitly defined. Conclusions regarding which aspects of the court experience influence outcome are hard to establish. Caution is expressed regarding rapid proliferation of this specialty court model with little hard evidence of its effectiveness. Research is needed to establish evidence-based best practices.

Available outcome studies point to the promise of the juvenile drug court model. An evaluation of a Summit City, Ohio court randomly assigned youth to either drug court or traditional adjudication. Drug court participants averaged one rearrest, whereas traditional court participants averaged 2.3 rearrests. Additionally, 11 percent of drug court clients, compared to 46 percent of traditional clients, had new charges within six months after court entry (Belenko, 2001). This study is limited by small sample size.

A 2001 review of judicial drug courts, noted that 80 percent of youth enrolled either returned to or remained in school. Retention rates in the court programs ranged between 56–77 percent. Most courts reported a significant decrease in recidivism, substantial decline in drug use as measured by urinalysis, improved family functioning, and development of skills that might enable drug-free, crime-free life (Blumenthal Guigui *et al.*, 2004). Anecdotally, juvenile drug courts claim to offer a remarkable potential to rehabilitate youth considered to be at high risk for escalating delinquency and substance use.

Caution is voiced by some, regarding possible risks ensuing from rapid proliferation of juvenile drug courts, despite lack of quality outcome data. Concerns include the possibility that these courts have a net-widening effect. Substance use among teens is common, and courts may be labeling, stigmatizing, or criminalizing youth, who might otherwise grow out of a normative, risk-taking phase. Police, schools, and parents may view drug courts as a readily available means of addressing teen substance use. To guard against entry of low-risk substance users into an intensive, unnecessary, possibly iatrogenic intervention, assessment tools must be developed that reliably identify youth at risk (Blumenthal Guigui et al., 2004).

An alternative, less intensive prevention program has been developed for 10- to 17-year-old first time offenders, charged with possession of alcohol, marijuana, or drug paraphernalia. Youth referred by school or by court are diverted to a chemical abuse awareness class. For four hours, the youth and his/her parent are taught skills for communicating and for making decisions regarding substance use. Class participation leads to dismissal of charges, whereas non-compliance results in traditional adjudication. This Juvenile Alcohol and Marijuana Diversion Program offers a less stigmatizing, preventive, and educational alternative for low-risk substance using youth (Gramckow & Tompkins, 1999).

Conclusion

Juvenile drug courts, mental health courts, and peer courts are innovative responses to justice-involved youth that restore the rehabilitative mission of the juvenile justice system. They promise to avoid the economic, and more importantly, the human cost of detention and punishment. Their success ultimately rests upon communities' commitment to provide therapeutic, vocational, recreational, and educational resources to their youth in need of support.

References

Anderson, D. (1999). *Kids, Courts and Communities: Lessons from the Red Hook Youth Court.* New York, NY: Center for Court Innovation.

Arredondo, D., Kumli, K., Soto, L. et al. (2001). Juvenile mental health court: rationale and protocols. *Juvenile and Family Court Journal*, Fall 2001, 1–19.

Belenko, S. (2001). *Research on Drug Courts: A Critical Review.* New York, NY: The National Center on Addiction and Substance Abuse at Columbia University.

Blumenthal Guigui, R., Michael, D., Schedler, S. et al. (2004). *Best Practice Number Fourteen: An Analysis of the Efficacy of Juvenile Drug Courts for Memphis and Shelby County.* Memphis, TN: Memphis Shelby Crime Commission.

Bureau of Justice Assistance (2000). *Emerging Judicial Strategies for the Mentally Ill in the Criminal Caseload: Mental Health Courts.* Washington, DC: US Department of Justice, Office of Justice Programs.

Bureau of Justice Assistance (2003). *Juvenile Drug Courts: Strategies in Practice.* Washington, DC: US Department of Justice, Office of Justice Programs.

Butts, J. & Buck, J. (2000). *Teen Courts: A Focus on Research.* Washington, DC: Office of Juvenile Justice and Delinquency Prevention, Juvenile Justice Bulletin.

Butts, J. & Buck, J. (2002). *The Sudden Popularity of Teen Courts.* Washington, DC: Urban Institute.

Butts, J., Buck, J. & Coggeshall, M. (2002). *The Impact of Teen Court on Young Offenders.* Washington, DC: The Urban Institute.

Cooper, C. S. (2001). *Juvenile Drug Court Programs.* Washington, DC: Juvenile Accountability Incentive Block Grants Program Bulletin.

Drug Court Clearinghouse and Technical Assistance Project (1999). *Looking at a Decade of Drug Courts.* Washington, DC: Report of Office of Justice Programs, Drug Court Technical Assistance Project at the American University.

Godwin, T. (1996). Teen courts: empowering youth in community prevention and intervention efforts. *Perspectives*, Winter 1996, 20–24.

Godwin, T., Steinhart, D. & Fulton, B. (1998). *Peer Justice and Youth Empowerment: An Implementation Guide for Teen Court Programs.* Washington, DC: American Probation and Parole Association.

Gramckow, H. & Tompkins, E. (1999). *Enabling Prosecutors to Address Drug, Gang, and Youth Violence.* Washington, DC: Juvenile Accountability Incentive Block Grants Program Bulletin # NCJ178917.

Harris, E. & Seltzer, T. (2004). *The Role of Specialty Mental Health Courts in Meeting the Needs of Juvenile Offenders.* Washington, DC: Judge David L. Bazelon Center for Mental Health Law.

Kessler, C. (2000). Youth force in the South Bronx. *Newsletter of the American Academy of Child and Adolescent Psychiatry.* July/August 2000.

Kessler, C. (2005). Alternatives to traditional adjudication: drug courts, mental health courts, peer courts. *American Academy of Child and Adolescent Psychiatry Task Force on Juvenile Justice Reform: Recommendations for Juvenile Justice Reform.* Washington, DC: American Academy of Child and Adolescent Psychiatry.

Koppelman, J. (2005). *Mental Health and Juvenile Justice: Moving Toward More Effective Systems of Care.* Washington, DC: The National Health Policy Forum at the George Washington University, Issue Brief No. 805.

Makkai, T. (1998). Drug courts: issues and prospects. *Australian Institute of Criminology: Trends and Issues in Crime and Criminal Justice*, No. 95.

McGarrell, E. (2001). *Restorative Justice Conferences as an Early Response to Young Offenders.* Washington, DC: Office of Juvenile Justice and Delinquency Prevention Bulletin # 187769.

Pearson, S. (2003). *Youth Court: A Path to Civic Engagement.* Lexington, KY: National Youth Court Center Policy Brief.

Pearson, S. & Jurich, S. (2005). *Youth Court: A Community Solution for Embracing At-Risk Youth (A National Update).* Washington, DC: American Youth Policy Forum.

Peters, R. H. & Peyton, E. (May 1998). *Guideline for Drug Courts on Screening and Assessment.* Washington, DC: The American University, Justice Programs Office.

Roberts, M., Brophy, J. & Cooper, C. (1997). *The Juvenile Drug Court Movement.* Washington, DC: US Department of Justice, Office of Justice Programs, Office of Juvenile Justice and Delinquency Prevention.

South Bronx Community Justice Center (1999). *This is the Deal on Youth Court.* New York, NY: Youth Force.

Steadman, H., Davidson, S. & Brown, C. (2001). Law and psychiatry. Mental health courts: their promise and unanswered questions. *Psychiatric Services,* **52,** 457–458.

Vickers, M. (May 2000). *National Youth Court Center.* Lexington, KY: National Youth Court Center.

19

Ethical issues of youthful offenders: confidentiality; right to receive and to refuse treatment; seclusion and restraint

Lilia Romero-Bosch and Joseph V. Penn

Introduction

A youth is held at a juvenile detention facility while awaiting legal disposition of his pending charges. The youth was recently prescribed multiple psychotropic medications in the community for "out of control" behaviors. The youth disclosed to detention staff that he was medication non-compliant and actively abusing illicit substances. The youth's urine drug screen was positive for cannabinoids and cocaine metabolites. There are no past mental health or medical records available. A clinical decision was made to hold all of the past psychotropic medications and establish a diagnostic baseline. A few days later, the youth was involved in an altercation with a peer and required physical restraint by staff and was placed in disciplinary "lock-up" status. The youth's family is upset that the psychotropic medications were discontinued. They blame the altercation, behavioral dyscontrol, and resulting disciplinary status on the lack of current psychotropic medication treatment. It remains unclear if the family is aware of the youth's recent substance abuse and medication non-compliance. The family is insistent that the youth's psychotropic medications be restarted. During a psychiatric evaluation, the youth does not appear motivated for mental health or substance abuse treatment, but is willing to comply with anything that will result in a more favorable legal disposition and shorter period of confinement.

Who has the right to make treatment decisions for this youth? Do the parents, youth's defense attorney, and the courts have a right to know the urine toxicology test results and to review the youth's mental health and/or medical records? What are some potential role and agency conflicts that may arise for clinical treaters or forensic evaluators in this correctional setting? How can mental health professionals, working with a youth across juvenile justice settings (i.e., probation, other court-mandated evaluation and treatment services, court clinic, jail or lock-up

The Mental Health Needs of Young Offenders: Forging Paths toward Reintegration and Rehabilitation, eds. Carol L. Kessler and Louis J. Kraus. Published by Cambridge University Press. © Cambridge University Press 2007.

facility, or other out-of-home placement), clarify their role, agency, and reporting duties to the courts? How do they balance these with state-mandated youth reporting requirements, and how do they determine optimal treatment options for the juvenile offender and their family? What are some other examples of patient confidentiality issues that may arise in these settings? What is the youthful offender's right to assent to or to decline treatment? This chapter will provide an overview of some relevant ethical issues – confidentiality, right to assent to and right to refuse treatment, seclusion, and restraint – that frequently arise in the context of evaluation and treatment of juvenile offenders. This chapter has applicability to psychiatry, psychology, social work, and other child mental health professionals. The terms, *clinician* or *forensic evaluator*, will apply to various disciplines in these settings.

Confidentiality

The issues of confidentiality in medicine, stem from ethical ideals existing since the time of Hippocrates. Due to the unique nature of the therapeutic relationship, and the potential for stigma, a clinician is particularly duty-bound to protect their patient's confidences and privacy. In *The Principles of Medical Ethics with Annotations Especially Applicable to Psychiatry*, based on the AMA's principles of medical ethics, guidelines of confidentiality, specific to psychiatry, are described (APA, 2001). Section 4, annotation 7 (APA, 2001) states:

Careful judgment must be exercised by the psychiatrist in order to include, when appropriate, the parents or guardian in the treatment of a minor. At the same time the psychiatrist must assure the minor proper confidentiality.

The ethics of privacy and confidentiality, as they arise in the forensic assessment versus clinical evaluation and treatment of youthful offenders, are not often addressed. Many argue that the same ethical guidelines from "traditional" clinical settings (outpatient, day treatment, inpatient) should apply equally or perhaps to a greater degree in juvenile justice settings (e.g., court-mandated outpatient treatment, court clinics, detention, and other secure settings). The American Psychiatric Association and the American Academy of Child and Adolescent Psychiatry do not currently provide specific recommendations for psychiatrists in their ethical guidelines (Schetky & Benedek, 2002). Paul Appelbaum (1997) suggested that "the primary value in forensic psychiatry should be justice based on the ethical principles of truth-telling and respect for persons." The American Academy of Psychiatry and the Law (AAPL) has promulgated the following *Ethical Guidelines for the Practice of Forensic Psychiatry* that specifically address the concept of confidentiality (AAPL, 2005):

Respect for the individual's right of privacy and the maintenance of confidentiality should be major concerns when performing forensic evaluations. Psychiatrists should maintain confidentiality to the extent possible, given the legal context. Special attention should be paid to the evaluee's understanding of medical confidentiality. A forensic evaluation requires notice to the evaluee and to collateral sources of reasonably anticipated limitations on confidentiality. Information or reports derived from a forensic evaluation are subject to the rules of confidentiality that apply to the particular evaluation, and any disclosure should be restricted accordingly.

The AAPL (2005) ethics guidelines also provide the following commentary on confidentiality and the practice of forensic psychiatry:

The practice of forensic psychiatry often presents significant problems regarding confidentiality. Psychiatrists should be aware of and alert to those issues of privacy and confidentiality presented by the particular forensic situation. Notice of reasonably anticipated limitations to confidentiality should be given to evaluees, third parties, and other appropriate individuals. Psychiatrists should indicate for whom they are conducting the examination and what they will do with the information obtained. At the beginning of a forensic evaluation, care should be taken to explicitly inform the evaluee that the psychiatrist is not the evaluee's "doctor." Psychiatrists have a continuing obligation to be sensitive to the fact that although a warning has been given, the evaluee may develop the belief that there is a treatment relationship. Psychiatrists should take precautions to ensure that they do not release confidential information to unauthorized persons.

Although not specifically addressing confidentiality issues for juvenile offenders, the AAPL (2005) ethics guidelines provide the following guidance regarding limitations of confidentiality in mandated treatment settings:

When a patient is involved in parole, probation, conditional release, or in other custodial or mandatory settings, psychiatrists should be clear about limitations on confidentiality in the treatment relationship and ensure that these limitations are communicated to the patient. Psychiatrists should be familiar with institutional policies regarding confidentiality. When no policy exists, psychiatrists should attempt to clarify these matters with the institutional authorities and develop working guidelines. Many mental health professionals have difficulty identifying the differences between the medico-legal concepts of confidentiality and privilege.

Thomas Gutheil (1998) has suggested that the first two letters of each word serve as a useful mnemonic to help differentiate the fundamental differences. **CO**nfidentiality is therefore the **C**linician's **O**bligation to keep material shared in a professional relationship confidential from third parties unless permitted; thus resulting in an ethical obligation with numerous legal expressions. Alternatively, **PR**ivilege is the **P**atient's **R**ight to bar the clinician from disclosing or testifying about professionally obtained material in legal or quasi-judicial settings (e.g., trials, depositions, hearings, administrative law reviews, tribunals); hence resulting in the alternative term "testimonial privilege." There are often many legal disagreements regarding the access to or admissibility of certain records in legal proceedings and the potential harm or risks of divulging this information. This typically results in an evidentiary concept usually expressed by conflicts between attorneys and is decided by a judge as to the inclusion or exclusion of this material in legal proceedings. Often additional questions may be raised regarding other aspects of confidentiality and disclosure of confidential records or health information. In these situations, consultation with colleagues, administrators, and risk management personnel is often invaluable, and if indicated, additional legal consultation is recommended.

Confidentiality in the child/adolescent forensic evaluation setting

The forensic evaluation of a court-involved minor is fundamentally different from a traditional clinical mental health evaluation for treatment purposes (Grisso, 1998; Haller, 2002). In a general adult forensic setting, the forensic evaluator's primary role is to answer a legal question. Specific aims of the child forensic evaluation are (1) to identify the stated reasons and factors leading to the referral, (2) to obtain an accurate diagnostic picture of the youth's developmental functioning and the nature and extent of the youth's behavioral difficulties, functional impairment, and/or subjective distress, and (3) to identify potential individual, family, school, peer, or other environmental factors that may account for problems that have resulted in the legal involvement or claimed impairment or distress. During the first meeting or phone contact with the retaining agency (private attorney, social service agency, or the family/juvenile court itself), the forensic evaluator should identify potential role conflicts, boundaries, and expectations of the proposed consulting (and specifically non-treatment) relationship to ensure that the evaluator will be able to complete an objective and comprehensive forensic evaluation. The forensic services provided may include record review only, examination of youth, verbal testimony such as in a deposition, preparation of a written report, and/or court testimony regarding the evaluation. A forensic evaluation may also involve critiquing the work that was previously done by another mental health professional or by a child protective services investigator (Penn, 2005).

During the initial meeting with a youth, the forensic evaluator has an ethical obligation to define their non-therapeutic role and to review the non-confidential nature of the evaluation. The forensic evaluator should be direct and clear regarding the evaluation purpose, process, outcome, and the absence of confidentiality. The traditional treater–patient relationship is not developed. The evaluator's role is that of fiduciary to the court or retaining agency (law firm, school department), and unlike the treating clinician, holds no fiduciary duty to the patient (Penn & Thomas, 2005). Table 19.1 illustrates some essential differences between clinical and forensic evaluations.

Table 19.1. Differences between clinical and forensic evaluations

	Traditional diagnostic "clinical evaluation"	Forensic evaluation
Purpose	Relieve suffering	Answer a legal question
Relationship	Doctor–patient	Evaluee–evaluant
Client	The patient	The court or retaining agency
Agency	Fiduciary duty to the patient; duty to the patient's best interests; patient's welfare first	Fiduciary duty to retaining source (e.g., attorney, court)
Objective	Help heal the patient	By report or testimony: inform and teach the fact-finder (e.g., judge, jury) or retaining agency
Process	Establish diagnosis and treatment plan	Conduct objective evaluation, diagnosis may be non-essential
Treatment	Treatment rendered	No treatment rendered
Sources of information	Self report, occasional some collateral records	Exhaustive attempt including serial interviews, interviews of additional historians, review of collateral data
Bias	Therapeutic bias exists: desire for patient to get better, serve as patient advocate	Attempt to be neutral and objective, lack of bias; no investment in outcome
End product	Establish a therapeutic relationship	Answer the referral question either in the form of a verbal or written report to retaining source, deposition, and or testimony

Source: Penn, 2005

When providing clinical evaluation and/or treatment to any juvenile justice-involved youth, it is recommended that mental health professionals clearly define and maintain their role as clinician to youthful offenders and their family members (Penn & Thomas, 2005). During a clinical evaluation, the mental health professional needs to be clear about their agency and non-forensic role. For example with an appropriate release of information, the treater might be able to provide factual information to attorneys or the courts regarding information that they have directly observed or experienced (examples include diagnoses, treatment modalities, medications dosage and schedule, duration and frequency of appointments, compliance with treatment). The treater should refrain from offering ultimate opinions or definitive statements regarding civil or criminal legal questions posed to them (i.e., causation, damages, psychic harm, and mitigating factors, criminal responsibility, and culpability, respectively). The youth evaluee and their families (parent or legal guardian) should be informed of the evaluator's role at the outset of any clinical evaluation or treatment (Schetky & Benedek, 2002).

The forensic evaluator should clarify role and agency issues (e.g., who has hired them, what the aim of their evaluation is, and who may have access to the interview and records). Additionally, evaluees should be made aware of the implications of data obtained during interviews. At the outset of the interview, the evaluator should review the following with the youth: purpose and process (solo evaluator versus team interview) of the evaluation, agency of the evaluator, whether the evaluation is being videotaped, what will happen to the information obtained (e.g., verbal reporting versus written report) as a result of the examination, and that the evaluation is not for treatment purposes.

As suggested by the AAPL (2005) ethics guidelines (described earlier), before beginning a forensic evaluation, psychiatrists should inform the evaluee that although they are psychiatrists, they are not the evaluee's "doctor," or clinical treatment provider. There is a continuing obligation to be sensitive to the fact that although a warning has been given, there may be slippage and a treatment relationship may develop in the mind of the examinee (AAPL, 2005). This issue may be particularly relevant with detained or pre-adjudicated (pre-trial, non-sentenced) incarcerated juveniles. It is also recommended that the examiner should provide these non-confidentiality warnings according to the youth's developmental maturity and identified cognitive abilities.

Although variable by jurisdiction, and not typically legally mandated, it is advisable to attempt to obtain a youth's assent to the interview process, and whenever possible, the same explanation should be provided to the parent or legal guardian. There is an exception to this in most emergency situations. The youth being evaluated should be able to demonstrate some understanding of the differences between information obtained for the purpose of therapeutic intervention and ongoing treatment, and information garnered for the purpose of a forensic or non-treatment evaluation. The following is an example of a possible confidentiality warning that might be explained and reviewed with a youth using basic and age appropriate terms: (1) the evaluation was for court purposes and did not involve treatment, (2) a report would be written based on the evaluation, (3) the forensic consultant may be asked to testify regarding the report, and (4) unless court-ordered, if a defense initiated evaluation, the youth's lawyer would determine whether the report would be introduced into evidence or not. Regarding the process and documentation of the confidentiality warning, some have asserted that a youth evaluee should be able to spontaneously recall each of these points or with some prompting by the examiner (and that this be included in the report). This non-confidentiality warning would be included in the body of a forensic report under the heading of *Confidentiality*. The following is suggested by way of example:

> Before the interview, Youth X was informed that the examination was being conducted pursuant to a court order, that a report would be prepared for the court, testimony may be required, and therefore the interview would not be confidential. Youth X stated that he/she understood this.

After the forensic evaluator's role has been established, the "work" of the evaluation begins. As in other child and adolescent psychiatry settings, collateral history is indispensable. Forensic evaluations typically include detailed review of all available records and, whenever possible, review of information from other collateral sources, serial interviews of the youth, and interviews with parents or other care providers.

One essential reason for attempting to gather and review collateral information from multiple sources is to assess the response style of the examinee. Whereas in clinical assessment, the response style is usually considered to be reliable, this is not to be assumed in forensic evaluations. Facing the prospect of incarceration, out-of-home placement, or other legal sanctions, it is not surprising that some youths may malinger, feign suicidality, or other psychiatric symptoms (National Commission on Correctional Health Care, 2003). This additional information will help forensic evaluators to identify inconsistencies and discrepancies in the youth's self report and to generate more reliable conclusions and recommendations.

During interviews with parents and other collateral historians, the struggle to maintain the confidentiality of certain information may present unique challenges. For example, when interviews/evaluations are conducted separately of a court-involved youth and parent (e.g., the youth is detained or in another out-of-home placement, the parent is not immediately available except via telephone), parents may ask the evaluator for details of the youth's past or recent alleged criminal behaviors, substance abuse, sexual activities, and other confidential issues. Furthermore, "... in forensic evaluations, parents' presentations may be colored by the nature of the legal issue, skewed memories, and their motives ... The forensic examiner is not expected to play detective" (Schetky & Benedek, 2002). However, it has been suggested that "forensic examiners need to be more aggressive than therapists in looking for contradictions and inconsistencies and probing for more detail" (Schetky & Benedek, 2002). In summary, although the ultimate goal of juvenile forensic evaluations is to conduct an optimal evaluation in order to best address the legal question posed, the child forensic evaluator must approach each evaluation with sensitivity to the youth's unique developmental vulnerabilities.

The conflict between the youth's right to confidentiality and a parent's right to know, often erupts when discussing the need for disclosure of certain medical (i.e., pregnancy status, HIV testing results, sexually transmitted diseases), substance abuse and toxicology test results, other mental health issues, or other identified risk taking behaviors. As a rule, the custodial parent, as legal guardian, has a fundamental legal right to the medical records of their children (Tillet, 2005). In some instances, states have granted the adolescent the right to privacy and confidentiality (Tillet, 2005). It is also common in some outpatient settings, for health care providers to establish at the outset of treatment an understanding with the parents and adolescent of ensured or explicit privacy except in emergency situations (see related section later in this chapter).

The issue of parental right to know versus the child/adolescent's right to privacy is hotly debated. The conflict centers on the main premise that barring an emergency, without consent from a legal guardian, evaluation and treatment of a minor is deemed unethical. However, clinicians suggest, and emerging literature supports the argument, that if minors do not feel that the information they provide is protected under the auspices of their doctor–patient relationship, they are not as forthcoming or engaged in the treatment alliance. And, as an extension of that "protected" relationship, minors, on occasion, have been given privacy over their medical records (Tillet, 2005).

The Health Insurance Portability and Accountability Act (HIPAA) of 1996 established minimum privacy standards for patients. The Act gives individuals more control over their personal information and establishes administrative procedures to ensure that medical information is confidential. However, HIPAA regulations specifically exempt minors from the national standard. The regulations specify that state statute still determines parental access to adolescent medical information. Where state law gives minors the right to confidentiality, such as treatment for STDs, HIPAA regulations are to be followed. (Tillet, 2005)

The need for sensitivity and care of written reports, records, and other health information is especially necessary with medical and, some would argue, even more so with mental health and/or substance abuse treatment records. There continues to be much debate regarding the issue of stigma and its effects on access to mental health and substance abuse treatment. This stigma may be further magnified in forensic, correctional, or other juvenile congregate care settings. When youths present with histories of sexual offending, and other perceived "deviant" behaviors, the clinician must make extra efforts to ensure that the juvenile offender's privacy is protected.

Although confidentiality and privilege issues are particularly relevant to pre-adjudicated youths (e.g., pre-trial youth with pending legal issues), they are also essential to post-adjudicated youths involved in mandated or court-ordered treatment. It is generally advisable to conduct the clinical assessment of a juvenile following adjudication with the intent of determining amenability to treatment, required level of care, and estimated risk of recidivism (Schetky & Benedek, 2002). The AAPL ethical guidelines described previously suggest that in a treatment situation, psychiatrists should be clear about any limitations on the usual principles of confidentiality in the treatment relationship and assure that these limitations are communicated to the patient (AAPL, 2005).

Psychiatrists and other mental health care professionals should take precautions to assure that none of the confidential information is disclosed to unauthorized persons (AAPL, 2005). Clinicians should be extremely careful regarding verbal or written communication with attorneys and other court personnel, and they should avoid inappropriate communication with the media. Responses to media requests regarding specific youth should be declined and instead directed to appropriate juvenile justice administrative personnel. If asked to evaluate youth who are charged with particularly heinous or high profile crimes, clinicians should be especially mindful of all communications to correctional and clinical staff, parents, and family members. Even confirmation of having seen a specific individual may represent a violation of confidentiality. After adjudication, the issues of any court ordered treatments, including the treater's role, agency, and mandated reporting to the court or probation, should be delineated for the youth and family (Penn & Thomas, 2005).

Exceptions to confidentiality

As highlighted earlier, the guiding ethical principles of confidentiality should apply to forensic evaluations and mandated treatment, as they do in general mental health evaluation and treatment. A conscientious clinician or forensic evaluator will make efforts to clearly define their role, and work diligently to avoid breaches of privacy. There are a few instances when confidentiality must be broken and disclosures be seriously considered regardless of the forensic versus clinical setting. These instances are common in regular clinical practice as well: (1) when the evaluee/patient is self-injurious or suicidal, (2) when the evaluee/patient is assaultive or homicidal, (3) when the evaluee/patient presents a clear and present risk of escape or the creation of disorder within the institutional facility (APA Task Force, 2000).

Superceding the ethical principle of confidentiality is the ethical principle of "first do no harm" and the duty to protect. A forensic evaluator or clinician utilizing these general principles in a judicious manner will likely avoid many common pitfalls when working with juvenile offenders, their families, and interfacing legal and other systems.

Consent

Barring an emergency situation a health care provider should, prior to offering services, first attempt to obtain informed consent. The issue of truly informed

Table 19.2. Elements of informed consent[a]

A complete informed consent process includes a discussion of the following elements:
The nature of the proposed care, treatment, services, medications, interventions, or procedures;
potential benefits, risks, or adverse effects, including potential problems related to recuperations;
the likelihood of achieving care, treatment, and service goals;
reasonable alternative to the proposed care, treatment, and service;
the relevant risks, benefits, and adverse effects related to alternatives, including the possible results of not receiving care, treatment, and services; and
when indicated, any limitations on the confidentiality of information learned from or about the patient.
Documentation of these elements may be in a form, progress note, or elsewhere in the record.

[a] Adapted with permission from Joint Commission for Accreditation of Healthcare Organizations (Grisso, 1998).
Source: Tillet, 2005

consent versus coerced treatment is particularly relevant in correctional settings and moreover in research settings. Informed consent is defined as "the agreement by a patient to a treatment, examination, or procedure after the patient receives the material facts about the nature, consequences, and risks of the proposed treatment, examination or procedure; the alternatives to it; and the prognosis if the proposed treatment is not undertaken" (National Commission on Correctional Health Care, 2003). The concept of informed consent has received much attention, and there has been much research, debate, and study regarding its definition and real-world application. There are many different policies and practices that clinicians can use to guide them in obtaining informed consent. The Joint Commission on Accreditation of Healthcare Organizations (JCAHO) offers one approach (see Table 19.2):

The Joint Commission on Accreditation of Healthcare Organizations (JCAHO) considers the informed consent process to include several components ... including the right to self-determination, shared decision-making power, and the ability or inability of individuals to comprehend information. (Tillet, 2005)

In reading the above description, or any other definitions and descriptions of informed consent, one immediately identifies the challenging question: "What about those who are underage, minors, not legally adults?"

Competency – mature minor

In the past, all minors were automatically considered, by the courts, to be incompetent, and therefore incapable of providing consent. This has become a hotly contested issue and has generated much research and discussion. Taking multiple factors into account, one considers who is the best decision-maker for the youth. Often it can be custodial parents, but if this is not a viable option, then most states execute the doctrine of parens patriae. Parens patriae is Latin for "parent of his or her country." Because the state has sovereignty over everything within its jurisdiction, parens patriae refers to "the power of the state to act as the parent of any child or, the authority over any individual who is in need of protection such as an incapacitated individual (sometimes called a person in need of protection) or a child whose parents are unable or unwilling to take care of the child." (Wikipedia, 2005)

The question of consent has its roots in the question of competency. Competency is often defined as an ability to understand the question at hand, and appreciate the various risks, benefits, and alternatives, so that a decision is deemed valid. Competency is seen as a situation specific state. For example, competency to stand trial is the present ability to appreciate the current legal proceedings and assist with one's legal defense. As mentioned earlier, minors were often categorically seen as incompetent to make decisions. However, recent literature has suggested that adolescents are as competent as adults in some regards. The ability to comprehend information is the difficult issue related to adolescent consent or the adolescent's capacity to make her own decisions. Weithorn and Campbell (1982) found that 14-year-olds were as competent as adults to make informed decisions about hypothetical situations, and other studies have found that adolescents understand the concepts of risk and benefit on the same level as adults (Tillet, 2005). Cognitively, adolescents may be able to comprehend the decision. However, psychologically, adolescents are not as good at making decisions that protect their best interests and well-being. Therefore, it may be developmentally normal for an adolescent to underestimate their vulnerability and risk.

There has been a recent trend towards considering certain minors in certain situations as being competent to make treatment decisions and offer consent. In such cases, they are often considered "mature minors." The mature-minor exception allows a physician to treat a minor based on the patient's consent if the minor demonstrates sufficient capacity to appreciate the nature, extent, and consequences of medical treatment (Simon, 1998). In juvenile and family court proceedings, youth offenders are presumed competent to stand trial unless they demonstrate some obvious evidence or history of impairment and deficiency, which may inhibit their ability to understand the legal proceedings and assist with their defense. The assessment of a juvenile's competency to stand trial (adjudicative competence) is a particularly intriguing area. The reader is encouraged to review the chapter by Geraghty, Fink, and Kraus in this volume, as well as the body of scholarly work by Grisso and colleagues (Grisso, 2005).

The question of "mature minor" takes a different turn, when a forensic specialist is asked to render an opinion regarding juvenile waiver, transfer, or bind-over to adult courts (i.e., whether or not the youth should be handled, by the courts, as a juvenile or an adult). In these cases, the forensic evaluator should perform a thorough assessment of the youth and be aware of the legal issues involved. In some settings, the evaluator will be asked to comment on the offender's mental health, substance use, and other relevant diagnoses and treatment needs; the youth's potential for rehabilitation; and their cognitive and emotional maturity. Careful assessment of these various domains is essential. The forensic evaluator's findings may carry significant weight in the decision-making of the court.

Consent is one of the core values of the ethical practice of medicine and psychiatry. It reflects respect for the person, a fundamental principle in the practices of pediatrics, medicine, psychiatry, and forensic psychiatry. Obtaining informed consent is therefore an expression of this respect. With regard to forensic evaluations, AAPL suggests that informed consent of the subject of a forensic evaluation be obtained whenever possible. Where consent is not required (for example, the evaluation is court-ordered), notice is still provided to the evaluee of the nature and context of the evaluation. If the evaluee is not competent to give consent, substituted consent may be obtained in accordance with the laws of the jurisdiction (AALP, 2005).

The American Academy of Psychiatry and the Law has proposed some additional suggestions with regard to the sensitive issue of consent in forensic settings. It is important to appreciate that in particular situations (such as court-ordered evaluations for competency to stand trial, clarification of the issues of forced medications or treatments), consent for the examination is not required. In such cases, the psychiatrist should inform the subject and explain that the evaluation is legally required and that if the subject refuses to participate in the evaluation, this fact will be included in any report or testimony. With regard to any person charged with criminal acts, ethical considerations preclude forensic evaluation prior to access to, or availability of, legal counsel. The only exception is an examination for the purpose of rendering emergency medical care and treatment. Finally, consent to treatment in a jail or prison, or other criminal justice setting, must be differentiated from consent to evaluation. The psychiatrists providing treatment in these settings should be familiar with the jurisdiction's rules in regard to the patient's right to refuse treatment (AAPL, 2005). The National Commission on Correctional Health Care (NCCHC) also provides guidance to clinicians in correctional settings (NCCHC, 2003).

Emergency consent

When a youth is deemed incompetent or the parent or custodial guardian is unable or unwilling to provide consent, barring an emergency setting, it is unethical to provide treatment without additional safeguards in place. There are, however, situations in which delays in securing consent or refusal of consent may place the minor in harm's way. In these situations, clinicians may have an ethical obligation to consider emergency consent or legal determination (i.e., judicial ruling or appointment of a temporary guardian to make decisions for the juvenile). Traditionally courts have upheld the health care provider's decisions to treat a youth in an acute or emergency setting if there exists a potential for harm from not intervening in a timely manner. Many challenging clinical scenarios arise in juvenile justice and forensic settings. Some examples include positive laboratory testing results for an STD, pregnancy, or other detected medical issues. Another common situation is the decision whether to initiate, continue, or discontinue non-emergency psychotropic medications without parental/guardian consent. There is often limited case law, immediate legal precedents, or other templates to guide clinicians and forensic evaluators with these real-world situations. It is therefore recommended that practitioners assessing or treating post-adjudicated youth, familiarize themselves with their local statutes, institutional policies, and seek professional and legal consultation when indicated. The issue of emergency consent may also arise during other interventions (i.e., voluntary or court-mandated treatments).

Right to treatment

As described above, US courts, historically, have not acknowledged the right of a minor to consent to treatment. More recently, however, there has been some movement towards establishing parameters for allowing minors some say in their *right* to treatment. Despite these advances, there is still no clear paradigm for understanding a minor's rights. The issue of a juvenile's right to treatment across different juvenile justice settings raises many questions. In most cases, clinicians and forensic specialists have looked to precedents in adult mental health for guidance.

In the modern legal and medical history of the United States, there has been much attention focused on the question of patient rights. As a result, the US government has established the *Patients' Bill of Rights*:

The *Patients' Bill of Rights* guarantees that consumers who face a medical emergency can get emergency care when and where they need it. It assures that people living with severe and chronic medical conditions can see a specialist of their choice. It guarantees a pregnant woman the right to see her doctor all the way through her pregnancy even if her health plan decides to drop that doctor from its network. It provides an independent and impartial appeals process that puts the final decision about care back in the hands of medical professionals where it belongs. And it protects patients against discrimination or violations of their confidentiality. (US Department of Health and Human Services, 2005a)

The establishment of a *Patient's Bill of Rights*, and court decisions in several landmark legal cases, has helped clarify the legal, clinical, and cultural standards of patients' rights to health care, even in the juvenile justice, and juvenile and adult correctional settings. In the cases of *Rouse vs. Cameron* (Bazelon Center for Mental Health Law, 2005), *Lake vs. Cameron* (Bazelon Center for Mental Health Law, 2005) and *Wyatt v. Stickney* (Treatment Advocacy Center, 2005a), the courts established that individuals suffering from mental illness had a right to treatment. Specifically, they were entitled to the *least restrictive* treatments that would best offer them a chance for rehabilitation and a return to their highest level of functioning. In *O'Connor v. Donaldson* (Schetky & Benedek, 2002; Stanford University, 2005), the court's decision went further to make clear the important connection between commitment and confinement. The court opined that a committed patient has a right to expect treatment. They further established that a patient, despite being ill, couldn't be confined unless they are deemed incompetent and pose a threat to themselves or others.

A State cannot constitutionally confine, without more, a non-dangerous individual who is capable of surviving safely in freedom by himself or with the help of willing and responsible family members or friends, and since the jury found, upon ample evidence, that petitioner did so confine respondent, it properly concluded that petitioner had violated respondent's right to liberty. (LSU Law Center, 2005a, pp. 573–576)

The issues regarding a patient's rights to treatment in general health care settings have become templates for questions regarding right to treatment in correctional medical and mental health care settings. These cases have served as the springboard for concerns over protecting inmates from undue punishment. The assertion has been that the denial of an inmate's right to medical and psychiatric treatment is indeed unethical and illegal. In the cases of *Estelle v. Gamble* (APA Task Force, 2000; LSU Law Center, 2005a; Cornell Law School, 2005) and *Farmer v. Brennan* (LSU Law Center, 2005b), these questions were examined and argued. As a result, there exists a current standard that, even in correctional settings, the right to treatment extends to include the precedent that denial of an inmate's health or safety concerns may constitute a denial of the patient's rights to treatment. Currently there is no established constitutionally based right to treatment standards for juveniles or juvenile offenders. The clinician or forensic evaluator must look at or extrapolate established precedents from adult cases.

Overall, the right to treatment movement can be characterized by the following types of legal solutions, largely based on the cases listed above: (1) judicial imposition of treatment for an individual patient such as in *Rouse v. Cameron*, (2) statistical standards as in the *Wyatt* approach, (3) malpractice suits as in the *Donaldson v. O'Connor* approach, (4) legislative bills of rights for patients (US Department of Health and Human Services, 2005b).

Right to refuse treatment

The establishment of the *right to refuse treatment* developed in parallel to the *right to treatment* movement. Many clinicians and forensic evaluators encounter clinical or forensic situations in which patients have refused treatment despite medical advice to the contrary. Many of these patients are seen as lacking insight, having impairments in their decision-making capacity, being legally incompetent, and potentially posing a risk of harm to self or others due to their lack of treatment compliance.

There have been several legal cases that provide a framework for guidance. In the cases of *Rogers v. Okin* (Treatment Advocacy Center, 2005b) and *Rennie vs. Klein* (Treatment Advocacy Center, 2005c), patients were found to have the right to refuse pharmacologic treatment despite being committed. The courts established that as long as they were deemed competent and the question at hand was non-emergent, the patient could refuse treatment and seek an independent psychiatric review of their case. However, this standard does not adequately address the question of right to refuse for *incompetent* individuals. When a patient is deemed by the clinician as being unable to make medical decisions, who has the right to decide for the patient? Who is deemed the best representative for the patient's interests? And how does that person balance the patient's best interests with the community's best interests?

These difficult questions were the core conflict in the case of Richard Roe III. Richard Roe III, (a pseudonym) was a successful young high school student who began to develop symptoms of schizophrenia. As his disease evolved, he became increasingly psychotic and assaultive. After several hospitalizations, and with the help of a mental health advocate, Richard Roe brought a suit against his treating facility, to seek the right to refuse treatment. After a year of legal proceedings, the court finally deemed Richard Roe incompetent to refuse treatment. More importantly, the court established the practice of "substitute (d) judgment" (Treatment Advocacy Center, 2005d).

Massachusetts' highest court, the Supreme Judicial Court, ruled that when a mentally ill individual who is incompetent to make his own treatment decisions refuses treatment, only a court can decide if he is to be treated, and must do so on the basis of substituted judgment, i.e. what the individual would choose, given what is known of his values and preferences, if he were competent." (Treatment Advocacy Center, 2005d)

As we have seen, inherent in the establishment of competence is the patient's right to refuse treatment. And similar to competence, the right to refuse treatment is a context specific privilege. The patient may refuse *specific* treatments, evaluations, or interventions but is not permitted to make blanket refusals. As with consents, each refusal must be an informed decision (National Commission on Correctional Health Care, 2003). In order for a patient to refuse treatment, the necessary information must be presented in a clear and developmentally appropriate way. Risks, benefits, and alternatives should always be provided in language that the patient could understand. With minors, development issues and cognitive capacity become even more salient. The clinician and forensic evaluator must keep in mind whether or not the youth fully understands the implications of their treatment decision(s). And, as indicated above, one must consider the juvenile's decreased ability to assess self-risk and vulnerability (Grisso, 2005).

To consider the nuances of right to refuse treatment is to provide the standard of care in clinical and forensic mental health settings. Everything becomes important to treatment, when the clinician is assessing their patient and their interactions in this comprehensive way. In fact, refusal of one or more treatment modalities (i.e., psychotherapy, psychotropic medications, substance treatment, or other treatment recommendations) itself can be considered a vital treatment issue for further exploration.

The clinician or forensic evaluator should be diligent in exploring the patient's specific questions and concerns regarding the evaluation or treatment recommendations that are offered. What has been that patient's experience in the past? How do they see their treatment relationship interfacing with the legal system? Do they truly understand the clinician or forensic evaluator's role? Are they mistrusting of treatment efforts or misinterpreting information provided, and if so, why?

Both the clinician and forensic evaluator should appreciate multiple explanations for the above concerns – there may be underlying conflicts of transference, counter-transference, miscommunication, power struggles, and disagreements with treatment staff or others. One should also consider what personal assigned meanings the patient may hold towards psychiatric treatment. The effects that the patient's religious, social, or cultural background may have on his view of mental health should also be explored. The acceptance of treatment implies the acknowledgment of being sick. This would entail the stripping of a youth's defenses against feeling vulnerable and disempowered (Simon, 1998).

So far, we have discussed interpretations of treatment refusal that consider psychotherapeutic, psychodynamic (unconscious), or other reasons for refusing treatment. But a clinician, and especially a forensic evaluator, should also be aware of more overtly conscious reasons for refusing treatment. The young offender may be garnering some real and concrete secondary gains from perpetuating the sick role (Simon, 1998). Structured interviews and objective measures from additional psychological testing (such as the MMPI-A validity scales) may be useful to assess response style. However, the mainstay of diagnosis remains a high index of suspicion combined with careful data collection, and ongoing assessment for discrepancies in historical inform-ation and for clinical inconsistencies in the mental status examination.

Restraints and seclusions

Definition

Consent/refusal, competence, and confidentiality are not the only issues of ethical importance in juvenile justice, correctional, and forensic mental health evaluation and treatment of juvenile offenders. The indications for and utilization of physical, mechanical, and/or chemical restraints requires careful weighing of the associated potential risks, benefits, and alternatives. In institutions where large numbers of individuals suffer from impaired impulse control, affect regulation, limited coping mechanisms, and other co-morbidities, it is often necessary to have defined policies and procedures regarding the seclusion and/or restraint of these patients, for multiple safety reasons.

"Seclusion is broadly defined as placing and retaining an inpatient in order to treat, contain and control emergency clinical conditions . . . A basic definition of restraint is restricting the patient's physical movements by the use of mechanical devices" (Simon, 1998). The implementation of seclusion and restraint in mental health settings has resulted in much controversy. And, in the same way, mental health systems, administrators, and professionals are often scrutinized for their intentions, ethics, and the practical application of these interventions. The clini-cian or forensic evaluator may be called upon to consult on or authorize the use of these interventions. This can be a very challenging and compromising position. The thoughtful clinician will realize that they should carefully consider all of the options, including other alternatives, and the inherent risk of harm to the youth and staff, before automatically agreeing with these serious intervention approaches.

Guidelines and policies

There has been research and some guidelines established for the use of seclusions and restraints. Both the American Correctional Association (ACA, www.aca.org) and the National Commission on Correctional Health Care (NCCHC, www.ncchc.org) have provided guidance for practitioners and administrators in correctional health settings. Each clinician should familiarize themselves with the specific policies of their institution. However, there are some basic principles common to all settings. First, the seclusions and restraints should be employed when there appears to be no other recourse. They are to be used for emergency reasons only, when the patient, other inmates, or staff are in danger.

Though the right to refuse treatment is inherent in the notion of informed consent, exceptions may arise in psych emergencies ... But as a rule, forced psychotropic medication is employed only when (1) the inmate is imminently dangerous to self or others, (2) all less restrictive or intrusive measures have been employed, (3) the physician or psychiatrist clearly documents ... (National Commission on Correctional Health Care, 2003)

Indications and contraindications

As a rule, these interventions should be discontinued as soon as it is safe to do so. There are risks and disadvantages unique to these measures that one should try to minimize. There have been many cases of minors being injured or dying when inappropriately restrained. There are even risks for seclusions, especially in the acutely suicidal patient. Tables 19.3 and 19.4 (Simon, 1998) provide some clinical guidelines for indications and contraindications.

The obvious physical and medical implications of seclusions and restraints are easy to understand. However, there are other more complex issues at hand. The clinician may often be called upon to order seclusion, or perhaps a chemical restraint. There may be requests and pressures from staff, and sometimes parents. The specialist needs to be mindful of the overt and covert reasons driving these requests.

Table 19.3. Indications for seclusion and restraint

1. To prevent clear, imminent harm to the patient or others
2. To prevent significant disruption to treatment program or physical surroundings
3. To assist in treatment as part of ongoing behavior therapy
4. To decrease sensory overstimulation[a]
5. To comply with patient's voluntary reasonable request[b]

[a] Seclusion only
[b] First seclusion; then, if necessary, restraint

Table 19.4. Contraindications for seclusion and restraint

1. For extremely unstable medical and psychiatric conditions[a]
2. For delirious or demented patients unable to tolerate decreased stimulation[a]
3. For overtly suicidal patients[a]
4. For patients with severe drug reactions, those with overdoses, or those requiring close monitoring of drug dosages[a]
5. For punishment of the patient or convenience of staff

[a] Unless close supervision and direct observation are provided.

Restraints should never be used to change or control a youth's behaviors. They should not be used unless they are part of a comprehensive treatment plan. The NCCHC, ACA, and other national organizations that develop health care standards for correctional facilities have created and promulgated national guidelines and standards for the use of punitive (restraints by properly trained direct care staff for immediate control of behavioral dyscontrol) versus therapeutic restraints (restraints for youths under treatment for mental illness) in juvenile correctional facilities. They specify the types of restraint that may be used and when, where, how, and for how long restraints may be used. A physician or other qualified health care professional, as allowed by the state health code, authorizes the use of therapeutic restraints in each case on reaching the conclusion that no other less restrictive treatment is appropriate (Penn & Thomas, 2005).

In a juvenile justice or correctional setting, chemical restraints and psychotropic agents should be employed in a highly judicious manner. It is recommended that as a general rule, without a court order, any use of psychotropic medications needs to be voluntary and not coerced or forced on a youth, except during psychiatric emergencies. The clinician would do well to be cognizant of these pitfalls, and aspire to work as an advocate for their patient. Furthermore, they should see their roles as educators for staff and families, who may be unaware of their reasons for requesting the use of restraints.

Implications for youths with histories of abuse, trauma and PTSD

The ethical significance behind the judicious use of chemical restraints does not overshadow the clinical importance. There are significant therapeutic ramifications of using chemical and physical restraints. The patient necessitating these interventions is often in an agitated distressed state. They may become disorganized and frightened. In addition, clinicians should be aware and use caution and discretion in using restraints in youths with histories of sexual abuse or other trauma history. Keeping this in mind, one can easily imagine the potential risks for retraumatization involved in restraining a minor. Thus, whenever possible, the treatment staff do not involve themselves in the non-medical or punitive restraint of incarcerated juveniles except for monitoring their health status (National Commission on Correctional Health Care, 2003). The clinician should work hard to minimize the likelihood of recalling a patient's past traumas in the process of assisting them in attaining present safety.

In summary, seclusions and restraints are often necessary in correctional settings. Although there are often particular institutional guidelines, the National Commission on Correctional Health Care, in a special appendix to their 2003 edition of *Correctional Mental Health Care*, addresses the issue of adolescents in correctional facilities in a broader way. The guidelines established in that appendix, echo much of the recommendations already listed. Specifically, they re-emphasize that restraints and seclusions should be used when no other intervention proves effective. Furthermore, they should be used infrequently and for short periods of time, as their research has shown that briefer periods of restraint and seclusion yield better results and decrease the chances of injury to the youth (National Commission on Correctional Health Care, 2003). These recommendations should serve as a reliable foundation and compass for the evaluation and treatment of juveniles in juvenile justice and correctional settings.

Conclusion

Numerous ethical challenges confront mental health professionals serving the needs of juvenile offenders. Issues of confidentiality, right to treatment, right to refuse treatment, and seclusions and restraints continue to serve as ongoing clinical and ethical struggles for clinicians, forensic evaluators, and the courts. In addition to these dilemmas, specific to correctional mental health, clinicians must also contend with difficulties often seen in general mental health inpatient or outpatient settings: effective screening, timely referral, and appropriately integrated treatments. Attempts to meet the needs of youth offenders rely on inter-agency collaboration and adherence to established standards of care. In addition, there needs to be continued development and validation of: (1) mental health screening for juveniles across juvenile justice and correctional settings, (2) further research on the prevalence of mental illness and the efficacy of various treatments for youth offenders, and (3) continued debate regarding legal and ethical implications of treatment specific to minors. Many ethical questions and challenges arise in the evaluation and treatment of this rapidly growing patient population, with limited resources. Addressing these questions can serve to continue the goal of rehabilitation for juvenile justice-involved and incarcerated youth, and nurture the hope of a healthier future for these young people, their families, and communities.

References

American Academy of Psychiatry and the Law (2005). *Ethical Guidelines for the Practice of Forensic Psychiatry*. Last revised 2005, http://www.aapl.org/ethics.htm.

American Psychiatric Association Task Force to Revise the APA guidelines on Psychiatric Services in Jails and Prisons (2000). *Psychiatric Services in Jails and Prisons*, 2nd edn. Washington, DC: American Psychiatric Association.

American Psychiatric Association (2001). *Opinions of the Ethics Committee on The Principles of Medical Ethics: With Annotations Especially Applicable to Psychiatry*. Washington, DC: American Psychiatric Association.

Appelbaum, P. S. (1997). A theory of ethics for forensic psychiatry. *Journal of the American Academy of Psychiatry and the Law*, **25**(3), 233–247.

Bazelon Center for Mental Health Law (2005). http://www.bazelon.org/about/judgebazelon.htm, accessed June 2005.

Cornell Law School (2005). http://straylight.law.cornell.edu/supct/html/historics/USSC_CR_0429_0097_ZS.html, accessed June 2005.

Grisso, T. (1998). *Forensic Evaluation of Juveniles*. Sarasota, FL: Professional Resource Press.

Grisso, T. (2005). *Evaluating Juveniles' Adjudicative Competence: A Guide for Clinical Practice*. Sarasota, FL: Professional Resource Press.

Gutheil, T. G. (1998). *The Psychiatrist in Court*. Washington, DC: American Psychiatric Press, Inc.

Haller, L. H. (2002). The forensic evaluation and court testimony. *Child and Adolescent Psychiatric Clinics of North America*, **11**(4) 689–704.

LSU Law Center (2005a). http://biotech.law.lsu.edu/cases/prisons/Estelle_v_Gamble.htm, accessed June 2005.

LSU Law Center (2005b). http://biotech.law.lsu.edu/cases/prisons/Farmer_v_Brennan.htm, accessed June 2005.

National Commission on Correctional Health Care (2003). Medical-legal issues. In *Correctional Mental Health Care, Standards and Guidelines*, 2nd edn. Chicago, IL: National Commission on Correctional Health Care.

Penn, J. V. (2005). Child and adolescent forensic psychiatry. *Medicine and Health Rhode Island*, **9**, 310–317.

Penn, J. V. & Thomas, C. R. (2005). AACAP Work Group on Quality Issues. Practice parameter for the assessment and treatment of youth in juvenile detention and correctional facilities. *Journal of the American Academy of Child and Adolescent Psychiatry*, **10**, 1085–1098.

Schetky, D. H. & Benedek, E. (ed) (2002). *Principles and Practice of Child and Adolescent Forensic Psychiatry*. Washington, DC: American Psychiatric Publishing, Inc.

Simon, R. (1998). *Concise Guide to Psychiatry and Law for Clinicians*, 2nd edn. Washington, DC: American Psychiatric Press.

Stanford University (2005). http://www.stanford.edu/group/psylawseminar/O'Connor.htm, accessed June 2005.

Tillet, J. (2005). Adolescents and informed consent: ethical and legal issues. *The Journal of Perinatal and Neonatal Nursing*, **19**(2), 112–121.

Treatment Advocacy Center (2005a). http://www.psychlaws.org/LegalResources/CaseLaws/Case5.htm, accessed June 2005.

Treatment Advocacy Center (2005b). http://www.psychlaws.org/LegalResources/CaseLaws/Case3.htm, accessed June 2005.

Treatment Advocacy Center (2005c). http://www.psychlaws.org/LegalResources/CaseLaws/Case6.htm, accessed June 2005.

Treatment Advocacy Center (2005d). http://www.psychlaws.org/LegalResources/CaseLaws/Case2.htm, accessed June 2005.

US Department of Health and Human Services (2005a). http://www.hhs.gov/asl/testify/t980721a.html, accessed June 2005.

US Department of Health and Human Services (2005b). http://aspe.hhs.gov/admnsimp/pl104191.htm, accessed September 2006.

Weithorn, L. A. & Campbell, S. B. (1982). The competency of children and adolescents to make informed treatment decisions. *Child Development*, **53**(6), 1589–1598.

Wikipedia (2005) http://en.wikipedia.org, accessed June 2005.

20

Post-adjudicatory assessment of youth

Louis J. Kraus and Hollie Sobel

Introduction

The first juvenile court in the United States was established in Chicago in 1899. With the realization that children had specific developmental needs different from adults, and in association with a rehabilitative as opposed to punitive focus, juvenile courts developed a parens patriae model. As time progressed, it became evident that such a model needed to be balanced with police power, that is, protecting the constituents of one's state. During this process there were a variety of developments within the juvenile court system. Many of these are not in the best interests of the child; do not take into account developmental and mental health needs; and do not use mental health services in assessing these issues. Examples of these issues include court-by-court variation in determining juvenile competency to stand trial or understand Miranda rights, transfer of youth to adult systems, and mandatory waiver to adult court. With regard to the latter, Grisso (1997) reports on evidence that youths' immaturity creates a substantial risk that they cannot approach their trials in adult court with the requisite understanding and decision-making capacities to assure a fair legal process.

At the present time, there is concern over a shift from juvenile court having a more rehabilitative model to the criminalization of juvenile court (Quinn, 2002). Intensified youth violence and a decrease in public support for youth offenders have contributed to a more punitive concept, certainly from a public perspective. However, jurisdictions are variable, with some juvenile courts continuing to focus heavily on rehabilitation. For instance, the North Carolina Willie M. program (*Willie M. et al. v. Governor James B. Hunt, Jr., State of North Carolina et al.*) focuses on identifying and strengthening protective factors in providing treatment for violent youth suffering from emotional, mental, or neurological handicaps (Kupersmidt *et al.*, 2004).

There continues to be a dichotomy within the US criminal justice system between courts designed for the adult system, and those attempting to address

The Mental Health Needs of Young Offenders: Forging Paths toward Reintegration and Rehabilitation, eds. Carol L. Kessler and Louis J. Kraus. Published by Cambridge University Press. © Cambridge University Press 2007.

juvenile offenders (Niarhos & Routh, 1992). Even though there is an attempt to develop a better understanding of juvenile offenders, consistency within courts is lacking.

The issue of consistent assessments has been addressed in the Netherlands. The Dutch system has a consistent pre-trial assessment, which answers specific questions including: (1) Why has the youngster committed the offense? (2) Is there a developmental and/or psychiatric disorder? (3) Was there a disorder at the moment of the offense? (4) What is the relation of the disorder to the offense and the degree of criminal responsibility? (5) What is the risk of recidivism and the prevention of favorable development? More specifically, issues of whether there should be a focus on treatment or punishment, waiver to adult court, and long-term expectations were addressed (Duits, 2005).

Males are over-represented within the justice system, with females accounting for 24 percent of juvenile arrests and 20 percent of juvenile court cases. However, the number of delinquent females is increasing at a faster rate than that of males. Within the US, there is also minority over-representation within both juvenile court and the juvenile correctional system (Arroyo, 2005). Assessments of reformatories as early as the nineteenth century showed significant differences in interventions for White versus Black youth. There continues to be significant concern (Piscotta, 1983).

The reality is that many communities simply cannot afford the treatment interventions necessary to help these wayward youth. With this caveat, there is an assumption in many systems that if these youth are not incarcerated, they will be at a significantly higher risk for reoffense (Kraus, 2005). In actuality, research has shown that court appearance for first-time offenders increases the likelihood of recidivism. In the United Kingdom, a cautioning response (formal warning by a police officer) to first offenders resulted in conviction over the following two years in only 11 percent of the sample (Home Office, 1995).

Both the most common and most complex assessments to make within juvenile court are post-adjudicatory evaluations. These assessments must always be held in a developmental framework, dependent on the age, cognition, and associated mental health issues of the youth being evaluated. In association with this, key issues such as recidivism, seriousness of offense, responsiveness to treatment, family systems, and age of the child all need to be taken into consideration (Kraus, 2005). In addressing these factors, referral for a comprehensive psychiatric assessment and psychological evaluation play an important role.

The post-adjudicatory evaluation serves to assess the child in association with review of all available collateral information. Mental health information should inform identification of both emergent risk and mental health service needs (Wasserman et al., 2003). The referral for this type of evaluation typically comes from the court, possibly probation, or any of the involved attorneys. Consistency in the evaluation, knowledge of available community resources, and expertise in juvenile delinquency, in the context of a developmental framework, are all necessary so that appropriate interventions can be put into place.

Court referral and structure of the evaluation

There are significant differences between juvenile court and adult court (Whitebread & Heilman, 1988). Records and proceedings are kept confidential. In addition, terminology is different. Children are taken into custody, not arrested. There is a disposition in place of a trial. Delinquents are typically placed in youth centers or juvenile facilities as opposed to their adult counterparts who are placed in jails or prisons. A youth, in lieu of standing trial, is adjudicated. Following adjudication, a delinquent disposition is made. Many dispositions are made without the use of mental health assessments of interventions. As better preliminary diagnostic evaluations are made of children, the need for post-adjudicatory assessments by qualified mental health professionals, including child and adolescent psychiatrists and pediatric psychologists, will be better understood.

Referral requests can be quite variable, dependent on the system in which one works. Typically, referrals will come through the court, either directly, or indirectly through the attorneys. There are times when the assessments will be contested, such as when a referral is made through the defense attorney. At other times the evaluation is done as a request from the court to better understand the needs of the child. The ultimate decision regarding placement and interventions are at the discretion of the judge. Evaluators should attempt to remain consistent in their assessment. Specific questions and concerns should be identified in writing. Appropriate releases and limits of confidentiality need to be documented. Available collateral information, including delinquency history, and school, mental health, and pediatric records should all be available prior to the evaluation commencing. Interviews with collateral sources are important as well. Well-structured assimilation of the collateral information is crucial in developing key recommendations. Ideally one should meet with the youth on at least two occasions, on one of those occasions preferably with his/her parents or guardians.

At the present time, there are no defined practice parameters in the United States for post-adjudicatory evaluations. The American Academy of Child and Adolescent Psychiatry is currently working on developing such parameters.

Twenty years ago, Jaffe *et al.* (1985) described the need for an assessment process in the London Family Court. Youth within this system received comprehensive assessments of their emotional, social, and educational needs. Other countries, such as Canada and the Netherlands, have begun to either assess this issue (Carrington & Moyer, 1995) or develop unified national assessments (Duits, 2005).

At times, an evaluator will be required to address whether or not a child needs to be incarcerated. At other times, this has already been determined. However, even with incarceration, questions regarding specific needs for the youth within their placement may be requested. One will need to have an understanding of the available services of a given facility, including educational interventions, mental health treatment, and other specialized services such as speech and language, occupational therapies (OT), etc. As mental health conditions may contribute to misbehavior, treatment may help prevent recontact with the justice system (Wasserman *et al.*, 2003).

There may be a need for additional evaluations (i.e., speech and language, OT, psychological, etc.) prior to placement. This should be clearly identified within the report. Services within correctional facilities are extremely variable. Internationally, many juvenile facilities will focus strictly on the punitive nature of the punishment with minimal rehabilitative services available.

Factors that affect disposition

The post-adjudicatory, or dispositional, stage is considered the most critical decision-making component of juvenile court. Sanborn (1996) assessed 100 juvenile court judges, prosecutors, defense attorneys, and probation officers from three juvenile facilities, and found that data differed regarding relevant factors that should have an effect on disposition.

Within Canada, a statistical analysis of eight provinces reported that the choice between a custodial and non-custodial disposition was determined mostly by the young offender's prior record. The seriousness of the offense was less important (Carrington & Moyer, 1995).

Hoge *et al.* (1995) examined the variables associated with post-adjudicatory dispositions within London Youth Court. Their analyses indicated that history of offending, as well as the seriousness of the offense, constituted the major predictors of incarceration. However, the study did not take into account mitigating circumstances associated with the delinquencies.

In the US, placement into a secure facility or waiver to adult court are directly related to the seriousness of the crime, chronicity of delinquency, culpability at the time of the offense, responsiveness, or for that matter, lack of responsiveness to prior mental health interventions, and whether or not there is a need for protection of the constituents of the state (police power). More serious violent offenses including murder, rape, assault with a deadly weapon, and attempted murder, will most likely result in incarceration regardless of the history. Non-violent offenses such as robbery, drug charges, and even home invasion, in association with younger age, will often lead to a question to the court regarding disposition. Typically, the most serious of charges result in the most restrictive disposition. Often when this is the case, there is little interest by the court in assessing the mental health of the defendant. As a result, we are left with a minimal understanding of children who likely have a variety of mental health and educational needs.

In a study conducted within Canada's youth justice system, Campbell and Schmidt (2000) reported that there was an overall concordance of 67.5 percent between clinicians' recommendations and court dispositions, with greater agreement for legal (88.2 percent) than mental health (52.5 percent) oriented suggestions. In addition, concordance was higher for male offenders (60 percent) compared to females (36 percent). Overall, suggestions made for counseling were twice as likely to be implemented than were those for psychiatric follow-up.

The study also revealed several mental health variables that predicted disposition above and beyond factors related to the crime. Youth offenders coming from problematic home environments (including dysfunctional relationships with parents, low parental supervision, inappropriate discipline techniques) and with high severity of substance abuse are more likely to receive a more restrictive disposition. An earlier study also conducted within Canada's youth justice system (Hoge *et al.*, 1995) identified antisocial attitude as a personality factor predictive of being disposed to custody.

In their final opinion, the authors reported that although the 2000 study results suggested mental health reports influence the disposition decision process through the court, the influence is more limited than expected given the purpose of these post-adjudicatory evaluations. Thus, in order to best serve these youth, while balancing their needs as well as safety and cost to the community, clinician reports must clearly state both the mental health issues confronting the individual, as well as the influence of such factors on their behavior.

Residential and community facilities

More often than not, requests for evaluation will be made when a child is going to be placed in either a community-based program or a residential program, and specific recommendations regarding treatment needs are required. An understanding of local and available facilities is important, including wraparound services, residential programs, and community-based services that can be included within the wraparound interventions. The child's specific needs and his/her amenability to mental health interventions as well as other services in less structured environments, in association with cost factors must be taken into account. It is also critical to consider the potential risk of harm to others the child may represent in a less structured environment. Mitigating factors regarding the juvenile's functioning should be flushed out in these evaluations. This can help the court better understand the complexities that led to the delinquency, for example, underlying depressive symptoms and other affective disorders, or in the case of younger individuals, undue influence.

In addition to assessing appropriate treatment, there is also a goal of reducing juvenile recidivism. Prior research has documented factors associated with repeat offenders (Chang *et al.*, 2003; Vermeiren *et al.*, 2002; Niarhos & Routh, 1992). Studies vary with regard to methodology, yielding some inconsistent results. Factors that have repeatedly been found to predict recurrence of unlawful behavior include prior offenses, drug use, diagnosis of conduct disorder, poor academic achievement, early age of onset of initial offense, and absence of a depressive disorder. These areas should be carefully assessed in the evaluation to help support the disposition recommendations.

Psychopathic offenders have been found to be both more likely to repeat criminal behavior (Hemphill *et al.*, 1998) and less amenable to treatment (Seto & Barbaree, 1999). However, psychopathy is difficult to assess in youth, as many of these traits can be considered transient features of relatively normal development (Seagrave & Grisso, 2002). In addition, characteristics such as impulsivity, sensation seeking, and irresponsibility overlap with symptoms of the disruptive behavior disorders, and therefore, can be considered separate from psychopathy (Corrado *et al.*, 2004). Furthermore, younger individuals may not yet have developed the cognitive capacity to think abstractly and to consider long-range consequences of their behavior (Keating, 1990). This is supported by research examining the functional development of regions of the brain in youth. For example, Segalowitz and Davies used event-related potentials in a 2004 study. Results demonstrated that the prefrontal cortex, associated with executive functions continues to mature into late adolescence (Segalowitz & Davies, 2004).

Although juvenile crime has plateaued, there was a significant increase in the 1980s and 1990s, which, among other issues, resulted in increased frequency of waiver to adult court in an attempt to decrease juvenile crime by increased incarceration (Snyder & Sickmund, 1999). However, by removing children from their community setting, they are also potentially being separated from those who could effect the strongest change (Carney & Bartell, 2003). The reality is that when these youth are released from correctional facilities they likely have not received the interventions necessary to help them improve educationally and to address mental health and developmental issues. In addition, returning youth to the same environment in which criminal behaviors were exhibited, without remediation of psychosocial factors, contributes to the likelihood of reoffending.

Developing comprehensive wraparound services are a component to the process of reducing recidivism rates. Recommendations for such services should follow from the psychiatric/psychological evaluation. They should be specific to the individual, and take into consideration the above variables associated in predicting future delinquent acts. Appropriate wraparound services may decrease conduct disordered behaviors in youth by providing family treatment to improve parental supervision and parent–child relationships (i.e., increasing warmth and structure). Promoting prosocial peer relations is also likely to decrease risk of reoffending. Interventions may also target academic functioning and school attendance, vocation, and mental health issues.

There is a huge diversity of treatment programs, some of which are community based; others which are specifically designed for delinquents and supported by state money for community-based delinquency programs; and others which simply can address some of the special needs of the youth. Ideally, juvenile courts will have knowledge of the available programs, their relative success rates, availability to enroll a particular youth, and which facilities are linked with each other.

Assessment of violent offenses, in association with better research documenting the complex and significant mental health needs of youthful offenders, has resulted in further interest in post-adjudicatory interventions. Although there is a paucity of long-term research in this area, community-based treatment techniques and programs have received attention (Hengler & Thomas, 2001). Research generally reveals advantages to participation in community-based services, although recidivism continues to be problematic (Carney & Buttell, 2003). (See Chapter 17 for an evaluation of community-based programs.)

Although there has been an interest in community-based treatment, the question of what type of treatment would be of most benefit remains. Two components to intervention include comprehensive wraparound services where treaters will often communicate with one another, in association with comprehensive educational interventions, which are often overlooked. Placing high numbers of delinquents in one group can potentially put them in a negative and high-risk environment. Alternatively, Feldman (1992) demonstrated that skill-building activity groups with combined delinquent and conventional peers yielded greater gains to the delinquent participants, with negligible negative effects to the prosocial youths.

Lyons *et al.* (2003) reported on the clinical and forensic outcomes from the Illinois Mental Health Juvenile Justice Initiative. In summary, this study reported, "By linking youths with significant mental health needs to existing community-based services, it appears possible both to emolliate psychopathology and to reduce delinquency." Forty-two percent of the delinquent youth who participated in the program were rearrested, compared to 72 percent of all youths detained in the sample. With increased duration of the intervention services, the rearrest rate fell to 29 percent. Many youth, surprisingly, go through the juvenile justice system without a mental health assessment. As such, there are youth with psychotic and depressive symptomatology who are not identified.

Many school systems, in particular in large metropolitan areas, will simply identify delinquent children as behavior disordered and are far less likely to look at underlying learning disabilities and emotional issues that could be affecting a child's basic educational needs. This is troubling due to the high rate of low academic achievement, truancy, and emotional difficulties among delinquent youth. In addition, Rutter *et al.* (1979) found that a high preponderance of low achieving students within a school is related to high levels of delinquency. Grande (1988) reported that up to 25–30 percent of a high-school population may need some type of psychological or educational assistance. Up to 42 percent of incarcerated delinquents are educationally handicapped. Yet, far fewer have had comprehensive educational assessments, and most do not have individualized educational plans (IEP).

Much recent research has focused on school prevention programs, and intervention strategies utilized with students whose level of inappropriate behavior has not reached criminal status (Hawkins & Herrenkohl, 2003). Earlier projects that have evaluated alternative school placements for delinquent youth have shown that individualized curricula, evaluation of student performance based on individual progress, vocational training, and focus on social skills led to decreased delinquent behaviors (Gold & Mann 1984; Kratcoski & Kratcoski, 1982).

When wraparound services are not available, or when the severity of a child's behavior, his/her developmental deficits, or mental health issues are so significant that a more restrictive environment is required, consideration of a therapeutic residential treatment program is warranted. Within the report, one must clarify whether this residential facility can be open or needs to be locked. A structured 24-hour environment with a specialized treatment program offers better consistency and treatment for those more severely mentally ill youth with other mental health issues such as alcohol and substance abuse.

Bailey (2005) has reported that for many young offenders in Britain, the greatest likelihood for consistent treatment, including education, is in a secure facility. Within the US, there is great variability of the clinical and educational services available. At the present time, numerous correctional facilities are the subject of civil rights investigations through the Department of Justice, Civil Rights of Institutional Persons Act (CRIPA). Much of this is related to the paucity of needed services available to youth within these facilities. At the same time, there can be a variety of services requested in a report and supported through the court that can potentially be accessed within correctional facilities. Many correctional facilities also have the ability to use consultative services when indicated. A need for more inter-agency agreements between state departments of mental health and youth corrections to collaborate in serving the mental health needs of those in custody has been identified (Grisso, 2000).

Abram *et al.* (2003) have reported on the increased mental health needs and diagnoses of incarcerated delinquents. This has been related to inadequate provision of mental health services to adolescents in the community (Grisso, 2000). Even though there is an increased incidence of affective disorders, alcohol and substance abuse, psychosis, and anxiety disorders including posttraumatic stress disorder, most correctional facilities do not offer services consistent with community norms (Kraus, 2005). This issue is further complicated by the concept that although these figures are becoming common knowledge, wraparound services and community-based programming continues to consistently lag behind community needs. A collaborative research program between the University of Manchester, the University of Central Lancashire, and clinical services at Bolton, Salford, and Trafford mental health and HS Trust is attempting to examine the level of mental health needs among young offenders and the level of continuity of care for those discharged into the community in association with current models of mental health service (Bailey, 2005).

Finally, a longitudinal study was conducted by Ryan *et al.* (2001) within the Michigan Department of Corrections. Results indicate that juveniles who received services while within a residential treatment facility, as well as community re-entry services, were less likely to be incarcerated as an adult.

Mental health professionals completing evaluations on delinquent youth are in the unique position of having the opportunity to add information and educate the court. Without this data, the court will only have an understanding of the youth's delinquency and not of his/her needs.

The evaluation

One part of the consultant question is to assist in determining the most appropriate environment for the youth. There can often be significant anxiety associated with this. There is no specific, all-inclusive tool that can definitively predict long-term risk of harm. As such, a comprehensive assessment of risk and resistance factors and background information, in association with a clinical assessment, is crucial.

After appropriate releases have been obtained, questions being requested by the court or attorneys have been identified and collateral information received, the evaluation is scheduled. It is not uncommon for a child to be resistant to an initial forensic evaluation. Working with the parent/guardian can often be of assistance with this process. In some cases, it is worthwhile to meet with the guardian or parent prior to the evaluation, and on other occasions it is appropriate to meet with the parent or guardian at the time of the initial evaluation. It is also useful to meet with the youth individually. This could create the opportunity to observe differences in the youth's behavior when they are with their parent/guardian and when they are alone. As well, it is not uncommon for the juvenile's presentation to vary over time. This may be related to a more realistic view of the offense committed, as well its impact on the youth's future, and his/her family. Conducting the evaluation across more than one session also allows for observing behavioral fluctuation.

If the youth appears agitated, either attempt to identify the problem or discontinue the evaluation for the day and resume it at a later time. In general, evaluating on different days will give a more global presentation of the child.

At times, a youth's attorney may request to be present during the evaluation or an evaluator may want him/her to attend. This issue always raises the question of whether or not this type of interaction may affect the evaluation per se. This should be at the evaluator's discretion, with a specific rationale that is relevant to the assessment.

It is important to identify one's role within the evaluation, and for the youth to realize that the purpose of the assessment is not for treatment, nor is it confidential. It is also important that the youth be able to identify the purpose of the evaluation and issues of non-confidentiality in his/her own words. This should be documented in writing.

As one is completing the evaluation, it is important to gain as much understanding as possible regarding the disposition questions, including the child's potential risk to others, risk for recidivism, ability to follow through with treatment interventions, and educational needs. To this end, collateral information plays a critical role. Documentation regarding prior delinquency, hospitalizations, head trauma, special education interventions, and outpatient treatment should be reviewed and discussed with the youth to gain a better understanding of his/her level of insight. Police reports and court documents will provide critical data related to the number and severity of any prior delinquent acts, as well as age at the time of previous detentions.

A comprehensive mental status exam with a specific emphasis on the youth's thought processes and thought content should be conducted as part of the evaluation. Potential malingering must also be assessed. Suicidal ideation should be evaluated, as risk for suicidal gestures may increase in the post-adjudication period when the youth is returned to confinement from the court (Hayes, 1999). An assessment of current and past substance use is also essential.

A solid diagnostic assessment, including interview and standardized rating scales completed by the offender and his/her parents and teachers, if possible, will offer important information regarding both contributing factors to the current offense, as well as likelihood of future criminal acts. Wasserman *et al.* (2005) presented assessment measures commonly used within a delinquent youth population. The Diagnostic Interview Schedule for Children: Present State Voice Version (Voice DISC; Shaffer *et al.*, 2000) was included among these. The Voice DISC is a diagnostic interview based on the fourth edition of the *Diagnostic and Statistical Manual of Mental Disorders* (DSM-IV; American Psychiatric Association, 1994) and is administered via computer with items presented both orally and in writing. A parent version is also available, without voice prompts. With regard to rating scales, the broad-band report measures of behavioral, emotional, and social functioning developed by Achenbach (Achenbach & Rescorla, 2001) were noted to be widely used. These include the youth self-report (YSR), child behavior checklist (CBCL), and teacher's report form (TRF), completed by the youth, parent, and teacher, respectively.

Personality functioning is additionally a critical area to assess in post-adjudicatory evaluations. Wasserman *et al.* (2005) reported that the *Minnesota Multiphasic Personality Inventory – Adolescent* (MMPI-A; Butcher *et al.* 1992) and the *Millon Adolescent Clinical Inventory* (MACI; Millon *et al.*, 1982) are both widely used in such assessments. The MMPI-A and MACI are objective measures of psychopathology structured in a true/false format, and completed by the adolescent.

In addition, intelligence and achievement testing may be appropriate, particularly, if no testing has been completed over prior years. In cases that are referred with questions regarding transfer to the adult court system, it is prudent to include an interview of adaptive functioning. An assessment of family functioning should also be administered. This may include both rating scales of the family environment as well as a clinical interview with the youth and caregivers to determine level of adult supervision, discipline methods, and parent–child relationships. Finally, information related to family history of criminal and psychiatric problems should be elicited.

Assessment of psychopathy can provide useful data related to amenability to treatment and risk of recidivism. However, as noted earlier, measurement of this construct is limited within a youth population. Several recent research projects have evaluated the utility of instruments that measure psychopathic characteristics within the juvenile justice system (Lee *et al.*, 2003; Murrie *et al.*, 2004; Corrado *et al.*, 2004). Seagrave and Grisso (2002) anticipate that juvenile psychopathy measures will become among the most widely used instruments in forensic assessment of delinquency cases.

The results of the clinician's evaluations and treatment recommendations have serious implications for the child's life. An adequate evaluation with direct treatment to reduce risk factors and enhance protective factors will help to minimize the possibility of further delinquency (DePrato & Hammer, 2002).

In summary, the post-adjudicatory evaluation is multifaceted. At its core is its focus on the best interests of the child with an understanding of the need to balance a parens patriae model and police power.

References

Abram, K. M., Teplin, L. A., McClelland, G. M. & Dulcan, M. K. (2003). Comorbid psychiatric disorders in youth in juvenile detention. *Archives of General Psychiatry*, **60**(11), 1097–1108.

Achenbach, T. M. & Rescorla, L. A. (2001). *Manual for the ASEBA School-Age Forms and Profiles*. Burlington: University of Vermont, Research Center for Children, Youth, and Families.

American Psychiatric Association (1994). *Diagnostic and Statistical Manual of Mental Disorders*, 4th edn. Washington, DC.

Arroyo, W. (2005). Disproportionate minority confinement. *American Academy of Child and Adolescent Psychiatry Juvenile Justice Reform Monograph*, October, 2005, 60–68.

Bailey, S. (2005). Meeting the mental health needs of "hard to reach" young offenders. IALMH Congress, Paris, 2005.

Butcher, J. N., Williams, C. L., Graham, J. R. *et al.* (1992). *Minnesota Multiphasic Personality Inventory – Adolescent (MMPI-A): Manual for Administration, Scoring, and Interpretation*. Minneapolis, MN: University of Minnesota Press.

Campbell, M. A. & Schmidt, F. (2000). Comparison of mental health and legal factors in the disposition outcome of young offenders, criminal justice and behavior. *Criminal Justice and Behavior*, **27**(6), 688–715.

Carney, M. M. & Bartell, F. (2003). Reducing juvenile recidivism: evaluating the wraparound services model research on social work practice. *Research on Social Work Practice*, **13**(5), 551–568.

Carrington, P. J. & Moyer, S. (1995). Factors affecting custodial dispositions under the Young Offender's Act. *Canadian Journal of Criminology*, April, 127–162.

Chang, J. J., Chen, J. J. & Brownson, R. C. (2003). The role of repeat victimization in adolescent delinquent behaviors and recidivism. *Journal of Adolescent Health*, **32**, 272–280.

Corrado, R. R., Vincent, G. M., Hart, S. D. & Cohen, I. M. (2004). Predictive validity of the psychopathy checklist: youth version of general and violent recidivism. *Behavioral Sciences and the Law*, **22**, 5–22.

DePrado, D. K. & Hammer, J. H. (2002). Assessment and treatment of juvenile offenders. In D. H. Schetky and E. P. Benedek, eds., *Principles and Practices of Child and Adolescent Forensic Psychiatry*. American Psychiatric Publishing Inc., pp. 267–278.

Duits, N. (2005). Quality of diagnostic assessments from juvenile court in the Netherlands. The IALMH Congress. Paris. Abstract.

Feldman, R. A. (1992). The St. Louis experiment: effective treatment of antisocial youths in prosocial peer groups. In J. McCord and R. E. Trembaly, eds., *Preventing Antisocial Behavior: Intervention from Birth Through Adolescence*. New York: Guilford Press, pp. 233–252.

Gold, M. & Mann, D. W. (1984). *Expelled to a Friendlier Place: A Study of Effective Alternative Schools*. Ann Arbor, MI: University of Michigan.

Grande, C. G. (1988). Educational therapy for the failing and frustrated student offender. *Adolescents*, **XXIII** (92), 889–897.

Grisso, T. (1997). The competence of adolescents as trial defendants. *Psychology, Public Policy, and Law*, **3**, 3–32.

Grisso, T. (2000). The changing face of juvenile justice. *Law and Psychiatry* , **51**(4), 425–427.

Hawkins, J. D. & Herrenkohl, T. I. (2003). Prevention in the school years. In D. P. Farrington & J. W. Coid, eds., *Early Prevention of Adult Antisocial Behavior*, pp. 265–291. United Kingdom: Cambridge University Press.

Hayes, L. M. (1999). *Suicide Prevention in Juvenile Correction and Detention Facilities: A Resource Guide for Performance-Based Standards for Juvenile Corrections and Detention Facilities*. Washington, DC: Council of Juvenile Correctional Administrators.

Hemphill, J. F., Hare, R. D. & Wong, S. (1998). Psychopathy and recidivism: a review. *Legal and Criminological Psychology*, **3**, 141–172.

Hengler, S. & Thomas, C. (2001). Recommendations for juvenile justice reform. *American Academy of Child and Adolescent Psychiatry Task Force on Juvenile Justice Reform*, **14**, 67–72.

Hoge, D. H., Andrews, D. A. & Leschied, A. W. (1995). Investigation of variables associated with probation and custody dispositions in a sample of juveniles. *Journal of Clinical Child Psychology*, **24**(3), 279–286.

Home Office, Department of Health, Welsh Office (1995). *National Standards for the Supervision of Offenders in the Community*. London, UK: HMSO.

Jaffe, P. G., Leschied, A. W., Sas, L. & Austin, G. W. (1985). A model for the provision of clinical assessment and service brokerage for young offenders; the London Family Court Clinic. *Psychologie Canadienne*, **26**(1), 54–61.

Keating, D. (1990). Adolescent thinking. In S. Feldman and G. Elliott, eds., *At the Threshold: The Developmental Adolescent*, Cambridge, MA: Harvard University Press, pp. 54–89.

Kratcoski, P. E. & Kratcoski, L. E. (1982). The Phoenix Program: an educational alternative for delinquent youths. *Juvenile and Family Court Journal*, **33**, 17–24.

Kraus, L. J. (2005). Juvenile justice reform: post adjudicatory assessment. *American Academy of Child and Adolescent Psychiatry. Recommendations for Juvenile Justice Reform Monograph*, October, 2005.

Kupersmidt, J. B., Coie, J. D. & Howell, J. C. (2004). Resilience in children exposed to negative peer influences. In K. I. Maton, C. J. Schellenbach, B. J. Leadbeater and A. L. Solarz, eds., *Investing in Children, Youth, Families, and Communities: Strengths-Based Research and Policy*. Washington, DC: American Psychological Association, pp. 251–268.

Lee, Z., Vincent, G. M., Hart, S. D. & Corrado, R. R. (2003). The validity of the antisocial process screening device as a self-report measure of psychopathy in adolescent offenders. *Behavioral Sciences and the Law* **21**, 771–786.

Lyons, J. S., Griffin, G., Quintenz, S., Genuwine, M. & Shasha, M. (2003). Clinical and forensic outcomes from the Illinois Mental Health Juvenile Justice Initiative. *Psychiatric services*, **54**(12), 1629–1634.

Millon, T., Green, C. J. & Meagher, R. B. (1982). *Millon Adolescent Clinical Inventory Manual*. Minneapolis, MN: National Computer Service.

Murrie, D. C., Cornell, D. G., Kaplan, S., McConville, D., & Levy-Elkon, A. (2004). Psychopathy scores and violence among juvenile offenders: a multi-measure study. *Behavioral Sciences and the Law*, **22**, 49–67.

Niarhos, F. J. & Routh, D. K. (1992). The role of clinical assessment in the juvenile court: predictors of juvenile dispositions and recidivism. *Journal of Clinical Child Psychology*, **21**(2), 151–159.

Piscotta, A. (1983). Race, sex, and rehabilitation: a study of differential treatment in the juvenile reformatory – 1825–1900. *Crime and Delinquency*, **29**(2), 254–269.

Quinn, K. (2002). Juveniles on trial. *Child and Adolescent Psychiatric Clinics of North America*, **11**(4), 719–730.

Rutter, M., Maughan, B., Mortimore, P., Ouston, J. & Smith, A. (1979). *Fifteen Thousand Hours: Secondary Schools and their Effects on Children*. London: Open Books; Cambridge, MA: Harvard University Press.

Ryan, J. P., Davis, R. K. & Yang, H. (2001). Reintegration services and the likelihood of adult imprisonment: a longitudinal study of adjudicated delinquents. *Research on Social Work Practice*, **11**(3), 321–337.

Sanborn, J. B. (1996). Factors perceived to affect delinquent dispositions in juvenile court: putting the sentencing decision into context. *Crime and Delinquency*, **42**(1), 99–113.

Seagrave, D. & Grisso, T. (2002). Adolescent development and the measurement of juvenile psychopathy. *Law and Human Behavior*, **26**, 219–239.

Segalowitz, S. J. & Davies, P. L. (2004). Charting the maturation of the frontal lobe: an electrophysiological strategy. *Brain and Cognition*, **55**, 116–133.

Seto, M. C. & Barbaree, H. E. (1999). Psychopathy, treatment behavior, and sex offender recidivism. *Journal of Interpersonal Violence*, **14**, 1235–1248.

Shaffer, D. M., Fisher, P. W., Lucas, C., Dulcan, M. K. & Schwab-Stone, M. E. (2000). NIMH Diagnostic Interview Schedule for Children Version IV (NIMH:DISC-IV): description, differences from previous versions, and reliability of some common diagnoses. *Journal of the American Academy of Child and Adolescent Psychiatry*, **39**, 28–38.

Snyder, H. & Sickmund, M. (1999). *Juvenile Offenders and Victims; 1999 National Report*. Washington, DC: Office of Juvenile Justice and Delinquency Prevention.

Vermeiren, R., Schwab-Stone, M., Ruchkin, V., De Clippele, A. & Deboutte, D. (2002). Predicting recidivism in delinquent adolescents from psychological and psychiatric assessment. *Comprehensive Psychiatry*, **43**(2), 142–149.

Wasserman, G. A., McReynolds, L. S., Fisher, P. & Lucas, C. P. (2005). The Diagnostic Interview Schedule for Children: Present State Voice Version. In T. Grisso, G. Vincent and D. Seagrave, eds., *Mental Health Screening and Assessment in Juvenile Justice*, New York, NY: Guilford Press, pp. 224–239.

Wasserman, G. A., Jensen, P. S., Ko, S. J. *et al.* (2003). Mental health assessments in juvenile justice: report on the consensus conference. *Journal of the American Academy of Child and Adolescent Psychiatry*, **42**(7), 752–761.

Whitebread, C. H. & Heilman, J. (1988). An overview of the law juvenile delinquency. *Behavioral Sciences and the Law*, **6**(3), 285–305.

Index